Neurobehavioral Manifestations of Neurological Diseases: Diagnosis and Treatment

Editors

ALIREZA MINAGAR
GLEN R. FINNEY
KENNETH M. HEILMAN

NEUROLOGIC CLINICS

www.neurologic.theclinics.com

Consulting Editor
RANDOLPH W. EVANS

February 2016 • Volume 34 • Number 1

ELSEVIER

1600 John F. Kennedy Boulevard ● Suite 1800 ● Philadelphia, Pennsylvania, 19103-2899

http://www.theclinics.com

NEUROLOGIC CLINICS Volume 34, Number 1
February 2016 ISSN 0733-8619, ISBN-13: 978-0-323-41702-0

Editor: Lauren Boyle
Developmental editor: Donald Mumford

Neurologic Clinics (ISSN 0733-8619) is published quarterly by Elsevier Inc., 360 Park Avenue South, New York, NY 10010–1710. Months of issue are February, May, August, and November. Periodicals postage paid at New York, NY, and additional mailing offices. Subscription prices are $300.00 per year for US individuals, $578.00 per year for US institutions, $100.00 per year for US students, $375.00 per year for Canadian individuals, $701.00 per year for Canadian institutions, $415.00 per year for international individuals, $701.00 per year for international institutions, and $210.00 for Canadian and foreign students/residents. To receive student/resident rate, orders must be accompanied by name of affiliated institution, date of term, and the *signature* of program/residency coordinator on institution letterhead. Orders will be billed at individual rate until proof of status is received. Foreign air speed delivery is included in all *Clinics* subscription prices. All prices are subject to change without notice. **POSTMASTER:** Send address changes to *Neurologic Clinics*, Elsevier Health Sciences Division, Subscription Customer Service, 3251 Riverport Lane, Maryland Heights, MO 63043. **Customer Service: Telephone: 1-800-654-2452 (U.S. and Canada); 314-447-8871 (outside U.S. and Canada). Fax: 314-447-8029. E-mail: journalscustomerservice-usa@elsevier.com (for print support); journalsonlinesupport-usa@elsevier.com (for online support).**

Reprints. For copies of 100 or more of articles in this publication, please contact the Commercial Reprints Department, Elsevier Inc., 360 Park Avenue South, New York, New York, 10010-1710; Tel.: +1-212-633-3874; Fax: +1-212-633-3820, and E-mail: reprints@elsevier.com.

Neurologic Clinics is also published in Spanish by Nueva Editorial Interamericana S.A., Mexico City, Mexico.

Neurologic Clinics is covered in *Current Contents/Clinical Medicine, MEDLINE/PubMed (Index Medicus), EMBASE/Excerpta Medica, and PsycINFO, and ISI/BIOMED.*

Contributors

CONSULTING EDITOR

RANDOLPH W. EVANS, MD
Clinical Professor, Department of Neurology, Baylor College of Medicine, Houston, Texas

EDITORS

ALIREZA MINAGAR, MD, FAAN, FANA
Professor and Chairman, Department of Neurology, Louisiana State University Health Sciences Center - Shreveport, Shreveport, Louisiana

GLEN R. FINNEY, MD
Director, Geisinger Health System Neurology, Wilkes-Barre, Pennsylvania

KENNETH M. HEILMAN, MD, FAAN, FANA
The James E. Rooks Jr. Distinguished Professor of Neurology, University of Florida College of Medicine, Department of Neurology and the Veterans Medical Center, Gainesville, Florida

AUTHORS

NADEJDA ALEKSEEVA, MD
Department of Neurology, Louisiana State University Health Sciences Center - Shreveport, Shreveport, Louisiana

OLEG CHERNYSHEV, MD
Assistant Professor, Department of Neurology, Louisiana State University Health Sciences Center - Shreveport, Shreveport, Louisiana

DEBRA E. DAVIS, MD
Associate Professor, Department of Neurology, Louisiana State University Health Sciences Center - Shreveport, Shreveport, Louisiana

ELIZABETH A. DISBROW, PhD
Associate Professor, Department of Neurology, Louisiana State University Health Sciences Center - Shreveport, Shreveport, Louisiana

RAMY EL-KHOURY, MD
Assistant Professor, Department of Neurology, Tulane University School of Medicine, New Orleans, Louisiana

GLEN R. FINNEY, MD
Director, Geisinger Health System Neurology, Wilkes-Barre, Pennsylvania

KENNETH M. HEILMAN, MD, FAAN, FANA
The James E. Rooks Jr. Distinguished Professor of Neurology, University of Florida College of Medicine, Department of Neurology and the Veterans Medical Center, Gainesville, Florida

VIJAYAKUMAR JAVALKAR, PhD
House Officer 4, Department of Neurology, Louisiana State University Health Sciences Center - Shreveport, Shreveport, Louisiana

ROGER E. KELLEY, MD
Chairman, Department of Neurology, Tulane University School of Medicine, New Orleans, Louisiana

BETH A. LEEMAN-MARKOWSKI, MD, MA, MMSc
Adjunct Assistant Professor, Department of Neurology, Emory University, Atlanta, Georgia

SAMANTHA E. MARIN, MD
Department of Neurosciences, University of California, San Diego (UCSD), La Jolla, California

VICTOR W. MARK, MD
Associate Professor, Departments of Physical Medicine and Rehabilitation, Neurology, and Psychology, University of Alabama at Birmingham, Birmingham, Alabama

JEANIE McGEE, DHEd
Assistant Professor of Neurology Research; Director of Neurology Clinical Trials, Department of Neurology, Louisiana State University Health Sciences Center - Shreveport, Shreveport, Louisiana

ALIREZA MINAGAR, MD, FAAN, FANA
Professor and Chairman, Department of Neurology, Louisiana State University Health Sciences Center - Shreveport, Shreveport, Louisiana

SAI KRISHNA J. MUNJAMPALLI, MBBS
Neurology Resident, Department of Neurology, Louisiana State University Health Sciences Center – Shreveport, Shreveport, Louisiana

ABDORREZA NASER MOGHADASI, MD
MS Research Center, Neuroscience Institute, Tehran University of Medical Sciences, Tehran, Iran

MARYAM NOROOZIAN, MD
Professor of Neurology; Director, Memory and Behavioral Neurology Division, Department of Psychiatry; Chair, Department of Geriatric Medicine, Tehran University of Medical Sciences (TUMS), Tehran, Iran

SHADI POURMAND, MD
MS Research Center, Neuroscience Institute, Tehran University of Medical Sciences, Tehran, Iran

MOHAMMAD ALI SAHRAIAN, MD
MS Research Center, Neuroscience Institute, Tehran University of Medical Sciences, Tehran, Iran

RUSSELL P. SANETO, DO, PhD
Head of the Program for Mitochondrial Medicine, Professor of Neurology and Adjunct Professor Pediatrics, Departments of Neurology and Pediatrics, Seattle Children's Hospital, University of Washington, Seattle, Washington

STEVEN C. SCHACHTER, MD
Professor of Neurology, Beth Israel Deaconess Medical Center, Massachusetts General Hospital – CIMIT, Harvard Medical School, Boston, Massachusetts

MARYAM SHARIFIAN, MD
MS Research Center, Neuroscience Institute, Tehran University of Medical Sciences, Tehran, Iran

ELYSE J. SINGER, MD
Director, NeuroInfectious Diseases Program; Director, University of California, Los Angeles National Neurological AIDS Bank; Professor of Neurology, David Geffen School of Medicine at University of California, Los Angeles, Los Angeles, California

APRIL D. THAMES, PhD
Assistant Professor of Psychiatry and Biobehavioral Sciences, David Geffen School of Medicine at University of California, Los Angeles, Los Angeles, California

RICHARD M. ZWEIG, MD
Professor, Department of Neurology, Louisiana State University Health Sciences Center - Shreveport, Shreveport, Louisiana

Contents

Assessing the mental status of patients with neurobehavioral disorder is a critical element in the diagnosis and treatment of these patients. This assessment should always be performed after the patient's history is taken and general physical as well as neurologic examination are completed. The mental status examination commences with observing the patient's appearance and determining level of consciousness. The examiner should also pay attention to patient's social behavior, emotional state, and mood. There are 3 major means of assessing a patient's mental status. One type attempts to determine if the patient is demented and the severity of the dementia as it pertains to their ability to perform activities of daily living as well as instrumental activities. A second type of assessment utilizes what may be termed as "screening tests" or "omnibus tests". These brief tests are performed independent of the patient's history and examination. The two most frequently used screening tests are the Mini-Mental Status Examination (MMSE) and the Montreal Cognitive Assessment (MoCA). The third means of assessing a patient's mental status is by using specific neuropsychological tests that focus on specific domains of cognition, such as frontal executive functions, attention, episodic verbal and visuospatial memory, declarative knowledge such as language (speech, reading and writing) and arithmetical, as well as visuospatial and perceptual abilities. These neurobehavioral, neuropsychiatric and neuropsychological assessments of patients with a cognitive decline and behavioral abnormalities should often be accompanied by laboratory tests, and neuroimaging that can help determine the underlying pathologic process so that effective therapeutic and management approaches can be provided.

Multiple sclerosis (MS) is the most common nontraumatic cause of physical disability in young adults. Cognitive and neuropsychiatric problems are common in this disease independent of motor disability. Such problems especially in mild cases are ignored by physicians, although they may have a major impact on quality of life. Neurobehavioral changes may affect the adherence to treatment and worsen the ultimate prognosis. Although many studies have been performed in this regard, it seems that combining cognitive evaluations with other outcome measures in MS will enhance the understanding of neurobehavioral changes in MS.

Behavioral disorders are common in persons infected with human immunodeficiency virus (HIV). The differential includes preexisting psychiatric diseases, substance abuse, direct effects of HIV infection, opportunistic infection, and the adverse effects of medical therapies. Many patients have more than one contributing or comorbid problem to explain these behavioral changes. The differential should always include consideration of psychosocial, genetic, and medical causes of disease. Treatment strategies must take into account the coadministration of antiretroviral therapy and the specific neurologic problems common in patients infected with HIV.

Traumatic brain injury (TBI) is a complex neurologic and neuropathologic process that may affect the patient's behavior permanently. Clinically, TBI is associated with a wide gamut of neurologic and psychiatric disorders, such as amnesia, cognitive decline, seizures, attention and concentration deficits, depression, manic behavior, psychosis, hostile and violent behavior, and personality alterations. Therapy and rehabilitative efforts should be designed based on the type of injury and the patient's specific needs. Gaining familiarity with the behavioral disorders outlined in this article and understanding how to identify and treat them plays a significant role in the management of patients with TBI.

It is important for neurologists to become more familiar with neuropsychological evaluation for Alzheimer's disease. The growth of this method in research, as an available, inexpensive, and noninvasive diagnostic approach, which can be administered even by non–specialist-trained examiners, makes this knowledge more necessary than ever. Such knowledge has a basic role in planning national programs in primary health care systems for prevention and early detection of Alzheimer's disease. This is more crucial in developing countries, which have higher rates of dementia prevalence along with cardiovascular risk factors, lack of public knowledge about dementia, and limited social support. In addition compared to the neurological hard signs which are tangible and measurable, the concept of cognition seems to be more difficult for the neurologists to evaluate and for the students to understand. Dementia in general and Alzheimer's disease as the prototype of cognitive disorders specifically, play an important role to explore all domains of human cognition through its symptomatology and neuropsychological deficits.

Commonly used medications can have neuropsychiatric and behavioral effects that may be idiosyncratic or metabolic in nature, or a function of interactions with other drugs, toxicity, or withdrawal. This article explores an approach to the patient with central nervous system toxicity, depending on presentation of sedation versus agitation and accompanying physical signs and symptoms. The effects of antihypertensives, opioids, antibiotics, antiepileptic agents, steroids, Parkinson's disease medications, antipsychotics, medications for human immunodeficiency virus infection, cancer chemotherapeutics, and immunotherapies are discussed. A look at the prevalence of adverse reactions to medications and the errors underlying such occurrences is included.

Frontotemporal dementia (FTD) is a not-uncommon explanation for progressive cognitive deficit in patients who often have a genetic susceptibility for such a neurodegenerative process. However, FTD does not seem to identify one particular pathogenetic mechanism but rather a spectrum of pathologies with particular predilection for the frontal and temporal lobes of the brain. There have been various subcategorizations of this form of dementia that have a tendency to be of earlier onset than typical Alzheimer disease and heralded by behavioral or communication manifestations. There is a behavioral variant and a language variant, referred to as primary progressive aphasia.

Cognitive deficits, including attention, language, memory, and executive dysfunction, are common in the setting of epilepsy and can greatly impair quality of life. The etiology is often multifactorial and may be due to the underlying seizure disorder, adverse effects of treatment, and psychiatric comorbidities, among other factors. Management of cognitive deficits aims to address these underlying etiologies as well as provide rehabilitative strategies. Several investigational therapies are also currently under study. This article examines current and future treatments for cognitive dysfunction in epilepsy.

 Videos of various behavioral changes caused by stroke accompany this article

Most patients who have endured a stroke sustain behavioral changes, although in many instances these effects can be subtle. Although

NEUROLOGIC CLINICS

THE CLINICS ARE AVAILABLE ONLINE!
Access your subscription at:
www.theclinics.com

Preface

Neurobehavioral Manifestations of Neurological Diseases: Diagnosis and Treatment

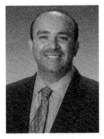
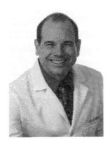
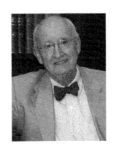

Alireza Minagar, MD, FAAN, FANA   Glen R. Finney, MD   Kenneth M. Heilman, MD, FAAN, FANA

Editors

Diseases that affect the central nervous system, including vascular, infectious, metabolic, endocrine, deficiency, trauma, and degenerative, often alter these patients' ability to function normally because they often cause neurobehavioral disorders. There are many forms of neurobehavioral disorders including deficits of memory, language, emotions, attention, perception, executive functions, visuospatial skills as well as others. Behavioral neurology is the specialty that focuses on assessment, diagnosis, and treatment of patients with acquired as well as developmental neurobehavioral disorders. The study of patients with neurobehavioral disorders, however, has also allowed behavioral neurologists to help understand how the brain mediates these various cognitive activities. The modern history of behavioral neurology starts with Gall, who posited localization of function now called modularity, and Paul Broca, who provided support for Gall's hypothesis by revealing that the left hemisphere mediates speech and language. A few years after Broca's reports, Karl Wernicke introduced information-processing models of brain function, and subsequently, Alois Alzheimer and Arnold Pick introduced the concept of degenerative diseases causing dementia. After the First World War, there was a hiatus in the development of behavioral neurology until the 1960s, when neurologists, such as Norman Geschwind, and neuropsychologists, such as Arthur Benton, initiated a renaissance in the subspecialties of neurology and psychology.

This issue presents some of the most recent knowledge about behavioral neurology and neurobehavioral disorders. Rather than focusing on specific neurobehavioral disorders, such as aphasia or neglect, this issue concentrates on how various diseases affect the patient's behavior, and how a clinician can diagnose these diseases as well as treat or manage these diseases and disorders. The authors who have

Neurol Clin 34 (2016) xiii–xiv
http://dx.doi.org/10.1016/j.ncl.2015.10.001
0733-8619/16/$ – see front matter © 2016 Published by Elsevier Inc.

neurologic.theclinics.com

contributed to this issue have attempted to write for readers who are general neurologists, behavioral neurologists, neuropsychiatrists, as well as neuropsychologists. During the preparation of this text, we benefited from generous contributions from the neurologists and neuroscientists who wrote these articles, and we acknowledge their effort and appreciate their input. We also want to acknowledge the hard work and unconditional support given to us by the developmental editor, Mr Donald Mumford, as well as the diligent and supportive staff at Elsevier, Inc, who assisted us at every step of the way toward publishing this issue.

Finally, we are heavily indebted to our patients and their caregivers from whom we learned so much. We wish that this issue of *Neurologic Clinics* will help improve patient care as well as entice our readers to continue their clinical, basic science, and neuroimaging research to unravel the basic pathophysiologic mechanisms and treatments of neurobehavioral disorders.

Alireza Minagar, MD, FAAN, FANA
Department of Neurology
LSUHSC - Shreveport
Shreveport, LA 71130, USA

Glen R. Finney, MD
Geisinger Health System Neurology
1000 East Mountain Boulevard
Wilkes Barre, PA 18711, USA

Kenneth M. Heilman, MD, FAAN, FANA
University of Florida College of Medicine
Department of Neurology and the Veterans Medical Center
Gainesville, FL 32610, USA

E-mail addresses:
aminag@lsuhsc.edu (A. Minagar)
gfinney@geisinger.ufl.edu (G.R. Finney)
heilman@neurology.ufl.edu (K.M. Heilman)

Assessment of Mental Status

Glen R. Finney, MD[a], Alireza Minagar, MD[b],*, Kenneth M. Heilman, MD[c]

KEYWORDS

- Behavioral neurology • Neuropsychiatry • Neuropsychology • Mental status
- Examination • Memory loss • Dementia

KEY POINTS

- Assessment of mental status is one the most important parts of a neurologic or psychiatric examination. This assessment includes the evaluation of the level of consciousness as well as the assessment of multiple neurobehavioral domains, including appearance, mood and emotional state, frontal executive functions, attention, episodic verbal and visuospatial memory, declarative knowledge such as language, as well as visuospatial and perceptual abilities.
- A comprehensive clinical interview of patients with neuropsychiatric disorders and cognitive decline focuses on presenting complaint(s), time course of development of disease process, individual characteristics such as gender, and cultural and educational background, family history of the same pathology and role of genetic factors, history of traumatic brain injury, presence of any medical conditions as well as sleep disorders and medicinal effects.
- Advanced neuroimaging of brain utilizing various MRI sequences and PET scan in combination with clinical manifestations of behavioral disorders and neuropsychological abnormalities have significantly improved our objective understanding of the underlying neuropathological processes.

INTRODUCTION

Neuropsychiatric assessment of a patient with behavioral disorder is a complex and multidimensional process which utilizes neurologic, psychological, and psychiatric approaches to determine how a neurologic or psychiatric disease can affect patient's behavior. With growth of our knowledge about dementing diseases and traumatic brain injury and with giant advances in the world of neuroimaging the borders between

[a] Geisinger Health System Neurology, Wikes-Barre, PA 18711, USA; [b] Department of Neurology, Louisiana State University Health Sciences Center - Shreveport, 1501 Kings Highway, Shreveport, LA 71130, USA; [c] University of Florida College of Medicine, Department of Neurology and the Veterans Medical Center, Gainesville, FL 32610, USA
* Corresponding author.
E-mail address: aminag@lsuhsc.edu

Neurol Clin 34 (2016) 1–16
http://dx.doi.org/10.1016/j.ncl.2015.08.001
0733-8619/16/$ – see front matter © 2016 Elsevier Inc. All rights reserved.
neurologic.theclinics.com

neurology and psychiatry are dissolving and the new subspecialty of "behavioral neurology and neuropsychiatry" is emerging. A deep understanding of how certain brain lesions clinically translate into fascinating neuro-behavioral abnormalities enables neurologists and psychiatrists to better formulate diagnostic and treatment approaches.

HISTORY AND PHYSICAL

As the case of almost all medical evaluations, the assessment should be consistent of three main components of history, general physical examination, and neurologic examination. The standard history initiates with recording of the "Chief complaint" and continue with obtaining information about history of present illness, past medical history, family history, social history, and review of symptoms. This part is followed by detailed general and then neurologic examination and assessment.

HISTORY

Obtaining a comprehensive history of the patient's mental, cognitive, and social capabilities and how and over what time period he or she has deteriorated is very important. It is of utmost significance to demonstrate that how the patient's cognitive abilities have evolved and deteriorated from its original status to the present time. Another significant point to bear in mind is that just like certain symptoms such as hemiplegia which point toward specific neuroanatomic pathways involvement such as corticospinal tract, certain findings such as aphasia and apraxia carry localizing values. Most patients with neuropsychiatric diseases such as Alzheimer disease (AD) are poor history givers and one should also interview the relatives and caregivers for certain details. The term dementia comes from two morphemes, "de" meaning a decrease and "mentia" meaning mentation. According the Diagnostic and Statistical Manual of Mental Disorders (3rd Edition Revised) to be considered to have dementia a person must have defects in mentation in at least two domains for example, episodic memory and naming and this patient's decline in cognitive functions must be sufficient to cause a functional disability that interferes with their daily functions. Currently, if patients have a cognitive disorder in one domain of cognition, such as episodic memory, many clinician term this disorder "mild cognitive impairment".[1]

One particular point about obtaining history of neuropsychiatric issues is that in many cases the patient may not even know why he or she is being interviewed. Patients with memory loss and no insight into the nature of their problem, as seen in patients with AD or traumatic brain injury, provide the best example. One the opposite end of this spectrum are the patients with mood disorders (particularly depression) and anxiety disorder who may be too much exaggerating about their cognitive issues. The issue of insight to the depth of one's neurocognitive issues is very significant since an individual who is clueless about his or her own deficits is more likely to be heedless to certain restrictions imposed by treating physician or being compliant with medical orders and medications.

Paying attention at the speed of onset (acute vs chronic) and pattern of evolution of the disease process and its course (static vs deteriorating) is necessary. History of hereditary factors should be obtained. For example, in a young patient with a family history of chronic headaches, young-onset dementia and recurrent strokes, who presents with recent onset memory loss, a diagnosis such as CADASIL should be entertained. A review of all medications which can affects someone's cognition adversely such as anti-cholinergic, anti-epileptic, and GABAergic medications is required and the interviewer should specifically inquire about any history of substance abuse. Seeking history of any civilian or military traumatic brain injury is imperative. Lastly, the history of neuropsychiatric disorders should also include sleep disturbances such as sleep apnea or rapid eye movement behavioral disorder (which points toward certain neurodegenerative diseases such as Parkinson's disease).

GENERAL PHYSICAL EXAMINATION

In many patients, their dementia may be related to diseases of their body that affect brain function. Thus, the evaluation of patients with dementia should always include a physical examination. Failure of any major organ such as the liver, lungs, heart or kidney may induce dementia and patients with organ failure often reveal signs on their physical examination. For example, a male patient with hepatic encephalopathy may have an enlarged spleen, palmer erythema and three or more spider angioma as well as palpable breasts. Similarly, endocrine disorders may also induce a dementia. For example, hypothyroidism may cause a dementia and patients with this disorder may be cold and shivering, have a hoarse voice, and have thickened skin.

NEUROLOGIC EXAMINATION

In addition to the mental status examination, that will be discussed below, a detail neurologic examination that includes examining: (a) all the cranial nerves, including all the olfactory nerve, since this can be impaired in parkinsonian disorders and AD; (b) a motor examination for strength, tone, and abnormal movements, speed of movement, accuracy of movement, size of movements, and precision of movements; (c) sensory examination; (d) gait; (f) reflexes including: deep tendon jerks, plantar (Babinski) response, grasp reflex, and glabella reflex.

Whereas patients with some forms of dementia such as AD may have a normal neurologic examination, patients with other forms of dementia show abnormalities on the neurologic examination. For example, patients with progressive supranuclear palsy may show abnormal vertical eye movements, as well as alterations in tone and gait and patients with corticobasal degeneration may show asymmetrical myoclonus, and an alien upper limb. Patients with hydrocephalus may show grasp reflexes, paratonia, and abnormalities of gait.

Whereas history, general physical examination and neurologic examination, may help in the diagnosis of dementia, often the most important part of the examination to determine the presence of dementia and the possible type of dementia is mental status testing.

MENTAL STATUS EXAMINATION

Assessment of mental status is a multifaceted and fascinating component of neurologic and psychiatric examinations and consists of an organized clinical approach to determine and report the patient's state of mind with heavy concentration on a number of cognitive domains such as level and content of consciousness, speech and comprehension, following orders, thought process and contents of thought, degree of insight and understanding of the self and surrounding events, and judgment. A detailed mental status examination combined with neuropsychiatric history of the patient along with other positive findings of the neurologic examination enables the clinicians to reach a reasonable diagnosis and design an appropriate therapeutic approach. Indeed, mental status examination is a fundamental skill in neurologic examination and plays a crucial role in determination of clinical manifestations of neurologic and psychiatric diseases. Mental status examination commences with observing and documenting the patient's appearance including hygiene, dress, and grooming. Whether the clothing is dull or colorful may indicate patient's mood and personality traits. The examining physician should always search for certain physical features indicative of nicotine smell and stains, alcoholism, malnutrition, substance abuse, needle tracks, and other unique findings which can serve as a window to the patient's state of mind.

Next, the treating physician should focus on the level of consciousness and determine the state of arousal and level of alertness. The level of consciousness covers a gamut of states from full orientation to self and others, location, and time to profound coma when patient is unresponsive even to painful stimuli. Somewhere in this wide spectrum one may find a patient in an acute confusional status or delirium when the patient is drowsy and disoriented but is able to answer to some questions in a meaningful manner. Terms such as obtundation are inaccurate and should be avoided. One should use the state of patient's response to verbal, motor, or painful stimuli as indicators of level of consciousness. The other component consists of determining the content of the patient's consciousness. A number of neuropathological processes may affect one's content of consciousness without touching the level of consciousness. Dementing diseases such as Alzheimer disease constitute an excellent example of this situation. During this phase of assessment of mental status one can also determine the level of concertation and attention. Simple bedside tests such as serial 7s, counting backwards, determination of digit span and the spelling the word "world" forward and backward are examples of tests designed to achieve this goal.

Following this stage, the examiner should pay attention to patient's social behavior and focus on certain features such as to whether the patient is being hostile, aggressive and rude, or polite, calm and shy, defensive or oppositional, seductive or exhibitionist, uncaring and apathetic as well as whether the patient makes good eye contact.

Meticulous assessment of patient's six communication skills comes next and includes speech fluency, comprehension, reading, writing, naming and repetition. Determination of the presence of aphasia and dysarthria are of prime significance and certain conditions such as stuttering and mutism should be excluded. Then, the examiner should focus on the rate and volume of the speech as well as its content.

Another component of mental status examination consists of assessment of mood and affect. Mood is what patient feels in his/her own words such as being happy, angry, depressed, or irritable, and affect is the apparent emotion carried by non-verbal behavior such as being anxious or angry. The examiner should specifically pay attention to the patient's facial and emotional prosody expression as clues to the underlying neurologic or psychiatric disease. While assessing mood and affect, one should seek for any clues to suicidal and homicidal ideas, risks for violent and aggressive behavior, irritability and impulsivity, and the presence of anxiety. Every detail can guide the physician toward a reasonable and accurate diagnosis.

Mental status examination, then proceeds with evaluation of the thought process and thought content. The examination of thought process focuses on the amount, the flow, and the logical coherence of the thought. The examiner should seek for key elements such as flight of ideas, ability to understand and reason, presence of confabulation, tangential thinking, poverty of thought and circumstantial thinking. Assessment of the thought content targets detection of abnormalities such as delusions, obsessions, phobias, and preoccupations.

Evaluation of the perceptions, insight and judgment, and abstract thinking are additional components of mental status examination. Abnormalities of perception include hallucinations, pseudo-hallucinations, and illusions. Patient's insight is determined by assessing how much he/she knowns about the nature and depth of their condition and their knowledge of the therapeutic approaches. Whether the patient is capable to make reasonable and accountable decisions reflects the patient's judgment. During the mental status assessment the physician should talk to the patient about famous sayings and proverbs and ask them to interpret them. Such bedside test roughly reflects patient's abstract thinking.

Although the mental status examination thus far has described observations, it is also possible to perform a more comprehensive approach such as that done by experts in behavioral neurology, neuropsychology and neuropsychiatry. Though doing all parts of this assessment may be beyond what the general practitioner could perform, a familiarity with this approach will provide some additional tools for the clinician's tool box as well as familiarity with this more in depth mental status assessment when reviewing reports from cognitive subspecialists.

There are three major means of assessing a patient's mental status in more depth. One type attempts to determine if the patient is demented and the severity of the dementia as it pertains to their ability to perform activities of daily living as well as instrumental activities. As mentioned dementia is in part defined as having a decline in cognitive functions that are sufficient to cause a functional disability that interferes with peoples' daily functions. The most frequently used scale for determining dementia induced disability is the "Clinical Dementia Rating Scale".[2] In addition to memory and orientation, this scale assesses the patient's judgment and problem solving skills such as financial affairs, their ability to successfully engage in community affairs, perform activities at home as well as their hobbies and their ability to perform self-care.

A second type of assessment utilizes what may be termed as "screening tests" or "omnibus tests". These tests are given to patients with complaints of decreased mental abilities and these tests are performed independent of the patient's history and examination findings. The two most frequently used tests that are used for screening are the Mini-Mental Status Examination (MMSE)[3] and the Montreal Cognitive Assessment (MoCA). These tests which usually take are carried out in a short period, allow clinicians to separate people who are well from those who have a reduction in the mental capacity. The Mattis Dementia Rating Scale takes about 30 minutes. Each of these screen tests will be briefly described below and the strengths and weaknesses of these tests will also be discussed.

The third means of assessing a patient's mental status is by using specific neurologic tests that focus on specific domains of cognition. Some define cognition as knowledge-understanding, but in this article we will use this term, as it is now more often used, for the brain mediated processes that account for perceiving and understanding as well as thinking, planning, and performing meaningful activities. These specific tests that are selected can be based on the patient's history and neurologic examination, as well as their performance on a screening test. The specific tests can test episodic memory, working memory, procedural memory, and declarative memory. They can assess executive functions, language abilities (speech, reading and writing) and include tests for fluency, naming, comprehension, and repetition, as well as tests that assess calculations, knowledge of one's own body, visuospatial abilities (copying, drawing, route finding), and ability to perform purposeful skilled actions. Each of these will also be discussed below.

OMNIBUS-SCREENING TESTS

A number of tests and scales for office-based assessment of cognition exist. Two of better recognized are MMSE and MoCA. MMSE is a short screening test with 30 items and provides examiner with a rapid and global view of the patient's cognitive function and covers various areas of certain cognitive capabilities consisting of orientation, registration, attention, calculation, recall, and language skills. Highest MMSE score is 30 and it serves as a useful screening tool for dementia as a global diagnosis and cannot be used as a tool to differentiate various forms of dementia from each other. The other brief neuropsychology test is MoCA, which consists of a one-page 30 points scale which concentrates on short-term memory recall, visuospatial skills, language, constructions, and executive functions. It is useful for early detection of mild cognitive impairment, early stages of Alzheimer disease, vascular dementia, and dementia associated with Parkinson disease.[4,5] Several other commonly utilized neuropsychological tests are presented in **Box 1**.

Mini-Mental Status Examination (MMSE): This brief test, that is, widely used, tests patient's episodic memory by determining if they are oriented as well as their ability to recall three words after a delay. The three word test is also used to test working memory since the patient is also asked to immediately repeat the three words they just heard. Both working memory and the ability to calculate is assessed by having patients perform serial sevens. To test speech and language patients are asked to name a pencil and watch as well as to repeat a sentence. The patient is also tested for agraphia and alexia by asking them to write a sentence and to read and follow the command, "Close your eyes." Finally, the patients are tested for constructional apraxia by asking them to copy intersecting pentagons.

MMSE can usually be given in about 10 to 15 minutes. Although this is a widely used screening test there are several shortcomings. First of all the test is now copyrighted and must be purchased. Secondly, this screening test does not adequately assess frontal-subcortical executive functions. The two objects that subjects are asked to name are high frequency and even in the presence of a naming deficit they may perform normally on this test. Finally, a score of 27 or even 25 are considered normal. However, patients who score 27 may have a cognitive impairment that does need further evaluation. For example, if a patient is disoriented to month and is able to recall one of three objects their score will be 27, but there is a good chance this patient has some disorder such as mild cognitive impairment and needs to be evaluated.

Box 1
Examples of common neuropsychological tests used for assessment of cognitive decline

Hopkins Verbal Learning Test

Trails A & B

Digits Forward and Backward

Judgment of Line Orientation

Benton Facial Recognition

Florida Apraxia Standardized Test

Controlled Oral Word Association Test

Boston Naming Test

Stroop Test

Wisconsin Card Sorting Test

Dementia Rating Scale

Rey-Osterrieth Complex Figure

Montreal Cognitive Assessment (MoCA): The MoCA initiates with an abbreviated version of the Trial Making Test, Part B. This test requires searching (spatial attention), engagement and disengagement as well as working memory and has been found to often be impaired in patients with frontal executive dysfunction. Then the patients are asked to draw a cube, which tests patient's visuo-constructive abilities. The next test, the Clock Drawing Test with setting the hand at 10 minutes past eleven, not only assesses visuospatial abilities, but also spatial-inattention (spatial neglect) and planning a frontal-executive function. The MoCA tests language function by having patients name three animals, (1) lion, (2) rhinoceros or rhino, and (3) a dromedary, but credit is given if the patient states "camel." Next the test assesses memory by asking the patient to recall 5 words provided by the examiner. After the examiner provides these three works the patient is asked to repeat these words. The examiner then again presents these five words and the patient is again asked to repeat these words, Then the patients is told, "I will ask you to recall those words again at the end of the test" and patients verbal episodic memory is tested at the end of the test when the patient is asked to recall these words. The patient's working memory is tested by the digit span forward (five digits) and backward (three digits). Auditory attention and vigilance is tested by asking the patient to tap their hand when they hear a target letter while the examiner speaking a series of letters. The serial sevens task assesses working memory and calculations. In addition to the naming test mentioned above speech-language is also tested by having the patient repeat sentences, to provide as many words as they can, in 1 minute that start with the letter F as well as performing a semantic test of similarities (eg, "How are a train and a bicycle alike?").

The MoCA examines many more cognitive domains than does the MMSE, and thus the MoCA has greater sensitivity and specificity. The MoCA can also be obtained free of charge. However, the MoCA is a brief screening test and it does not asses all cognitive functions and in addition it does not intensely examine several domains of cognition. For example, some patients with Alzheimer disease in addition to having an amnestic disorder have an ideomotor apraxia, but the MoCA does not assess for apraxia. In addition, many patients with AD also have naming deficits and the MoCA has only three animals that subjects are asked to name. Patients with Alzheimer's disease often also have finger agnosia and cannot even name their index finger (also called pointer and forefinger). Thus, dependent on the patient's history, physical and neurologic examination as well as their performance on this or the other screening tests further specialized test should be performed.

Mattis Dementia Rating Scale: The third test, the Mattis Dementia Rating Scale, unlike the MMSE and MoCA, usually takes about 30 minutes to perform and about 10 minutes to score. This test investigates 5 major domains, Attention, Initiation/Perseveration, Construction, Conceptualization and Memory. Like the MoCA and MMSE, this test assesses memory by determining the patient's orientation, word and visual recognition memory, but unlike these other screening test it also assesses story recall as well as word and visual memory. This test also assesses visuospatial function and assesses frontal-subcortical executive function by using of Luria's tests for perseveration and initiation.

Monsch and coworkers[6] revealed that the Mattis Dementia Rating Scale was sensitive for detecting patients with Alzheimer disease, and Llebaria and colleagues[7] reported that it was also useful for discriminating between Alzheimer disease and Parkinsonian syndromes, the latter patients revealing more evidence for frontal-subcortical-executive dysfunction on the initiation/perseveration subtests. Paul and colleagues[8] also found that the initiation/perseveration subtests was also valuable in detecting subcortical white matter changes associated with vascular dementia.

There are several other screening tests such as the Addenbrooke's Cognitive Examination (Revised), The Blessed Dementia Scale, The 7 Minute Screen and the St. Louis University Mental Status Examination; however, in general these screening test do not offer any advantages over the tests mentioned above and are not as frequently used.

SPECIAL TESTS

There are many special neuropsychological tests that can help diagnose the type of dementia and help specify the functional neurobehavioral disabilities associated with the large variety of diseases that induce dementia. A review of most of these tests is discussed in Lezak and colleagues' text,[9] Neuropsychological Assessment, which contains more than 1000 pages describing neuropsychological tests. In this section, we will briefly mention some of the tests that we have found to be helpful in assessing patient's functional abilities in specific domains.

EPISODIC MEMORY

Almost all patients who have dementia have, as a major complaint, a deficit in memory. The screening tests mentioned above test for episodic memory by investigating orientation as well as word learning or story recall. However, often more sensitive tests are required and there are several word learning and recall tests such as the Hopkins Verbal Learning Test[10] and the California Verbal Learning Test.[11] In addition to testing memory, these tests allow the examiner, uncaring and apathetic to discriminate between deficits of learning, encoding and recall. This may be important because patients with frontal-subcortical dysfunction may have impaired recall but relatively intact learning and encoding and thus be able to recognize words that they did not spontaneously recall. The Wechsler Memory Scale has patients recall stories and also tests visuospatial memory.[12]

PROPOSITIONAL LANGUAGE

Many forms of dementia are associated with word finding difficulty, including AD, and the primary progressive aphasias (eg, logopenic primary progressive aphasia, and semantic dementia). One of the most commonly used tests for assessing patients naming abilities is the Boston Naming Test.[13] However, patients with language disorders also frequently have problems with spontaneous speech (eg, reduced fluency, paraphasic errors, and agrammatism), impairments of repetition, and comprehension. One of the most commonly used brief tests of propositional language is the Western Aphasia Battery. The Boston Diagnostic Aphasia Examination-Third Edition also has many valuable tests for assessing language.

Patients with dementia that impair frontal lobe functions may have subtle reductions of fluency and one of the best means of assessing fluency is with the Controlled Oral Word Association Test.[14] When performing this test patients are asked to name as many different words as they can that start with the letter F, A and S, but not to use proper names or numbers. The MoCA does test patient's ability to produce words that start with the letter F, but a recent study suggests that the using the letter A, may be more sensitive for the presence of dementia.[15]

Patients with AD may be impaired in their letter production fluency, but they are often more impaired in semantic fluency. When testing semantic fluency patients are given a semantic category, such as animals and they are asked to name as many animals as possible in 1 minute.

Patients with diseases such as AD may have impairment in reading as well as writing; however, in one form of AD known as "posterior cortical atrophy" or Benson's syndrome, one of the first symptoms may be impairment in reading without other language deficits. The screening tests mention above do test reading comprehension: however, if more detailed testing is required both the Western Aphasia Battery and the Boston Diagnostic Aphasia Examination may be useful.

ATTENTION AND VIGILANCE

Patients with dementing diseases such as AD, may reveal unilateral or hemispatial neglect. In the screening tests mentioned above patients with neglect may on the Trail Making subtest of the MoCA fail to find targets on one side and on the clock drawing test they may put all the numbers on one side. However, these screening tests may not detect spatial neglect and the most frequently used tests to assess for spatial neglect are the line bisection test, the cancellation test and drawing tests. These tests, as well as others can be found in the Behavioral Inattention Test.[16]

Patients with dementing diseases often have impairments of vigilance and while the MoCA has a detection test that assesses vigilance, this test may not detect more subtle deficits. Therefore, for more sensitive testing clinicians may want to use a continuous performance test such as The Conners Continuous Performance Test III (CPT 3).[17] Working memory tests can also assess attention and vigilance and there are N-Back tests that are very sensitive for these deficits.

VISUOSPATIAL SKILLS

Patients with several forms of dementia, including AD have visuospatial deficits including an impairment of visuospatial memory. The screening tests mentioned above often do test some visuospatial skills. For example, the MoCA has people draw a cube and a clock. However, these tests do not assess patient's visuospatial memory. A more sensitive and specific test for visuospatial abilities is the Rey-Osterrieth Complex Figure Test.[18] When performing this test patients are asked to copy a complicated line drawing, and then to reproduce this drawing from memory (recall). Therefore, this test evaluates both visuospatial abilities and memory.

There are many other visuospatial skills, such as face recognition that may be impaired in certain forms of dementia but screening tests mentioned above do not test for these disorders and there is a paucity of standardized tests that assess for this type of dysfunction. The major problem with such tests is that facial recognition, unlike word recognition is very dependent upon an individual's personal experiences.

EXECUTIVE FUNCTIONS

The term "executive functions" includes a vast array of neurobehavioral functions, including the ability to disengage and think divergently, the ability to plan and initiate activities, the ability to persist until the goal is accomplished, the ability not to perform activities that are not related to goal-oriented activities and the ability to discontinue an activity when the goal is accomplished or is no longer relevant.

As mentioned whereas the MMSE does not adequately assess for executive dysfunctions, both the MoCA and the Mattis do assess for some of these functions. There are, however, many other neuropsychological tests that do assess for these functions. One of the major executive dysfunctions is abulia-apathy. Unfortunately, this terribly disability is difficult to assess with neuropsychological tests and the diagnosis of this disorder is often heavily dependent on history. However, fluency tests such as the Controlled Oral Word Association Test does test for verbal initiation (as well as persistence) and in the visuospatial domain the Design Fluency Test can be used.[19]

In regard to testing disengagement the Stroop Test, where subjects are provided with words that name colors and these words are printed in a colored font that is, not always the same as the written color. The patients are instructed to name the color of the print rather than read the name of color word and patients with disengagement disorders are impaired on this test.

The test most often used to assess patients for disengagement is the Wisconsin Card Sorting Test, where the patient selects a sorting strategy and then is requested by the examiner to alter the strategy and patients with impaired disengagement perseverate on this strategy. The continuation of a strategy when it is no longer useful is a form of perseveration. There are several brief motor tests for perseveration including Dubois and colleagues'[20] clapping test, Luria's[21] triple loop test, and Luria's ramparts test. In the triple loop test the examiner draws a triple loop and then asks the patient to copy this, but does not let the patient see the example. The patient with motor perseveration will make more than triple loops. In the ramparts test the examiner shows the patient a series of connected alternating triangle and squares that are open on the bottom and asks the patient to draw these ramparts. Patients with perseveration will often repeat these figures rather than alternating them.

When testing for persistence and defective response inhibition, people will use the eyes closed, mouth open test of Miller Fisher[22] or Kertesz and colleagues[23] where patients are asked to maintain a posture over a period of time. Another form of defective response inhibition is "echopraxia." AR Luria[21] developed a test for echopraxia where the patient is told when the examiner lifts one finger the patient is to hold up two fingers and when the examiner holds up two fingers the patient is to hold up one finger. Patients with echopraxia copy the examiner. To examine defective response inhibition of the fingers, Luria used a 'go no-go paradigm' where the patient is told that if the examiner puts up one finger the patient is to put up two fingers, and if the examiner puts up two fingers the patient is not to put up any fingers.[21] Lhermitte[24] placed objects in front of patients with frontal dysfunction (eg, a pitcher or water and an empty glass) and without being instructed, these patients used these objects (eg, filled the glass with water and drank the water); a phenomenon called "utilization behavior."

Some patients with frontotemporal dementia will have inappropriate impulsivity and risk taking, while history is an important part of making this diagnosis there are tests such as ecological delay-discounting test[25] and the Iowa Gambling Test[26] where subjects with dementia will select from the stack of cards that have higher rewards, but even greater penalties.

Finally, one of the most important executive functions is planning ahead and one of the best means of examining planning is the Tower of London Test or Tower of Hanoi Tests. In its most simple form there are three rods and on one rod there are three disks piled on in ascending order, the largest on the bottom and the smallest at the top. The goal or objective of the puzzle is to move the entire stack to another rod so they are in the same order as they were initially; however, only one disk (the top disk) can be moved at a time to one or the other rods and no larger disk can be placed on a smaller disk. The score is the number of moves.

PERFORMANCE OF PURPOSEFUL SKILLED MOVEMENTS-PRAXIS

To successfully interact with our environment, as well as take care of ourselves and others, we need to perform purposeful skilled movements with our upper limbs. A loss of these skills is called apraxia.[27] There are 4 major forms of apraxia that may be associated with dementia and these are: (1) ideational apraxia, an inability to correctly sequence a series of acts leading to a goal; (2) conceptual apraxia, a loss of mechanical-tool knowledge; (3) ideomotor apraxia, a loss of the knowledge of how, when making transitive and intransitive movements to correctly posture and move the forelimb in space; (4) limb-kinetic apraxia, a loss of hand-finger deftness.

Patients with AD will often show evidence of ideomotor apraxia and conceptual apraxia.[28] Ideomotor apraxia as well as limb kinetic apraxia is also seen with Parkinson's disease and parkinsonian syndromes such as corticobasal degeneration and in this disorder the ideomotor and limb-kinetic apraxia is often asymmetrical.

One of the easiest means of assessing patients for limb-kinetic apraxia is the coin rotation task.[29,30] The tests for conceptual apraxia are discussed by[28]; however, one of the simplest tests to use is the alternative tool test.[31] Whereas the Florida Apraxia Battery[27] is an excellent means of assessing patients for ideomotor apraxia, a more brief test is the Apraxia Screen of TULIA (AST).[32] This test consists of twelve gestures, some transitive, some intransitive, and some meaningless. Half of the gestures are performed to verbal command and half to imitation. Finally, ideational apraxia, a deficit in sequencing a series of acts leading to a goal can be tested by providing patients with sets of pictures that show the steps in completing a task, but the steps are out of order. The participants are required to point to the pictures in the correct sequence to complete each task.[33]

One should bear in mind that the tests used to assess a patient's mental status are not a perfect test and a number of variables such as patient's cultural background, level of education, and religious beliefs may affect the test outcome.

FUNCTIONAL AND BEHAVIORAL ASSESSMENT

There are several different definitions for disease, but one of the most practical is that disease is that which causes dysfunction (problems in life). Dementias are a family of diseases that by definition requires a decline in function in real life, not just being outside of the cut-off for some neuropsychological measure. Indeed, some people, for example, those with learning disabilities or low level of education, may fall below standard cut-offs for 'normal', but function normally in their day-to-day lives. Conversely, there are people who have had a high level of ability prior to developing a cognitive problem, that though they are declining, they still might score in the 'normal' range. There are also types of dementias, such as frontotemporal lobar degenerations, that early in their course don't affect the areas of the brain that are commonly tested with cognitive screens or neuropsychological instruments, but do have a profound impact on function in the world outside of the clinic. These are just some of the reasons why it is vital to include functional and behavioral measures in the evaluation of patients for cognitive deficits, especially in the case of dementias. Screening for symptoms of dysfunction and behavioral disturbance is mandatory, but the use of standardized measures for function and behavior provides more reliable information for making a clinical diagnosis and counseling regarding the severity of cognitive disorders.

A number of tools have been developed to transform qualitative information regarding function and behavior from patients and caregivers into quantitative measures, either using a survey or structured interview format. In 2011, the dementia performance measurement set was released, a group of quality measures for dementias that was developed by a consortium of the American Academy of Neurology, American Geriatrics Society, American Medical Directors Association, and American Psychiatric Association for the Physician Consortium for Practice Improvement. Measure # 3 calls for a functional status assessment at least once every 12 months. Measure # 4 indicates that a neuropsychiatric symptom assessment be performed at least once every 12 months as well.

FUNCTIONAL ASSESSMENT

The Alzheimer's Association and the Physician Consortium for Practice Improvement recommend as a quality measure ascertainment of function yearly for those patients with a diagnosis of dementia. National guidelines recommend that at minimum yearly conducting an assessment of both instrumental activities of daily living (IADL) and activities of daily living (ADL). Examples of the more elementary ADLs include participation in bathing, dressing, feeding, mobility, and toileting. The more advanced independent IADLs include such activities as cooking, handling finances, medication management, and shopping. There are numerous validated, reliable instruments available in the medical literature for this purpose, though there is no front-runner for clinical use. Many of these tools can be given to caregivers to answer not just patients, an important consideration given the amount of anosognosia (literally absence of knowledge of illness) that is, commonly found in dementia patients. Examples include but are not limited to:

- Barthel Activities of Daily Living Index[34]
- Modified Blessed Dementia Scale[35]
- Functional Activities Questionnaire (used by the National Alzheimer's Coordinating Center)[36]
- Index of Independence in Activities of Daily Living[37]
- Instrumental Activities of Daily Living Scale[38]

BEHAVIORAL ASSESSMENT

Behavioral symptoms can occur with any of the dementias, and as an early or presenting symptom, especially in those under the age of 65, they are the hallmark of frontotemporal dementia. They are also a frequent finding in those who have suffered a traumatic brain injury. These symptoms are often more distressing and disabling than cognitive symptoms. It is a quality measure to assess for behavioral symptoms yearly. Symptoms recommended for assessment, and those often are included in behavioral surveys or structured interviews, are:

Activity disturbances:

- Agitation
- Apathy
- Appetite
- Diurnal/sleep-wake cycle disturbances
- Eating disturbances
- Impulsiveness
- Purposeless hyperactivity
- Repetitive behavior
- Resistiveness with care
- Sleep problems
- Socially inappropriate behaviors
- Verbal or physical aggressiveness
- Wandering

Mood disturbances:

- Anxiety
- Dysphoria
- Euphoria
- Irritability
- Mood lability/fluctuations

Thought & perceptual disturbances:

- Fixed false beliefs (delusions)
- Hearing or seeing things not there (hallucinations)
- Paranoia

There are a few instruments available for quantifying the type and severity of behavioral symptoms in this group of patients, examples of which are listed here:

- Behavioral and Psychological Symptoms of Dementia[39]
- Dementia Signs and Symptoms Scale[40]
- Frontal Systems Behavior Scale[41]
- Neuropsychiatric Inventory[42]

DIAGNOSTIC WORK UP

Diagnostic work up for neuropsychiatric diseases begins with an inclusive bedside or office interview, with screening questionnaires, a detailed general physical and neurologic examination, a detailed and comprehensive neuropsychology examination along with MR or CT scan of brain, brain functional imaging, as well as blood and serologic tests. In some cases additional tests such as EEG and lumbar puncture with examination of cerebrospinal fluid (CSF) may be needed.

MRI and CT scan of brain are used routinely to assess the patient's brain for any specific structural lesion(s) or disease process which can cause cognitive decline and dementia. Generally, MRI is superior to CT scan since it provides more detailed imaging information about the brain than does the CT scan and does not include ionizing radiation. However, patients with metal in their body and pacemakers may not be able to undergo MRI. In patients with cognitive impairment certain structural pathologies such as stroke, multiple sclerosis, hydrocephalus, and cancers can be eliminated using MRI or CT scan of brain. In those patients with degenerative dementia the patterns of atrophy may also help with the diagnosis. For example, patient with AD will often show atrophy of their medial temporal lobe, patients with logopenic primary progressive aphasia will show atrophy of the left parietal lobe, and those with semantic dementia their left anterior temporal lobe.

The blood studies should include complete blood count, comprehensive metabolic panel, thyroid function tests, vitamins B1, B6, B12, D, and folate levels, HBA1c, ESR and CRP. In those patients who may have infections, blood tests such as those for syphilis fluorescent treponemal antibody absorption (FTA-ABS), HIV, and Lyme titer, should be obtained. In cases suspicious for underlying occult malignancies paraneoplastic panel, particularly anti-N-methyl-D-aspartate receptor (NMDAR) antibodies, antibodies directed against voltage-gated potassium channels and against voltage-gated calcium channels should be checked.

In patients with cognitive decline and memory loss electroencephalography (EEG) is ordered on a case-by-case basis to exclude seizures, encephalopathy, and certain diseases such as Creutzfeldt-Jakob disease. Nerve conduction studies and needle electromyography are utilized to confirm certain diseases such as amyotrophic lateral sclerosis and myotonic dystrophy which also include cognitive impairment and dementia. Sleep studies are indicated in certain patients with sleep disorders, particularly with sleep apnea, since apnea may contribute to memory and thinking decline. Spinal tap and examination of CSF is another informative test which should be on selective cases. CSF can be examined for certain biomarkers such protein 14-3-3, total tau, and RT-QuIC for diagnosis of Creutzfeldt-Jakob disease or longitudinal assessment of CSF for total tau protein, hyperphosphoryalted tau protein 181, beta-amyloid (1-42) protein levels for diagnosis of Alzheimer disease, as well as test for infectious agents, including fungi (eg, Cryptococcus), syphilis, bacteria, and viruses (eg, herpes).

SUMMARY

The present article provided our readers with a succinct and practical guide for conducting neurobehavioral assessment of patients with cognitive decline and behavioral abnormalities. The clinical interview and neurologic examination combined with neuropsychological assessment as well as laboratory tests, and neuroimaging have enhanced our capabilities to better characterize neurobehavioral disorders and design more effective therapeutic and management approaches.

REFERENCES

1. Petersen RC, Smith GE, Waring SC, et al. Mild cognitive impairment: clinical characterization and outcome. Arch Neurol 1999;56(3):303–8.
2. Morris JC. The Clinical Dementia Rating (CDR): Current vision and scoring rules. Neurology 1993;43:2412–4.
3. Folstein MF, Folstein SE, McHugh PR. "Mini-mental state". A practical method for grading the cognitive state of patients for the clinician. J Psychiatr Res 1975; 12(3):189–98.
4. Hoops S, Nazem S, Siderowf AD, et al. Validity of the MoCA and MMSE in the detection of MCI and dementia in Parkinson disease. Neurology 2009;73(21):1738–45.
5. Chou KL, Lenhart A, Koeppe RA, et al. Abnormal MoCA and normal range MMSE scores in Parkinson disease without dementia: cognitive and neurochemical correlates. Parkinsonism Relat Disord 2014;20(10):1076–80.
6. Monsch AU, Bondi MW, Salmon DP, et al. Clinical validity of the Mattis Dementia Rating Scale in detecting Dementia of the Alzheimer type. A double cross-validation and application to a community-dwelling sample. Arch Neurol 1995; 52(9):899–904.
7. Llebaria G, Pagonabarraga J, Kulisevsky J, et al. Cut-off score of the Mattis Dementia Rating Scale for screening dementia in Parkinson's disease. Mov Disord 2008;23(11):1546–50.
8. Paul R, Moser D, Cohen R, et al. Dementia severity and pattern of cognitive performance in vascular dementia. Appl Neuropsychol 2001;8(4):211–7.
9. Lezak MD, Howieson DB, Bigler ED, et al. Neuropsychological assessment. 5th edition. New York: Oxford University Press; 2012.
10. Velayudhan L, Ryu SH, Raczek M, et al. Review of brief cognitive tests for patients with suspected dementia. Int Psychogeriatr 2014;26(8):1247–62.
11. Abwender DA, Swan JG, Bowerman JT, et al. Qualitative analysis of verbal fluency output: review and comparison of several scoring methods. Assessment 2001;8(3):323–38.
12. Tulsky DS. A new look at the WMS-III: new research to guide clinical practice. J Clin Exp Neuropsychol 2004;26(4):453–8.
13. Kaplan, Goodglass H, Weintraub S. Boston naming test. Philadelphia: Lea & Febiger; 1983.
14. Sumerall SW, Timmons PL, James AL, et al. Expanded norms for the Controlled Oral Word Association Test. J Clin Psychol 1997;53(5):517–21.
15. Behforuzi H, Burtis DB, Williamson JB, et al. Impaired initial vowel versus consonant letter-word fluency in dementia of the Alzheimer type. Cogn Neurosci 2013; 4(3–4):163–70.

16. Wilson B, Cockburn J, Halligan P. Development of a behavioral test of visuospatial neglect. Arch Phys Med Rehabil 1987;68(2):98–102.
17. Conners CK, MHS Staff, editors. Conners' continuous performance test II: computer program for windows technical guide and software manual. North Tonawanda (NY): Multi-Health Systems; 2000.
18. Loring DW, Martin RC, Meador KJ, et al. Psychometric construction of the Rey-Osterrieth Complex Figure: methodological considerations and interrater reliability. Arch Clin Neuropsychol 1990;5(1):1–14.
19. Baldo JV, Shimamura AP, Delis DC, et al. Verbal and design fluency in patients with frontal lobe lesions. J Int Neuropsychol Soc 2001;7(5):586–96.
20. Dubois B, Slachevsky A, Pillon B, et al. "Applause sign" helps to discriminate PSP from FTD and PD. Neurology 2005;64(12):2132–3.
21. Luria AR. Higher cortical functions in man. New York: Basic Books; 1966.
22. Fisher CM. Left hemiplegia and motor impresistence. J Nerv Ment Dis 1956; 123(3):201–18.
23. Kertesz A, Clydesdale S. Neuropsychological deficits in vascular dementia vs Alzheimer's disease. Frontal lobe deficits prominent in vascular dementia. Arch Neurol 1994;51(12):1226–31.
24. Lhermitte F. 'Utilization behaviour' and its relation to lesions of the frontal lobes. Brain 1983;106(Pt 2):237–55.
25. Manes F, Torralva T, Ibáñez A, et al. Decision-making in frontotemporal dementia: clinical, theoretical and legal implications. Dement Geriatr Cogn Disord 2011; 32(1):11–7.
26. Heilman KM, Rothi LJG. Apraxia. In: Heilman KM, Valenstein E, editors. Clinical Neuropsychology. Oxford: Oxford University Press; 2003. p. 215–35.
27. Heilman KM, Rothi LJG. Apraxia. In: Heilman KM, Valenstein E, editors. Clinical neuropsychology. Oxford (United Kingdom): Oxford University Press; 2003. p. 215–35.
28. Ochipa C, Gonzalez-Rothi LJ, Heilman KM. Conceptual apraxia in Alzheimers disease. Brain 1992;115:1061–71.
29. Hanna-Pladdy B, Mendoza JE, Apostolos GT, et al. Lateralised motor control: hemispheric damage and the loss of deftness. J Neurol Neurosurg Psychiatry 2002;73(5):574–7.
30. Quencer K, Okun MS, Crucian G, et al. Limb-kinetic apraxia in Parkinson disease. Neurology 2007;68(2):150–1.
31. Falchook AD, Mosquera DM, Finney GR, et al. The relationship between semantic knowledge and conceptual apraxia in Alzheimer disease. Cogn Behav Neurol 2012;25(4):167–74.
32. Vanbellingen T, Kersten B, Van de Winckel A, et al. A new bedside test of gestures in stroke: the apraxia screen of TULIA (AST). J Neurol Neurosurg Psychiatry 2011;82(4):389–92.
33. Qureshi M, Williamson JB, Heilman KM. Ideational apraxia in Parkinson disease. Behav Neurol 2011;24(3):122–7.
34. Wade DT, Collin C. The Barthel ADL Index: a standard measure of physical disability? Int Disabil Stud 1988;10(2):64–7.
35. Erkinjuntti T, Hokkanen L, Sulkava R, et al. The Blessed Dementia Scale as a screening test for dementia. Int J Geriatr Psychiatry 1988;3:267–73.
36. Pfeffer RI, Kurosaki TT, Harrah CH Jr, et al. Measurement of functional activities in older adults in the community. J Gerontol 1982;37(3):323–9.
37. Katz S, Ford AB, Moskowitz RW, et al. Studies of illness in the aged. The index of ADL: A standardized measure of biological and psychological function. JAMA 1963;185:914–9.

38. Lawton MP, Brody EM. Assessment of older people: self-maintaining and instrumental activities of daily living. Gerontologist 1969;9:179–86.

39. Cerejeira J, Lagarto L, Mukaetova-Ladinska EB. Behavioral and psychological symptoms of dementia. Front Neurol 2012;3:73.

40. Loreck DJ, Bylsma FW, Folstein MF. A new scale for comprehensive assessment of psychopathology in Alzheimer's disease. Am J Geriatr Psychiatry 1994;2(1): 60–74.

41. Grace J, Malloy PF. Frontal systems behavior scale (FrSBe): professional manual. Lutz (FL): Psychological Assessment Resources; 2001.

42. Cummings JL, Mega M, Gray K, et al. The Neuropsychiatric Inventory: comprehensive assessment of psychopathology in dementia. Neurology 1994;44: 2308–14.

Behavioral Neurology of Multiple Sclerosis and Autoimmune Encephalopathies

Abdorreza Naser Moghadasi, MD[a,1], Shadi Pourmand, MD[a,1],
Maryam Sharifian, MD[a], Alireza Minagar, MD[b],
Mohammad Ali Sahraian, MD[a,]*

KEYWORDS

- Multiple sclerosis • Cognition • Behavioral change • Depression

KEY POINTS

- Cognitive impairment may start at an early stage in multiple sclerosis (MS), and approximately 50% of the patients may face such difficulty.
- Different areas of cognitive domains are involved in MS patients, including memory, information-processing speed, attention, and executive function.
- Lability, irritability, inflexibility, aggression, impatience, and apathy are the most common behavioral symptoms among patients with MS.
- Management of cognitive and behavioral abnormalities in MS should include both pharmacologic and nonpharmacologic approaches to achieve the best results. Particular attention to diagnose and manage behavioral impairments should start immediately after diagnosis.
- Multicenter controlled studies aimed at treating cognitive and neurobehavioral problems in MS should be planned, and cognitive tests should be considered as an outcome measure in future disease-modifying trials.

INTRODUCTION

Multiple sclerosis (MS) is a chronic autoimmune disorder that usually affects young adults. The disease frequently starts in a relapsing course with different signs and symptoms that may lead to a progressive phase in which the patients experience progression of disability with or without exacerbations.[1] A diagnosis of MS often has

The authors have no conflict of interest to disclose.
[a] MS Research Center, Neuroscience Institute, Tehran University of Medical Sciences, Sina Hospital Hassan Abad Square, Tehran 1136746911, Iran; [b] Department of Neurology, Louisiana State University Health Sciences Center - Shreveport, 1501 Kings Highway, Shreveport, LA 71130, USA
[1] These authors contributed equally to this work.
* Corresponding author. MS Research Center, Neuroscience Institute, Sina Hospital, Hassan Abad Square, Tehran, Iran.
E-mail address: msahrai@tums.ac.ir

Neurol Clin 34 (2016) 17–31
http://dx.doi.org/10.1016/j.ncl.2015.08.002
0733-8619/16/$ – see front matter © 2016 Elsevier Inc. All rights reserved.

profound social and psychological impacts on the patient's life not only for physical disabilities but also for its special features. MS starts at the most productive years of life, and unpredictability of the clinical course, the impact on education, employment, sexual and family functioning, friendships, and activities of daily living are some of the features making MS different from other neurologic diseases.[2]

Neuropsychiatric symptoms are well documented in MS and can be divided into cognitive and behavioral symptoms. Although changes in cognitive abilities in MS are not universal and uniform, some cases may experience changes in cognitive abilities from the beginning of the disease even at the stage of clinically isolated syndrome, and many patients face this problem with a progression of physical disabilities.[3,4] Actually, most of the mild to moderate cognitive and neurobehavioral changes may be ignored or may receive less attention by the clinicians because of their special focus on the physical aspects of the disease and the misconception of intellectual abilities being spared in MS. Even most of the pivotal trials on approved medications did not consider this point seriously, and the major outcome measures were annual relapse rate and level of disability. During the last 2 decades, thanks to the development of more sensitive neuropsychological tests, many studies have demonstrated the high prevalence of cognitive problems in MS and its special impact on quality of life regardless of physical disabilities. Cognitive impairment has been reported in 40% to 60% of patients based on the type of home-based or community-based studies.[4,5]

Frank dementia is rare and may be seen in less than 10% of the patients.[6] Several aspects of life, such as driving, employment, and social activities, have been demonstrated to be affected by changes in cognitive performance.[7,8]

Different areas of cognitive domains are involved in MS patients, including memory, information processing, attention, and executive function.[9] Any disorder in the above-mentioned areas can affect the person's behavioral trends. Actually, cognitive impairment and behavioral changes are closely related and both of them should be taken into account in the management of such patients.

In this review, first a summary of most important cognitive domains that are involved in MS is provided and then some important aspects of behavioral changes in clinical practice are described. Also a brief review on the management of cognitive declines and behavioral problems in MS is provided.

COGNITIVE PROBLEMS
Information Processing

The information-processing speed is affected more frequently and at an earlier stage than other cognitive domains in MS.[10,11] It has been proven that there is a direct relationship between the information-processing speed and T2 lesion volume and brain atrophy.[12] In addition, it has been demonstrated that the extent of corpus callosum atrophy is directly correlated with information-processing speed disorder.[13] Information-processing speed disorder may directly affect the patient's behavior. These patients may find it difficult to learn new information.[14] Moreover, information-processing speed disorder can decrease the speed of planning and problem-solving.[15] Furthermore, it has been reported that information-processing speed has a direct relationship to anxiety, depression, and apathy in MS.[16–18]

Memory

Memory disorders, especially in long-term memory, have been reported in MS patients. Memory disorder is associated with reduced hippocampal activity and male gender.[19] Memory disorder is usually due to the disturbance in acquiring new information. Different aspects of memory may be involved in this disease; the most common is the involvement of working memory.[20] One of the reasons for the high prevalence of this disorder is the information-processing speed disturbance and its role in working memory,[20] which affects working memory in the early stages of the disease because of the involvement of the network modularity.[21] Another affected aspect of memory is verbal memory.[22] Memory disorders may result in behavioral problems and impaired learning, which affect decision-making abilities.[23]

Executive Function

Executive functioning refers to the cognitive abilities that manage complex goal-directed behavior and adaptation to environmental changes or demands.

Different aspects of executive functions, like conceptual reasoning, semantic encoding, and temporal ordering, are disturbed in MS patients.[24] It seems that frontal lobe lesions and their size are associated with the extent of executive function disorder.[25,26] The involvement of the frontal lobe may result in accompanying behavioral problems like apathy and disinhibition.[27]

Emotional Intelligence

Emotional intelligence refers to the ability of a person to perceive and evaluate his and other people's emotions and manage them, which is one of the effective factors in coping with the human environment.[28] A study showed that MS patients experience more disturbances in emotional intelligence than normal individuals,[29] which can play an important role in the behavioral abnormalities of these patients.

Decision-Making

The ability to make decisions is an important factor in maintaining goals of life despite varying external and internal conditions of an individual. Any problem with decision-making can significantly affect many aspects of life, such as occupation as well as treatment adhesion. Decision-making alteration can lead to mood disorders.[30] Difficulty in information processing, executive performance, and working memory are among the causes of disorder in the ability of decision-making in such patients.

Disorder in decision-making ability may occur during the early phases of the disease and deteriorate with the time.[31] Interestingly, decision-making disorder can take place individually, despite normal functioning of the other cognitive domains; this is more pronounced in patients with secondary progressive (SP) MS compared with those with primary progressive and relapsing forms.[31]

PSYCHOLOGICAL AND BEHAVIORAL PROBLEMS

Psychological problems, such as depression, anxiety, euphoria, hallucination, and delusion, may cause behavioral abnormalities in patients with MS. It seems that the severity of these disorders is related to the social stresses and volume of lesions on MRI.[32] Patients with an SP course suffer more frequently from psychological disorders compared with others.[33] In a meta-analysis of 23 studies, Rosti-Otajärvi and Hämäläinen concluded that the most common behavioral symptoms among patients with MS are lability (41%), irritability (38%), inflexibility (26%), aggression (23%), impatience (22%), and apathy (22%). They also found that adjustment disorder (17%) is the most frequent behavioral impairment in such patients.[34] Some of the most important psychological disorders are discussed briefly.

Depression

The relationship between depression and MS has been well established in various studies.[35,36] Although different prevalence has been reported in various communities, it seems that up to 65% of the patients suffer this disorder.[37,38] Studies have even shown a direct relationship between the extent of disability and depression.[39,40] Moreover, depression is one of the exacerbating factors of fatigue[41] and is a risk factor for suicide[42,43] due to its effect on the quality of life.[44] The rate of suicide due to depression is also high in MS; in one study, it is the leading cause of death in up to 15% of MS clinic patients.[45]

Anxiety

Although anxiety is less frequent than depression in MS patients, its prevalence is higher than the normal population.[38] The prevalence is higher in female patients, those with a lower age of onset, and if the disease is accompanied by pain or fatigue.[46,47] Anxiety has also a direct relationship with disability.[48]

As for the type of anxiety, panic disorder has the highest prevalence followed by obsessive-compulsive and generalized anxiety disorders.[49] Contrary to depression, functional imaging studies have shown no direct relationship between anxiety and abnormal MRI findings,[50] which could indicate that in contrast to the depression (as a biological event), anxiety has no biological basis and is probably a psychological response to the conditions produced by the disease.[50]

Personality Disorders

Personality disorders are common in patients with MS.[51] It has been shown that these patients have a lower self-esteem than the control group, are less capable of coping with stressful conditions, and are less competent.[52] It has also been demonstrated that personality disorders have a direct relationship with mood and anxiety disorders, and that depressed/anxious patients are less agreeable, less extroverted, and more neurotic than other patients.[53] Functional MRI (fMRI) has showed that the personality traits of the patients may be associated with the pattern of neural activity on fMRI.[54] Furthermore, it has been reported that cortical atrophy may result in personality disorders.[55,56] Personality disorders can in turn affect the disease trend. Personality disorders, especially low conscientiousness and neuroticism, can be accompanied by poor treatment adherence,[57] which in turn may worsen the prognosis.

Psychotic Disorders

Psychotic disorders may be seen in MS patients, and the reported prevalence of psychosis and bipolar disorder is around 5%.[58] Different psychotic disorders are reported in these patients, including euphoria, hallucination, and delusion.[59] In rare cases, psychosis can be the first manifestation of the disease.[60,61] It seems that there is a relationship between psychosis with the amount of lesions in the periventricular area, especially lesions around the temporal horns.[62]

Substance Abuse

A history of substance abuse has been reported in 19% of the patients[63] and is more prevalent in younger patients with less disability.[63] The most commonly abused substance is alcohol.[64] However, there is no correlation between alcohol consumption and risk of MS development.[65]

MANAGEMENT OF COGNITIVE AND BEHAVIORAL ABNORMALITIES IN MULTIPLE SCLEROSIS

Treatment of cognitive impairment in MS should include disease-modifying therapies (DMT) in combination with pharmacologic and nonpharmacologic cognitive-enhancement strategies.[66]

Although cognitive aspects were not considered as an outcome measure in MS, follow-up single- or multicenter studies demonstrated that different types of DMTs may be effective in preventing cognitive declines in MS. Interferon (IFN) -β-1a[67,68] and IFN-β-1b[69] were both shown to be effective, but in a single study, it was demonstrated that IFN-β-1a preparations are more helpful in resolving the cognitive impairments in MS patients compared with IFN-β-1b.[70]

Although glatiramer acetate was shown to guard against rapid memory decline during in experimental autoimmune encephalomyelitis,[71] it failed to show any significant effect on cognitive function in a 2-year longitudinal study on relapsing MS.[72]

Natalizumab was shown to reduce cognitive changes, fatigue, and brain atrophy rate in relapsing-remitting MS.[73–75]

SYMPTOMATIC PHARMACOTHERAPY

Different agents and cognitive enhancers, such as acetyl choloine receptor inhibitors, have been used to prevent cognitive decline or improve this function with different results. Donepezil (10 mg daily), a reversible inhibitor of acetyl cholinesterase, showed its effectiveness in primary studies,[76,77] but failed to demonstrate the same effect in placebo-controlled trials, especially in mild cases.[78–80] Rivastigmine, another cholinesterase inhibitor (1.5 mg once a day increment to 3 mg twice daily), used in Alzheimer disease showed a nonsignificant increase in total recall score in MS patients.[81] It is safe and well tolerated, but clinical trials did not show a significant improvement in cognition of MS patients compared with placebo.

Memantine (10 mg twice a day), acting on the glutamatergic system by blocking N-methyl-D-aspartate (NMDA) receptors, was used for treatment of cognitive impairment in MS. Overall, it is a safe and well-tolerated medication with limited adverse effects. Despite these advantages, placebo-controlled clinical trials did not show any significant improvement in cognition of MS patients.[82]

Primary studies on ginkgo biloba reported modest beneficial effects on select functional measures in MS without any significant adverse effects.[83,84] Again, other studies showed that treatment with ginkgo biloba extract does not improve cognitive performance in MS.[85]

NONPHARMACOLOGIC COGNITIVE-ENHANCEMENT STRATEGIES

Neuropsychological rehabilitation or behavioral memory interventions (eg, modified Story Memory Technique) may have favorable effects on patients' cognitive performance and coping with cognitive impairments.[86–88]

In a Cochrane Review, the authors found a low level of evidence for neuropsychological rehabilitation to reduce cognitive symptoms in MS. Cognitive training was also found to improve memory span and working memory. A combination of cognitive training with other neuropsychological rehabilitation methods was found to improve attention, immediate verbal memory, and delayed memory.[89]

DEPRESSION

Depression should be treated properly in these patients because it may have a direct effect on the morbidity and mortality of the disease.[90] Depression may affect cognition, fatigue, sleep, and even adhesion to prescribed medications; this means that clinicians should plan for a comprehensive treatment of depression using pharmacotherapy or psychotherapy at any stages of the disease.

PHARMACOTHERAPY

Use of antidepressants in depressed patients with MS is strongly recommended. Different types of antidepressant were studied in MS.

Selective serotonin reuptake inhibitors (SSRIs) are considered a well-tolerated first-line treatment of depression in MS. In this group, sertraline is usually the first option. Sertraline is usually started at 25 mg/d and can increase up to 50 mg/d. It is important to wait a few weeks to assess the drug's effects before increasing the dose. A maximum dose of sertraline is generally 200 mg/d in a single dose.[91]

More than antidepressive effects, one study showed immune-modulatory effects of sertraline on an experimental autoimmune encephalomyelitis mouse model.[92]

The second choice among SSRIs is Paroxetine. It is usually started at 10 mg/d for the first 5 days and then is increased up to 20 mg/d. The maximum dose of Paroxetine is about 50 mg/d in a single dose.[91,93]

Fluvoxamine is another choice, starting with 25 mg/d and then increasing 25 mg/d every 5 days until 200 mg/d is reached. The important consideration about fluvoxamine is the risk of increasing the blood level of corticosteroids and cyclophosphamide as MS treatments.[91]

Fluoxetine is effective in both depression and MS fatigue.[94] More than routine antidepressant effects, some studies showed neuroprotective effects of fluoxetine in MS by the observed partial normalization of the structure-related magnetic resonance spectroscopy parameter N-acetylaspartate in white matter lesions.[95] Fluoxetine also tends to reduce the formation of new enhancing lesions.[96] However, a single study reported exacerbation of symptoms of MS in a patient taking fluoxetine.[97]

Tricyclic antidepressants (TCAs) are generally reserved for second-line treatment in MS-related depression due to sedating and anticholinergic side effects, such as fatigue, orthostatic hypotension, imbalance, cognitive disturbances, and bladder problems. However, these anticholinergic properties may be helpful to patients with symptoms of bladder spasticity or chronic pain. In this group, amitriptyline, desipramine, or other TCAs are used at 25 to 100 mg/d.[91,98]

Serotonin noradrenaline reuptake inhibitors, with the exception of duloxetine, and other newer antidepressants have failed to treat MS depression because of their side-effects profile and also their frequent interaction with other drugs.

With duloxetine, the initial dose for depression is 40 mg/d in 2 doses; it can increase to 60 mg/d in 1 to 2 doses if necessary. Duloxetine may increase the risk of liver problems in patients who received other medications for MS treatment.[91] Valporic acid has also been used in MS patients with dysphoric mood disorders, depression, and panic attacks.[99,100]

PSYCHOTHERAPEUTIC INTERVENTIONS
Cognitive-Behavior Therapy

Several studies have demonstrated the valuable effect of cognitive-behavior therapy (CBT) on MS-related depression by assisting the patients to correct distorted cognitive appraisal of the environment and also core beliefs that lead to malformed behaviors.[90,101,102] It changes the connection between life events and learned reactions, such as depression beliefs. CBT can help the subjects to achieve better coping skills in reaction to the environmental stresses.[90,101] Computerized forms of CBT and telephone-administered CBT are particularly appealing because of the frequent physical disability in MS patients, which is an obstacle to receiving sufficient therapy.[103]

Problem-Solving Therapy

Internet-based problem-solving therapy was shown to be a new possibility to reach and treat MS patients with depressive symptoms. It also improves the quality of care, especially in patients who experience disease-related or other barriers to participate in face-to-face counseling.[104,105]

Electroconvulsive Therapy

Electroconvulsive therapy (ECT) can be used in the treatment of severe drug-refractory depression. However, neurologic relapse after ECT was seen in 20% of the patients. The presence of active brain lesions on MRI before ECT may be a potential risk factor for relapse.[106–108]

Others

The association of modifiable lifestyle factors with depression risk was shown in an international sample of people with MS.[109] This study demonstrated that poor diet, low levels of exercise, obesity, smoking, marked social isolation, and taking IFN all were associated with greater risk of depression. Patients who supplemented with ω-3s, frequent fish consumption, vitamin D, and those who meditated or who had moderate alcohol consumption had significantly reduced depression risk.[109] Music and music therapy were shown to be effective in mood disorders of MS too.[110]

Psychosis

There are reports of coincidence of psychosis and MS.[62] Treatment of psychosis in MS was not studied in trials, but low doses of atypical antipsychotics such as risperidone or clozapine can be considered the treatment of choice. A combination of benzodiazepines may also be useful for sedation.[111,112] ECT was shown to be effective in some case reports.[113,114]

BEHAVIORAL NEUROLOGY OF AUTOIMMUNE ENCEPHALOPATHIES

Different kinds of autoimmune encephalitis are increasingly recognized causes of neurologic dysfunction. A combination of various manifestations, such as behavioral changes, psychosis, movement disorders, seizures, autonomic instability, and coma, may be the initial symptom or present during the course of the disease. Several types of idiopathic or paraneoplastic autoimmune encephalitis have been reported in the literature.[115]

In anti-NMDA receptor encephalitis, the antibodies are detected in the cerebrospinal fluid or the serum of patients, especially young women with ovarian teratoma. It has also been reported in teratoma of other locations (such as mediastinum, testis) or with other cancers.[116,117]

These patients typically develop schizophrenia-like psychiatric symptoms, usually preceded by fever, headache, or viral infection-like illness. In the peak of psychosis, most patients developed seizures followed by an unresponsive/catatonic state, decreased level of consciousness, and central hypoventilation frequently requiring mechanical ventilation. Orofacial limb dyskinesias is very common; these included grimacing, masticatory-like movements, and forceful jaw opening and closing, which resulting in lip and tongue injuries or broken teeth.

Autonomic symptoms, cardiac dysrhythmias, and hypoventilation are the other symptoms. The highly characteristic syndrome evolved in 5 stages: First: the prodromal phase (fever, headache, or viral infection-like illness); second: the psychotic phase (schizophrenia-like psychiatric symptoms); third: the unresponsive phase; fourth: the hyperkinetic phase (most prolonged and crucial phase, which is usually severe and can be fatal, but potentially reversible); last: the gradual recovery phase. If patients overcome the hyperkinetic phase, gradual improvement is expected within months. Full recovery can be expected over 3 or more years.[117,118]

Limbic encephalitis was first identified as a clinicopathologic entity in 1968 as a paraneoplastic syndrome associated with small-cell lung cancer.[119] This disorder refers to an inflammatory process of the limbic system, including the medial temporal lobes, amygdala, and also cingulate gyrus. It is one of the most frequently misdiagnosed disorders.[120]

The disorder, which develops in a few days or weeks, is characterized by the development of severe short-term memory loss (typical of all limbic encephalitis), various types of seizures, including myoclonic-like movements, faciobrachial dystonic seizures and tonic seizures, confusion, and psychiatric features (cognitive decline and irritability).[121]

Despite several reports of association with cancer, most patients do not have cancer.[121]

The Ophelia syndrome is a form of limbic encephalitis that occurs in association with Hodgkin lymphoma in children and young adults and presents with learning and memory difficulties. The prompt recognition of this disorder is important because it usually precedes the diagnosis of lymphoma.[122,123]

Hashimoto encephalopathy (encephalopathy associated with autoimmune thyroid disease) is a relatively rare condition observed in a small percentage of patients presenting with autoimmune thyroid disease.[124]

It is a subacute, relapsing-remitting, steroid-responsive encephalopathy characterized by protean neurologic and neuropsychiatric symptoms.

Most clinical manifestations include altered mental status, hallucinations, delusional thinking, and often, epileptic seizures, neurologic diffuse or focal signs, headache, and altered cognitive function.[125]

It is diagnosed by the clinical syndrome, slowing in electroencephalogram, normal MRI, presence of elevated titers of antithyroid antibodies, the lack of another diagnosis based on clinical evaluation, and the response to corticosteroid and other immunosuppressant treatment.[126]

In cases with acute or subacute neurobehavioral changes, especially when they present in combination with seizures, myoclonus, abnormal movements, and other neurologic disorders, autoimmune encephalitis should be considered. Some of them may be preceded with upper respiratory tract infections and can be seen at all ages. Early diagnosis and proper management may be lifesaving for the patients, although residual behavioral, language, and cognitive problems may persist for the rest of life.

REFERENCES

1. Koch-Henriksen N, Sørensen PS. The changing demographic pattern of multiple sclerosis epidemiology. Lancet Neurol 2010;9:520–32.

2. Patti F, Vila C. Symptoms, prevalence and impact of multiple sclerosis in younger patients: a multinational survey. Neuroepidemiology 2014;42:211–8.
3. Calabrese P. Neuropsychology of multiple sclerosis: an overview. J Neurol 2006; 253(Suppl):10–5.
4. Jonsson A, Andresen J, Storr L, et al. Cognitive impairment in newly diagnosed multiple sclerosis patients: a 4-year follow-up study. J Neurol Sci 2006;245:77–85.
5. Amato MP, Zipoli V, Portaccio E. Multiple sclerosis-related cognitive changes: a review of cross-sectional and longitudinal studies. J Neurol Sci 2006;245:41–6.
6. Longley WA. Multiple sclerosis-related dementia: relatively rare and often misunderstood. Brain Impairment 2007;8:154–67.
7. Schultheis MT, Garay E, DeLuca J. The influence of cognitive impairment on driving performance in multiple sclerosis. Neurology 2001;56:1089–94.
8. Rao SM, Leo GJ, Ellington L, et al. Cognitive dysfunction in multiple sclerosis. II. Impact on employment and social functioning. Neurology 1991;41:692–6.
9. Rogers JM, Panegyres PK. Cognitive impairment in multiple sclerosis: evidence-based analysis and recommendations. J Clin Neurosci 2007;14:919–27.
10. Van Schependom J, D'hooghe MB, Cleynhens K, et al. Reduced information processing speed as primum movens for cognitive decline in MS. Mult Scler 2015;21:83–91.
11. Denney DR, Gallagher KS, Lynch SG. Deficits in processing speed in patients with multiple sclerosis: evidence from explicit and covert measures. Arch Clin Neuropsychol 2011;26:110–9.
12. Rao SM, Martin AL, Huelin R, et al. Correlations between MRI and information processing speed in MS: a meta-analysis. Mult Scler Int 2014;2014:975803.
13. Bergendal G, Martola J, Stawiarz L, et al. Callosal atrophy in multiple sclerosis is related to cognitive speed. Acta Neurol Scand 2013;127:281–9.
14. Chiaravalloti ND, Stojanovic-Radic J, DeLuca J. The role of speed versus working memory in predicting learning new information in multiple sclerosis. J Clin Exp Neuropsychol 2013;35:180–91.
15. Owens EM, Denney DR, Lynch SG. Difficulties in planning among patients with multiple sclerosis: a relative consequence of deficits in information processing speed. J Int Neuropsychol Soc 2013;19:613–20.
16. Niino M, Mifune N, Kohriyama T, et al. Apathy/depression, but not subjective fatigue, is related with cognitive dysfunction in patients with multiple sclerosis. BMC Neurol 2014;14:3.
17. Goretti B, Viterbo RG, Portaccio E, et al. Anxiety state affects information processing speed in patients with multiple sclerosis. Neurol Sci 2014;35:559–63.
18. Labiano-Fontcuberta A, Mitchell AJ, Moreno-García S, et al. Anxiety and depressive symptoms in caregivers of multiple sclerosis patients: the role of information processing speed impairment. J Neurol Sci 2015;349(1–2):220–5.
19. Hulst HE, Schoonheim MM, Van Geest Q, et al. Memory impairment in multiple sclerosis: relevance of hippocampal activation and hippocampal connectivity. Mult Scler 2015. [Epub ahead of print].
20. Brissart H, Leininger M, Le Perf M, et al. Working memory in multiple sclerosis: a review. Rev Neurol (Paris) 2012;168:15–27.
21. Gamboa OL, Tagliazucchi E, von Wegner F, et al. Working memory performance of early MS patients correlates inversely with modularity increases in resting state functional connectivity networks. Neuroimage 2014;94:385–95.
22. Lafosse JM, Mitchell SM, Corboy JR, et al. The nature of verbal memory impairment in multiple sclerosis: a list-learning and meta-analytic study. J Int Neuropsychol Soc 2013;19:995–1008.

23. Nagy H, Bencsik K, Rajda C, et al. The effects of reward and punishment contingencies on decision-making in multiple sclerosis. J Int Neuropsychol Soc 2006;12:559–65.
24. Arnett PA, Rao SM, Grafman J, et al. Executive functions in multiple sclerosis: an analysis of temporal ordering, semantic encoding, and planning abilities. Neuropsychology 1997;11:535–44.
25. Foong J, Rozewicz L, Quaghebeur G, et al. Executive function in multiple sclerosis. The role of frontal lobe pathology. Brain 1997;120(Pt 1):15–26.
26. Foong J, Rozewicz L, Davie CA, et al. Correlates of executive function in multiple sclerosis: the use of magnetic resonance spectroscopy as an index of focal pathology. J Neuropsychiatry Clin Neurosci 1999;11:45–50.
27. Chiaravalloti ND, DeLuca J. Assessing the behavioral consequences of multiple sclerosis: an application of the frontal systems behavior scale (FrSBe). Cogn Behav Neurol 2003;16:54–67.
28. Hoffmann M, Cases LB, Hoffmann B, et al. The impact of stroke on emotional intelligence. BMC Neurol 2010;10:103.
29. Ghajarzadeh M, Owji M, Sahraian MA, et al. Emotional intelligence (EI) of patients with multiple sclerosis (MS). Iran J Public Health 2014;43:1550–6.
30. Marvel CL, Paradiso S. Cognitive and neurological impairment in mood disorders. Psychiatr Clin North Am 2004;27:19–36.
31. Farez MF, Crivelli L, Leiguarda R, et al. Decision-making impairment in patients with multiple sclerosis: a case-control study. BMJ Open 2014;4(7):e004918.
32. Ron MA, Logsdail SJ. Psychiatric morbidity in multiple sclerosis: a clinical and MRI study. Psychol Med 1989;19:887–95.
33. Heaton RK, Nelson LM, Thompson DS, et al. Neuropsychological findings in relapsing-remitting and chronic-progressive multiple sclerosis. J Consult Clin Psychol 1985;53:103–10.
34. Rosti-Otajärvi E, Hämäläinen P. Behavioural symptoms and impairments in multiple sclerosis: a systematic review and meta-analysis. Mult Scler 2013;19(1):31–45.
35. Minden SL, Orav J, Reich P. Depression in multiple sclerosis. Gen Hosp Psychiatry 1987;9:426–34.
36. Sadovnick AD, Remick RA, Allen J, et al. Depression and multiple sclerosis. Neurology 1996;46:628–32.
37. Mrabet S, Ben Ali N, Kchaou M, et al. Depression in multiple sclerosis. Rev Neurol (Paris) 2014;170:700–2.
38. Joffe RT, Lippert GP, Gray TA, et al. Mood disorder and multiple sclerosis. Arch Neurol 1987;44:376–8.
39. Jones KH, Jones PA, Middleton RM, et al. Physical disability, anxiety and depression in people with MS: an internet-based survey via the UK MS Register. PLoS One 2014;9(8):e104604.
40. Chwastiak L, Ehde DM, Gibbons LE, et al. Depressive symptoms and severity of illness in multiple sclerosis: epidemiologic study of a large community sample. Am J Psychiatry 2002;159:1862–72.
41. Azimian M, Shahvarughi-Farahani A, Rahgozar M, et al. Fatigue, depression, and physical impairment in multiple sclerosis. Iran J Neurol 2014;13:105–7.
42. Lebrun C, Cohen M. Depression in multiple sclerosis. Rev Neurol (Paris) 2009; 165(Suppl 4):S156–62.
43. Feinstein A. Multiple sclerosis and depression. Mult Scler 2011;17:1276–81.
44. Salehpoor G, Rezaei S, Hosseininezhad M. Quality of life in multiple sclerosis (MS) and role of fatigue, depression, anxiety, and stress: a bicenter study from north of Iran. Iran J Nurs Midwifery Res 2014;19(6):593–9.

45. Chwastiak LA, Ehde DM. Psychiatric issues in multiple sclerosis. Psychiatr Clin North Am 2007;30:803–17.
46. Beiske AG, Svensson E, Sandanger I, et al. Depression and anxiety amongst multiple sclerosis patients. Eur J Neurol 2008;15:239–45.
47. Wood B, van der Mei IA, Ponsonby AL, et al. Prevalence and concurrence of anxiety, depression and fatigue over time in multiple sclerosis. Mult Scler 2013;19:217–24.
48. Askari F, Ghajarzadeh M, Mohammadifar M, et al. Anxiety in patients with multiple sclerosis: association with disability, depression, disease type and sex. Acta Med Iran 2014;52:889–92.
49. Korostil M, Feinstein A. Anxiety disorders and their clinical correlates in multiple sclerosis patients. Mult Scler 2007;13:67–72.
50. Zorzon M, de Masi R, Nasuelli D, et al. Depression and anxiety in multiple sclerosis. A clinical and MRI study in 95 subjects. J Neurol 2001;248:416–21.
51. Stathopoulou A, Christopoulos P, Soubasi E, et al. Personality characteristics and disorders in multiple sclerosis patients: assessment and treatment. Int Rev Psychiatry 2010;22:43–54.
52. Ozura A, Erdberg P, Sega S. Personality characteristics of multiple sclerosis patients: a Rorschach investigation. Clin Neurol Neurosurg 2010;112(7):629–32.
53. Bruce JM, Lynch SG. Personality traits in multiple sclerosis: association with mood and anxiety disorders. J Psychosom Res 2011;70:479–85.
54. Gioia MC, Cerasa A, Valentino P, et al. Neurofunctional correlates of personality traits in relapsing-remitting multiple sclerosis: an fMRI study. Brain Cogn 2009; 71(3):320–7.
55. Benedict RH, Hussein S, Englert J, et al. Cortical atrophy and personality in multiple sclerosis. Neuropsychology 2008;22:432–41.
56. Benedict RH, Carone DA, Bakshi R. Correlating brain atrophy with cognitive dysfunction, mood disturbances, and personality disorder in multiple sclerosis. J Neuroimaging 2004;14(3 Suppl):36S–45S.
57. Bruce JM, Hancock LM, Arnett P, et al. Treatment adherence in multiple sclerosis: association with emotional status, personality, and cognition. J Behav Med 2010;33:219–27.
58. Marrie RA, Reingold S, Cohen J, et al. The incidence and prevalence of psychiatric disorders in multiple sclerosis: a systematic review. Mult Scler 2015;21: 305–17.
59. Feinstein A, DeLuca J, Baune BT, et al. Cognitive and neuropsychiatric disease manifestations in MS. Mult Scler Relat Disord 2013;2:4–12.
60. Aggarwal A, Sharma DD, Kumar R, et al. Acute psychosis as the initial presentation of MS: a case report. Int MS J 2011;17:54–7.
61. Carrieri PB, Montella S, Petracca M. Psychiatric onset of multiple sclerosis: description of two cases. J Neuropsychiatry Clin Neurosci 2011;23(2):E6.
62. Feinstein A, du Boulay G, Ron MA. Psychotic illness in multiple sclerosis. A clinical and magnetic resonance imaging study. Br J Psychiatry 1992;161:680–5.
63. Bombardier CH, Blake KD, Ehde DM, et al. Alcohol and drug abuse among persons with multiple sclerosis. Mult Scler 2004;10(1):35–40.
64. Turner AP, Hawkins EJ, Haselkorn JK, et al. Alcohol misuse and multiple sclerosis. Arch Phys Med Rehabil 2009;90:842–8.
65. Massa J, O'Reilly EJ, Munger KL, et al. Caffeine and alcohol intakes have no association with risk of multiple sclerosis. Mult Scler 2013;19:53–8.
66. Patti F. Treatment of cognitive impairment in patients with multiple sclerosis. Expert Opin Investig Drugs 2012;21:1679–99.

67. Patti F, Amato MP, Bastianello S, et al, COGIMUS Study Group. Effects of immunomodulatory treatment with subcutaneous interferon beta-1a on cognitive decline in mildly disabled patients with relapsing-remitting multiple sclerosis. Mult Scler 2010;16:68–77.

68. Patti F, Amato MP, Trojano M, et al, COGIMUS Study Group. Longitudinal changes in social functioning in mildly disabled patients with relapsing-remitting multiple sclerosis receiving subcutaneous interferon β-1a: results from the COGIMUS (COGnitive Impairment in MUltiple Sclerosis) study (II). Qual Life Res 2012;21:1111–21.

69. Lacy M, Hauser M, Pliskin N, et al. The effects of long-term interferon-beta-1b treatment on cognitive functioning in multiple sclerosis: a 16-year longitudinal study. Mult Scler 2013;19(13):1765–72.

70. Mokhber N, Azarpazhooh A, Orouji E, et al. Cognitive dysfunction in patients with multiple sclerosis treated with different types of interferon beta: a randomized clinical trial. J Neurol Sci 2014;342:16–20.

71. LoPresti P. Glatiramer acetate guards against rapid memory decline during relapsing-remitting experimental autoimmune encephalomyelitis. Neurochem Res 2015;40:473–9.

72. Weinstein A, Schwid SR, Schiffer RB, et al. Neuropsychologic status in multiple sclerosis after treatment with glatiramer. Arch Neurol 1999;56:319–24.

73. Portaccio E, Stromillo ML, Goretti B, et al. Natalizumab may reduce cognitive changes and brain atrophy rate in relapsing-remitting multiple sclerosis—a prospective, non-randomized pilot study. Eur J Neurol 2013;20:986–90.

74. Iaffaldano P, Viterbo RG, Paolicelli D, et al. Impact of natalizumab on cognitive performances and fatigue in relapsing multiple sclerosis: a prospective, open-label, two years observational study. PLoS One 2012;7:e35843.

75. Wilken J, Kane RL, Sullivan CL, et al. Changes in fatigue and cognition in patients with relapsing forms of multiple sclerosis treated with natalizumab: the ENER-G Study. Int J MS Care 2013;15:120–8.

76. Noetzli M, Eap CB. Pharmacodynamic, pharmacokinetic and pharmacogenetic aspects of drugs used in the treatment of Alzheimer's disease. Clin Pharmacokinet 2013;52:225–41.

77. Krupp LB, Christodoulou C, Melville P, et al. Donepezil improved memory in multiple sclerosis in a randomized clinical trial. Neurology 2004;63:1579–85.

78. O'Carroll CB, Woodruff BK, Locke DE, et al. Is donepezil effective for multiple sclerosis-related cognitive dysfunction? A critically appraised topic. Neurologist 2012;18:51–4.

79. Krupp LB, Christodoulou C, Melville P, et al. Multicenter randomized clinical trial of donepezil for memory impairment in multiple sclerosis. Neurology 2011;76:1500–7.

80. He D, Zhang Y, Dong S, et al. Pharmacological treatment for memory disorder in multiple sclerosis. Cochrane Database Syst Rev 2013;(12):CD008876.

81. Mäurer M, Ortler S, Baier M, et al. Randomised multicentre trial on safety and efficacy of rivastigmine in cognitively impaired multiple sclerosis patients. Mult Scler 2013;19:631–8.

82. Lovera JF, Frohman E, Brown TR, et al. Memantine for cognitive impairment in multiple sclerosis: a randomized placebo-controlled trial. Mult Scler 2010;16:715–23.

83. Johnson SK, Diamond BJ, Rausch S, et al. The effect of Ginkgo biloba on functional measures in multiple sclerosis: a pilot randomized controlled trial. Explore (NY) 2006;2:19–24.

84. Lovera J, Bagert B, Smoot K, et al. Ginkgo biloba for the improvement of cognitive performance in multiple sclerosis: a randomized, placebo-controlled trial. Mult Scler 2007;13:376–85.
85. Lovera JF, Kim E, Heriza E, et al. Ginkgo biloba does not improve cognitive function in MS: a randomized placebo-controlled trial. Neurology 2012;79: 1278–84.
86. Hämäläinen P, Rosti-Otajärvi E. Is neuropsychological rehabilitation effective in multiple sclerosis? Neurodegener Dis Manag 2014;4:147–54.
87. Chiaravalloti ND, Wylie G, Leavitt V, et al. Increased cerebral activation after behavioral treatment for memory deficits in MS. J Neurol 2012;259: 1337–46.
88. Gich J, Freixanet J, García R, et al. A randomized, controlled, single-blind, 6-month pilot study to evaluate the efficacy of MS-Line!: a cognitive rehabilitation programme for patients with multiple sclerosis. Mult Scler 2015. [Epub ahead of print].
89. Rosti-Otajärvi EM, Hämäläinen PI. Neuropsychological rehabilitation for multiple sclerosis. Cochrane Database Syst Rev 2014;(2):CD009131.
90. Skokou M, Soubasi E, Gourzis P. Depression in multiple sclerosis: a review of assessment and treatment approaches in adult and pediatric populations. ISRN Neurol 2012;2012:427102.
91. Pérez LP, González RS, Lázaro EB. Treatment of mood disorders in multiple sclerosis. Curr Treat Options Neurol 2015;17:323.
92. Taler M, Gil-Ad I, Korob I, et al. The immunomodulatory effect of the antidepressant sertraline in an experimental autoimmune encephalomyelitis mouse model of multiple sclerosis. Neuroimmunomodulation 2011;18:117–22.
93. Ehde DM, Kraft GH, Chwastiak L, et al. Efficacy of paroxetine in treating major depressive disorder in persons with multiple sclerosis. Gen Hosp Psychiatry 2008;30:40–8.
94. Shafey H. The effect of fluoxetine in depression associated with multiple sclerosis. Can J Psychiatry 1992;37:147–8.
95. Sijens PE, Mostert JP, Irwan R, et al. Impact of fluoxetine on the human brain in multiple sclerosis as quantified by proton magnetic resonance spectroscopy and diffusion tensor imaging. Psychiatry Res 2008;164:274–82.
96. Mostert JP, Admiraal-Behloul F, Hoogduin JM, et al. Effects of fluoxetine on disease activity in relapsing multiple sclerosis: a double-blind, placebo-controlled, exploratory study. J Neurol Neurosurg Psychiatry 2008;79: 1027–31.
97. Browning WN. Exacerbation of symptoms of multiple sclerosis in a patient taking fluoxetine. Am J Psychiatry 1990;147:1089.
98. Schiffer RB, Wineman NM. Antidepressant pharmacotherapy of depression associated with multiple sclerosis. Am J Psychiatry 1990;147:1493–7.
99. Stip E, Daoust L. Valproate in the treatment of mood disorder due to multiple sclerosis. Can J Psychiatry 1995;40:219–20.
100. Marazziti D, Cassano GB. Valproic acid for panic disorder associated with multiple sclerosis. Am J Psychiatry 1996;153:842–3.
101. Larcombe NA, Wilson PH. An evaluation of cognitive-behaviour therapy for depression in patients with multiple sclerosis. Br J Psychiatry 1984;145: 366–71.
102. Hind D, Cotter J, Thake A, et al. Cognitive behavioural therapy for the treatment of depression in people with multiple sclerosis: a systematic review and meta-analysis. BMC Psychiatry 2014;14:5.

103. Beckner V, Howard I, Vella L, et al. Telephone-administered psychotherapy for depression in MS patients: moderating role of social support. J Behav Med 2010;33:47–59.

104. Boeschoten RE, Nieuwenhuis MM, van Oppen P, et al. Feasibility and outcome of a web-based self-help intervention for depressive symptoms in patients with multiple sclerosis: a pilot study. J Neurol Sci 2012;315(1–2):104–9.

105. Boeschoten RE, Dekker J, Uitdehaag BM, et al. Internet-based self-help treatment for depression in multiple sclerosis: study protocol of a randomized controlled trial. BMC Psychiatry 2012;12:137.

106. Krystal AD, Coffey CE. Neuropsychiatric considerations in the use of electroconvulsive therapy. J Neuropsychiatry Clin Neurosci 1997;9(2):283–92.

107. Coffey CE, Weiner RD, McCall WV, et al. Electroconvulsive therapy in multiple sclerosis: a magnetic resonance imaging study of the brain. Convuls Ther 1987;3:137–44.

108. Mattingly G, Baker K, Zorumski CF, et al. Multiple sclerosis and ECT: possible value of gadolinium-enhanced magnetic resonance scans for identifying high-risk patients. J Neuropsychiatry Clin Neurosci 1992;4:145–51.

109. Taylor KL, Hadgkiss EJ, Jelinek GA, et al. Lifestyle factors, demographics and medications associated with depression risk in an international sample of people with multiple sclerosis. BMC Psychiatry 2014;14:327.

110. Raglio A, Attardo L, Gontero G, et al. Effects of music and music therapy on mood in neurological patients. World J Psychiatry 2015;5:68–78.

111. Chong SA, Ko SM. Clozapine treatment of psychosis associated with multiple sclerosis. Can J Psychiatry 1997;42:90–1.

112. Sharma E, Rao NP, Venkatasubramanian G, et al. Successful treatment of co-morbid schizophrenia and multiple sclerosis. Asian J Psychiatr 2010;3:235–6.

113. Pontikes TK, Dinwiddie SH. Electroconvulsive therapy in a patient with multiple sclerosis and recurrent catatonia. J ECT 2010;26:270–1.

114. Urban-Kowalczyk M, Rudecki T, Wróblewski D, et al. Electroconvulsive therapy in patient with psychotic depression and multiple sclerosis. Neurocase 2014;20: 452–5.

115. O'Toole O, Clardy S, Lin Quek AM. Paraneoplastic and autoimmune encephalopathies. Semin Neurol 2013;33:357–64.

116. Irani SR, Bera K, Waters P, et al. N-methyl-D-aspartate antibody encephalitis: temporal progression of clinical and paraclinical observations in a predominantly non-paraneoplastic disorder of both sexes. Brain 2010;133(Pt 6): 1655–67.

117. Dalmau J, Tüzün E, Wu HY, et al. Paraneoplastic anti-N-methyl-D-aspartate receptor encephalitis associated with ovarian teratoma. Ann Neurol 2007;61: 25–36.

118. Armangue T, Petit-Pedrol M, Dalmau J. Autoimmune encephalitis in children. J Child Neurol 2012;27:1460–9.

119. Corsellis JA, Goldberg GJ, Norton AR. Limbic encephalitis and its association with carcinoma. Brain 1968;91:481–96.

120. Graus F, Saiz A. Limbic encephalitis: a probably under-recognized syndrome. Neurologia 2005;20:24–30.

121. Machado S, Pinto AN, Irani SR. What should you know about limbic encephalitis? Arq Neuropsiquiatr 2012;70:817–22.

122. Lancaster E, Martinez-Hernandez E, Titulaer MJ, et al. Antibodies to metabotropic glutamate receptor 5 in the Ophelia syndrome. Neurology 2011;77: 1698–701.

123. Carr I. The Ophelia syndrome: memory loss in Hodgkin's disease. Lancet 1982; 1(8276):844–5.
124. Kirshner HS. Hashimoto's encephalopathy: a brief review. Currneurolneurosci Rep 2014;14(9):476.
125. Tamagno G, Federspil G, Murialdo G. Clinical and diagnostic aspects of encephalopathy associated with autoimmune thyroid disease (or Hashimoto's encephalopathy). Intern Emerg Med 2006;1:15–23.
126. Hoffmann F, Reiter K, Kluger G, et al. Seizures, psychosis and coma: severe course of Hashimoto encephalopathy in a six-year-old girl. Neuropediatrics 2007;38:197–9.

Neurobehavioral Manifestations of Human Immunodeficiency Virus/AIDS

Diagnosis and Treatment

Elyse J. Singer, MD[a],*, April D. Thames, PhD[b]

KEYWORDS

- Brain • Infection • Delirium • Encephalitis • Behavior • HIV • AIDS

KEY POINTS

- Behavioral disorders are an important problem in patients with human immunodeficiency virus (HIV)/acquired immunodeficiency syndrome even in the current era of antiretroviral therapy.
- Behavioral disorders can be caused by preexisting psychosocial problems, substance abuse, or major psychiatric disorders, or by HIV infection itself, opportunistic infections, or effects of medications that treat HIV and related conditions.
- Physicians who evaluate behavioral changes in patients infected with HIV should screen for underlying medical disease, substance abuse, adverse effect of medications, and suicide risk.

INTRODUCTION

More than 34 million persons worldwide are infected with human immunodeficiency virus (HIV) type 1, which is the cause of acquired immunodeficiency syndrome (AIDS). An estimated 20% of the more than 1 million individuals infected with HIV (HIV+) in the United States are unaware of their HIV serostatus, and do not receive treatment with antiretroviral therapy (ART). Among those who are aware of their serostatus, more than 50% receive no ART or receive only inadequate treatment, which places them at high risk for morbidity and mortality,[1] including central nervous system (CNS) disorders.

Disclosures: This work was supported by 1U24MH100929 (E.J. Singer), and K23MH095661 (A.D. Thames). The authors have nothing to disclose.
[a] NeuroInfectious Diseases Program, UCLA National Neurological AIDS Bank, David Geffen School of Medicine at UCLA, 710 Westwood Plaza, Room A129, Los Angeles, CA 90095, USA;
[b] Department of Psychiatry and Biobehavioral Sciences, David Geffen School of Medicine at UCLA, 740 Westwood Plaza, C8-746, Los Angeles, CA 90095, USA
* Corresponding author.
E-mail address: esinger@mednet.ucla.edu

Neurol Clin 34 (2016) 33–53
http://dx.doi.org/10.1016/j.ncl.2015.08.003
0733-8619/16/$ – see front matter © 2016 Elsevier Inc. All rights reserved.

neurologic.theclinics.com

HIV invades the CNS early, during the first days to weeks of primary infection. Approximately 24% of patients with primary HIV infection have symptoms of an aseptic meningitis. HIV infection can result in progressive cognitive, motor, and behavioral abnormalities, particularly in persons who receive no ART, begin ART late in their disease, or receive inadequate ART that does not fully suppress HIV.[1]

The neuropsychiatric effects of HIV can mimic idiopathic psychiatric disorders, delaying diagnosis and treatment of the underlying cause. The differential diagnosis of behavioral disorders in HIV+ persons includes preexisting psychiatric disease, infections, and medication-related causes. Because the processes that underlie such behavioral changes can be varied, this article first describes some important HIV-related behavioral symptoms (**Box 1**) and then describes the clinical features of the most common underlying conditions.

BEHAVIOR DISORDERS CAUSED BY PREEXISTING PSYCHIATRIC ILLNESS

Behavioral disorders are common among both HIV+ and at-risk HIV-seronegative (HIV−) persons. Depression and anxiety receive the most attention, but delirium, apathy, mania, and severe mental illness (SMI) are also important. Although the presence of pre-HIV mental disorder is the strongest predictor of psychiatric diagnosis after knowledge of seropositivity,[2] it can be difficult to disentangle the effects of premorbid psychiatric illness from the biological effects of HIV, CNS opportunistic infections (OI), prescribed medications, or substance abuse. However, these distinctions are important in order to provide accurate diagnoses and treatments.

SEVERE MENTAL ILLNESS

Individuals with SMI, such as schizophrenia, bipolar disorder, and major depressive disorder (MDD), are at increased risk for contracting HIV. Once infected, they are at higher risk for suicide attempts, substance abuse, and failure to adhere to ART.[3] Adults with SMI are disproportionately at risk because they are more likely to have multiple sexual partners, fail to use condoms, and engage in needle sharing. They are more resistant to risk reduction efforts because most of these programs assume that they have the cognitive capacity to make informed decisions about their behavior. Individuals with substance use disorders and victims of physical and sexual abuse also have specific risks for acquiring HIV.[4]

Persons with a premorbid history of idiopathic SMI are characterized as having primary psychosis, whereas those with new SMI associated with medical illness, HIV disease, OI, or metabolic encephalopathies are characterized as having secondary psychosis.[5] There are phenotypic differences between primary psychosis and the

---

Box 1
Presentation of behavioral disorders in persons affected by HIV/AIDS

I. Preexisting psychiatric disease

II. Depression

III. Anxiety

IV. Mania

V. Apathy

VI. Delirium

secondary psychosis associated with HIV. Persons with HIV-associated secondary psychosis are reported to show more disorders of consciousness, orientation, attention, and memory than patients with primary SMI.[5] They also tend to report fewer delusions, have a more variable course, and are more likely to have eventual remission of their psychosis.[6]

MOOD DISORDERS AND DEPRESSION

Almost 50% of a large, nationally representative HIV+ sample screened positive for a mental health disorder, primarily MDD and dysthymia.[7] In part, these high rates of MDD may be caused by premorbid psychiatric illness. Some populations at high risk for HIV, such as men who have sex with men (MSM) or intravenous (IV) drug users, have high baseline rates of MDD, which may inflate the prevalence of MDD in HIV+ individuals. Alternatively, MDD may be a reaction to an HIV diagnosis, medical illness, HIV stigma, or the direct CNS effects of HIV as mediated by altered cytokine and neurotransmitter metabolism.[8] Identifying and treating MDD is important to long-term management because prolonged MDD is associated with decreased adherence to ART.[9]

The diagnosis of MDD in HIV+ persons may be difficult, because the neurovegetative symptoms of premorbid MDD (such as lack of energy, fatigue, anorexia, and sleep disturbances) may also be caused by the biological effects of HIV. HIV infection stimulates increasing levels of proinflammatory cytokines such as interleukin-6, interleukin-1 beta, tumor necrosis factor-alpha, and interferon-gamma, which are associated with sickness behavior (fever, hypersomnia, anorexia, decreased motor activity, and loss of interest in the environment).[10] In differentiating between preexisting MDD and the neurovegetative symptoms of HIV, it may be useful to remove the somatic depression symptoms included in diagnostic instruments such as the Beck Depression Inventory II[11] and the Center for Epidemiologic Studies Depression Scale.[12] For example, HIV+ persons may be screened using the Beck Depression Inventory for Primary Care, a tool that focuses on nonphysical symptoms.[13] HIV+ patients are also at risk for hypothyroidism, adrenal insufficiency, and hypogonadism, which may present with neurovegetative symptoms.[14]

Double-blind, randomized clinical trials (RCTs) indicate that serotonin-specific reuptake inhibitors (SSRIs) and tricyclic antidepressants (TCADs) are useful in treating the symptoms of MDD in HIV+ patients.[15] Because of the lower incidence of anticholinergic side effects, SSRIs such as fluoxetine and paroxetine are typically used as first-line agents, whereas TCADs are sometimes used for patients with both depression and neuropathic pain. The atypical antidepressant bupropion, which has been studied in open-label trials, can have significant interactions with the ART drugs ritonavir and efavirenz, and cannot be used in patients with seizure disorders.[16] Modafinil, a psychostimulant, reduced fatigue in HIV+ patients in an RCT,[17] although its effects on other MDD symptoms was unclear. The monoamine oxidase inhibitor selegiline did not improve cognition in an RCT of HIV+ persons with neurocognitive deficits.[18] Use of other monoamine oxidase inhibitors in HIV+ patients is limited because of the potential for serious adverse effects.

MANIA

Primary mania typically presents in young adulthood and is characterized by persistently increased or irritable mood, increased physical activity, pressured speech, flight of ideas, racing thoughts, grandiosity, a decreased need for sleep, distractibility, and excessive high-risk activities. In contrast, secondary mania can present suddenly at any age in a previously normal person with no history of mood disorder, and it is frequently associated with brain disease.[19] HIV+ patients with secondary mania, or so-called HIV mania, are described as being agitated, disruptive, sleepless, having high levels of energy, and being excessively talkative. They have a high rate of psychotic symptoms such as auditory or visual hallucinations and paranoia.[20] HIV mania is reported to be associated with irritability rather than euphoria. Unlike primary mania, cognitive deficits are usually present.[20]

A first episode of HIV mania typically occurs in the context of a CNS disorder, such as HIV-associated neurocognitive disorder (HAND) or a CNS OI. The mechanisms are poorly understood; however, the HIV *nef* protein is reported to alter CNS dopamine metabolism leading to hyperactive, maniclike behaviors in animal models.[21]

Reports of HIV mania have decreased coincident with the widespread use of ART, but it remains a problem among untreated and undertreated persons.

The differential diagnosis of brain disorders underlying suspected HIV mania includes substance use (especially stimulants), alcohol withdrawal, metabolic abnormalities (eg, hyperthyroidism), and CNS OI. Evaluations should include a neurologic and mental status examination, brain MRI scan with and without contrast, serology for syphilis, urine toxicology, and cerebrospinal fluid (CSF) examination (if medically safe), including tests for OI and a quantitative HIV CSF polymerase chain reaction (PCR) (viral load in CSF).

The choice of psychotropic drugs to treat HIV mania is based on case reports and open-label studies, rather than RCTs, as well as the desire to avoid adverse drug interactions, and the avoidance of HIV-specific side effects. HIV mania may improve with an approach that combines resolution of the underlying CNS process, use of a mood stabilizing drug, and/or addition of an antipsychotic drug. For example, the mood stabilizer and antiepileptic drug valproic acid has been used to successfully treat mania in HIV+ patients.[16] The disadvantages to valproic acid use are as follows: valproic acid is metabolized in the liver, and liver disease is common in HIV+ persons; further, valproic acid has interactions with many ART drugs.[22,23] This disadvantage must be weighed against the potential disadvantages of other mood stabilizers, such as lithium, which can exacerbate renal disease, or carbamazepine, which can induce bone marrow suppression, hepatotoxicity, and induce the metabolism of ART (particularly protease inhibitors).[22,24,25] Likewise, the older, high-potency dopamine receptor 2–blocking agents have been reported to cause serious extrapyramidal movement disorders and neuroleptic malignant syndrome in patients with AIDS.[26,27] Atypical antipsychotics, such as risperidone, clozapine, ziprasidone, quetiapine, and olanzapine, are frequently used to manage psychosis in HIV+ patients[28,29]; however, they are associated with development of metabolic syndrome, cardiac problems, and obesity, and may require dose adjustment if they are used with the protease inhibitor ritonavir.[30,31] Interactions between clozapine and ritonavir may increase clozapine levels and lead to bone marrow toxicity.[16]

APATHY

Apathy is a common symptom of HIV and other neurodegenerative diseases. Apathy is characterized by a lack of interest in life activities, loss of interest in interacting with others, and decreased motivation. Apathy can be dangerous if it results in failure to pursue medical care.[32] This behavior is associated with impaired function of the subcortical regions and frontostriatal circuits, which are prime targets for HIV.[33] The emergence of apathy in HIV+ patients is often associated with the onset of deficits in attention, working memory, learning, psychomotor, and executive function, such as characterize HAND.

Apathy may be diagnosed from a history, or by use of diagnostic inventories such as the Apathy Evaluation Scale,[34] the apathy subscale of the Neuropsychiatric Inventory,[35] and the Frontal Systems Behavioral Scale.[36] Rivastigmine[37] and methylphenidate[38] have been studied in neurodegenerative disease as palliative treatments for apathy, but there are no studies in HIV+ patients.

DELIRIUM

Delirium is an acute change in mental state characterized by fluctuating cognitive, perceptual, and behavioral disturbances; altered level of consciousness; inattention; sleep-wake cycle disturbance; and delusions. Historically, delirium is associated with elderly, hospitalized patients. However, delirium is also common in HIV+ young adults and children, and is associated with increased mortality in HIV+ patients.[39–41] Risk factors include polypharmacy, substance use and withdrawal, and underlying CNS disease. Other factors that may trigger delirium include hypoxia, sepsis, thyroid disease, adrenal insufficiency, recent changes in medications, and end-organ failure.

The treatment of delirium includes environmental management to reorient the patient and reduce agitation, and psychotropic medication to control aberrant behavior. There is only 1 controlled study of delirium treatment in AIDS, which dates to the pre-ART era. Breitbart and colleagues[42] compared the use of low-dose haloperidol, low-dose chlorpromazine, and lorazepam in hospitalized patients with AIDS with delirium. The groups treated with low-dose haloperidol and chlorpromazine showed improvement (although mild extrapyramidal symptoms were noted) but patients treated with lorazepam had a significant increase in their delirium, to such a degree that the lorazepam arm of the study was terminated. Open-label studies and case reports suggest that the atypical antipsychotics clozapine, risperidone, and ziprasidone benefit patients with AIDS with psychosis and/or delirium.[16] Some clinicians argue that the use of older, D2-blocking antipsychotics should be avoided as first-line treatment in patients with AIDS, because of reports of neuroleptic malignant syndrome and extrapyramidal movement disorders.[26]

ANXIETY

Anxiety is common in HIV+ patients, estimated to occur in 22% to 47%.[43,44] Posttraumatic stress disorder (PTSD) is a common anxiety disorder in HIV+ persons, estimated at 10% to 54% among populations such as MSM, minority women, and those with persistent pain.[45,46] A study of HIV+ patients revealed that death anxiety was associated with overall PTSD symptom severity scores, as well as severity scores for reexperiencing, avoidance, and arousal symptoms of PTSD.[47]

Generalized anxiety disorder has been found to range between 6.5% and 20% in HIV+ samples.[7,48] Physiologic manifestations of anxiety, such as dyspnea, chest pain, tachycardia, and dizziness, may be misattributed to HIV, cardiovascular disease, or seizure disorder (caused by syncope from hyperventilation) in HIV+ persons. In contrast, HIV-related infections, and substance intoxication or withdrawal, may mimic anxiety symptoms in patients with tremors, rigors, or chills. The symptoms of anxiety may affect performance on cognitive testing, potentially leading to a misdiagnosis of HAND. A reduction of up to 1 standard deviation (SD) in test performance has been documented in studies of healthy minority populations who have anxiety about test taking.[49,50]

There is an emerging body of literature that has linked anxiety sensitivity (a fear of anxiety symptoms) to suicide[51,52]; in particular, cognitive concern (eg, "I fear that I will lose my mind") is linked to suicidal thoughts.[53] Anxiety also interferes with ART adherence.[48,54]

Assessment of an anxiety disorder requires a history of symptoms (particularly before HIV infection), family history, substance use history (especially stimulants), and the use of over-the-counter medications, herbal supplements, and caffeine. HIV+ patients with subclinical or overt neurocognitive impairment are more sensitive to the side effects of anxiolytic medications and should start at low doses.[55] Drug-drug interactions have been reported with anxiolytics and AIDS medications; for example, there are case reports of HIV+ patients on protease inhibitors who experienced prolonged sedation when given midazolam.[56] Buspirone, a popular antianxiety agent and 5-hydroxytryptamine (5HT) 1A agonist, has been reported to cause extrapyramidal signs when given with protease inhibitors such as ritonavir.[57]

HUMAN IMMUNODEFICIENCY VIRUS–ASSOCIATED NEUROCOGNITIVE DISORDER

HAND (previously known as HIV encephalopathy, HIV-associated dementia, or AIDS dementia complex)[2,3] is the most common CNS disorder caused by HIV infection. It is characterized by the subacute onset of cognitive deficits, central motor abnormalities, and behavioral changes. Although cognitive decline is the defining feature in HAND, many patients have mild deficits that are detectable only by neuropsychological testing, and do not reach the functional criteria required to diagnose a dementia (eg, inability to perform activities of daily living). The mildest form of HAND is classified as asymptomatic neurocognitive impairment, and is determined by a lack of significant cognitive complaints, neuropsychological test performance of which at least 2 cognitive domains are greater than 1 SD less than the mean of demographically adjusted normative scores, and no evidence of functional decline. The next is mild neurocognitive disorder, classified by self-report or proxy report of declines in at least 2 instrumental activities of daily living, such as (1) financial management; (2) unemployment or a significant reduction in job responsibilities caused by reduced cognitive abilities; (3) decline in vocational functioning (eg, increased errors, decreased productivity, or greater effort is required to achieve prior levels of productivity); (4) self-report or proxy report of increased problems in at least 2 cognitive ability areas in day-to-day life (this is not reliable among individuals with depression); or (5) scores at least 1 SD less than the mean on a performance-based laboratory measure of everyday functioning (eg, medication management). The most severe form of HAND, HIV-associated dementia (HAD) is marked by at least moderate to severe cognitive impairment (ie, at least 2 SDs less than demographically adjusted normative means) in at least 2 cognitive domains along with marked ADL declines that are not fully attributable to comorbidities or delirium. The neurocognitive profile of HIV has been characterized by deficits in attention, psychomotor speed, episodic memory, working memory, and executive functions,[58,59] reflecting frontal-subcortical compromise. For example, patients with HAND frequently complain of slowed thinking and problems with learning new information (**Box 2**).

Box 2
Infectious disorders associated with behavioral disorders in patients with HIV

HAND

I. Cryptococcal meningitis

II. Toxoplasmosis encephalitis

III. Herpes simplex virus encephalitis

IV. Neurosyphilis

V. Progressive multifocal leukoencephalopathy

The use of ART has attenuated the most severe aspects of HAND such as HAD,[60] but cases still occur in HIV+ persons who are untreated, inadequately treated, or in persons who have so-called CNS escape (a phenomenon in which ART controls HIV in the periphery but not in the CNS).[61] Patients who develop HAND despite taking adequate ART are likely to have higher CD4+ counts, lower or undetectable plasma viral loads, and lower or absent levels of CSF biomarkers of HAND than patients with HAND in the pre-ART era.[62] However, HAND is associated with a lower nadir (lowest ever) absolute CD4+ level both pre-ART and post-ART.

In some patients with HAND, cognitive deficits are overshadowed by behavioral/psychiatric features. Common behavioral symptoms associated with HAND include apathy, irritability, inertia, lack of spontaneity, social withdrawal, psychomotor slowing, complaints of diminished attention and concentration, emotional lability, and occasionally HIV mania. Many of these symptoms are not specific to HAND and occur in mood disorders and in other CNS diseases.

The differential diagnosis of behavioral changes associated with HAND includes an exacerbation of a premorbid psychiatric disease, neurosyphilis, CNS OI or tumor, adverse effects of medications, and the effects of substance abuse. The work-up should include neuroimaging, preferably brain MRI with and without contrast. In most cases this is normal or shows cerebral atrophy with or without white matter changes, characteristic of HIV encephalitis. If not contraindicated, a CSF examination should be conducted to exclude OI, malignancy, and neurosyphilis. If available, an HIV quantitative PCR in CSF (also called a CSF viral load) may point to CNS escape that may respond to a change in ART. Urine toxicology for drugs of abuse; screening for alcoholism and related disorders; and routine tests for thyroid disease, B_{12} deficiency, and folate deficiency are essential. A neuropsychological examination is extremely useful in staging the degree of impairment and identifying any psychiatric disorders that confound the diagnosis of HAND.

HAND is treated by starting ART (if the patient is treatment naive) and ensuring that the patient fully adheres to the regimen and attains suppression of plasma and CSF viral load.[63] If the ART regimen is not controlling HIV replication, particularly in the CNS, it may be intensified by adding or substituting drugs with a higher CSF penetration effectiveness (CPE) score.[64] However, this approach is controversial,[61,63] because higher CPE scores correlate with lower HIV RNA load in CSF but do not necessarily correlate with better cognition.[65] Individual case reports indicate that concurrent behavioral disorders may also improve with ART.[66] The results of small RCTs indicate that psychostimulants such as methylphenidate may improve depression, neurocognitive test scores, and fatigue in HIV+ patients.[67–69]

CRYPTOCOCCAL MENINGITIS

Cryptococcal meningitis (CM), caused by the fungus *Cryptococcus neoformans*, is the most common meningitis in AIDS. Typical patients with AIDS/CM have absolute CD4+ counts of less than 100 cells/μL and present with a subacute course of fever, malaise, and headache, with or without meningismus or photophobia. Behavioral symptoms such as personality changes, psychosis, or AIDS mania can also herald the onset of AIDS/CM.[70] The diagnosis of AIDS/CM is made by showing cryptococcal infection by cryptococcal antigen testing or fungal culture in blood and/or CSF. India ink examination of CSF is also useful but is no longer performed by many laboratories. Patients with AIDS may have minimal or no CSF lymphocytic pleocytosis, but increased opening pressure, increased total protein levels, and low-normal CSF glucose levels are common. The preferred treatment of AIDS/CM includes either IV liposomal amphotericin B, in a dosage of 3 to 4 mg/kg/daily, and flucytosine at a dosage of 100 mg/kg daily in 4 divided doses for at least 2 weeks in patients with normal renal function.[71] Fluconazole can be used for induction therapy at a starting daily dosage of 1200 mg/day but is inferior to amphotericin and should be used only when standard treatment is unavailable or cannot be tolerated. Especially in low-resource settings, it may be necessary to delay ART treatment of AIDS/CM in order to avoid immune reconstitution inflammatory syndrome. Most patients require continued maintenance treatment with daily oral fluconazole until their CSF is sterilized and their CD4+ levels improve. Individual case reports indicate the amelioration of behavioral symptoms in AIDS/CM with atypical antipsychotics such as olanzapine.[72] A retrospective study indicates that substantial numbers of AIDS/CM survivors have persistent neurocognitive deficits.[73]

TOXOPLASMOSIS ENCEPHALITIS

Toxoplasmosis encephalitis (TE), the most common cause of a CNS mass lesion in AIDS, is caused by the parasite *Toxoplasma gondii*.[74] This organism is usually acquired in early life and remains in latent (cystic) form within the brain. TE typically occurs when the cysts reactivate; for example, in patients with AIDS with CD4+ cell counts less than 100 cells/μL. These TE lesions are highly inflammatory, producing cerebral edema and destruction of brain tissue. Typical symptoms of AIDS/TE include headache; seizures; fever; decreased cognition; altered level of consciousness; and focal neurologic signs such as hemiparesis, visual field deficits, or aphasia.[74] Behavioral symptoms in AIDS/TE are of 2 types: nonfocal symptoms such as delirium,[75] psychosis,[75,76] or mania[77]; and focal deficits such as aphasia,[78] parkinsonism,[79] or unilateral movement disorders.[80] Note that latent toxoplasmosis in HIV-negative, immunologically intact patients has also been associated with psychiatric diseases and behavioral disorders.[81]

The diagnosis of TE is supported when a patient with AIDS presents with typical clinical symptoms and brain neuroimaging shows at least 1 contrast-enhancing mass lesions, often surrounded by a ring of edema.[74] These lesions are commonly found in the cerebral cortex, basal ganglia, cerebellum, or brain stem.[74] The most important differential diagnosis is CNS lymphoma. Many patients with AIDS/TE are at risk for cerebral herniation, so CSF studies may be unobtainable. When obtained, CSF typically shows a low-grade pleocytosis, increased total protein levels, and sometimes increased red blood cell levels. Toxoplasmosis cannot be cultured by conventional means. Direct molecular detection by PCR is highly specific (96%–100%) but is not sensitive enough (50%) to reliably detect TE in CSF.[71,82] Detection of the organism requires a brain biopsy. Thus, CSF is important mainly to exclude alternative diagnoses. Patients with AIDS with typical clinical and imaging features of TE coupled with positive serum toxoplasmosis serology (serum immunoglobulin G) and no alternative explanation for their symptoms are usually treated empirically with antitoxoplasmosis therapy, and followed carefully. The absence of toxoplasmosis antibodies makes a diagnosis of AIDS/TE unlikely (although not impossible).[71] The typical choice of drugs includes pyrimethamine in combination with sulfadiazine and leucovorin, adjusted for body weight.[71] Pyrimethamine plus clindamycin plus leucovorin is the preferred alternative regimen for patients with TE who cannot tolerate sulfadiazine or do not respond to first-line therapy.[71] Atovaquone is an alternative in patients unable to tolerate either sulfonamides or clindamycin.[83] Steroids should not be administered unless needed to treat a mass effect causing increased intracranial pressure, because they may obscure the diagnosis. Improvement typically occurs within 14 days with anti-TE therapy and supports an empiric diagnosis of TE.[83] If the patient fails to improve or worsens, a brain biopsy may be needed to reach a diagnosis.

NEUROSYPHILIS

Syphilis, caused by the spirochete *Treponema pallidum*, is a sexually transmitted infection, so co-occurrence with HIV is common. HIV causes impaired cell-mediated immunity, which accelerates the progression of syphilis, so that HIV+ persons have a greater frequency of neurosyphilis.[84]

As with HIV, syphilis enters the CNS early in infection. Up to half of individuals with early syphilis have CSF abnormalities that indicate neuroinvasion, and up to a quarter have treponemes in their CSF. Most healthy patients clear the organisms. Failure to clear is the first step to neurosyphilis. Most patients with neurosyphilis have asymptomatic infection of the CSF and meninges; only a fraction of those, who go untreated, develop symptomatic neurosyphilis, and even fewer develop general paresis (GP), which is the form of neurosyphilis most likely to present with behavioral changes. The host immune response is key to this process.[84]

GP is caused by syphilitic infection of the brain parenchyma and is associated with neuronal loss. It typically occurs late in infection (20–30 years), although this process may be accelerated in HIV+ persons. Before the penicillin era, GP was a common reason for psychiatric hospitalization. Symptoms include dementia (which is not normally seen in primary psychiatric disease), emotional lability, anhedonia, grandiosity, paranoia, hallucinations, and mood changes that mimic mania and depression. Other features associated with GP include headache, seizures, pupillary abnormalities, and ataxia; patients with a concurrent tabes dorsalis (another form of late syphilis that affects the spinal cord) have loss of vibratory and position sense in the legs, incontinence, weakness, reflex changes, and lightninglike pains.[85]

In GP, the MRI may be normal, or may show frontal and temporal atrophy caused by neuronal loss. In HIV+ persons with GP, these changes may be overshadowed by concurrent HIV encephalitis. Gummas (syphilitic granulomas) may appear on MRI as space-occupying lesions.

The diagnosis of neurosyphilis can be challenging in HIV+ patients. Screening tests that use a nonspecific, nontreponemal antibody, such as the rapid plasma reagin (RPR), are usually reactive within 3 to 4 weeks of syphilis infection in HIV+ patients, although rare cases of failure to develop antibodies have been reported in extremely immunocompromised persons.[86] The RPR is sensitive but not specific, so is confirmed with a more specific treponemal test, such as the fluorescent treponemal antibody (FTA) absorption test, the microhemagglutination test for antibodies to *T pallidum*, or *T pallidum* particle agglutination assay.

At a minimum, HIV+ patients with syphilis and ophthalmologic, otologic, or neuropsychiatric signs or symptoms should be screened for neurosyphilis with a CSF examination to determine whether they have laboratory signs of neurosyphilis and to establish a baseline for treatment if this is the case. However, *T pallidum* is an obligate intracellular parasite and cannot be cultured by conventional means. Thus, laboratory diagnosis rests on 2 factors: the detection of CSF abnormalities (eg, increased CSF white blood cell count, increased total protein level), and reactive serologic testing (eg, the CSF Venereal Disease Research Laboratory [VDRL] test). The CSF PCR is investigational and not currently recommended for the diagnosis of syphilis.[71] However, a study that used the laborious rabbit inoculation method to directly culture spirochetes from CSF found that 33% of patients with untreated primary and secondary syphilis who had a nonreactive CSF VDRL test nonetheless had *T pallidum* isolated from their CSF.[87] This study and others suggest that the CSF VDRL test is specific but not very sensitive for neurosyphilis. An alternative method of diagnosing neurosyphilis in patients with syphilis with nonreactive CSF VDRL tests is to find CSF abnormalities, such as pleocytosis and increased CSF protein level, in a patient diagnosed with syphilis. However, low-grade lymphocytic pleocytosis and increased CSF protein level are common in asymptomatic HIV+ patients,[88] thus reducing the value of these tests in HIV+ persons when the CSF VDRL test is nonreactive. Some investigators report an association between serum RPR titers of at least 1:32 and/or CD4+ counts less than 350 cells/μL with neurosyphilis in HIV+ persons,[89] although cases of neurosyphilis have been reported that do not meet this criteria.

Another proposal is that a CSF FTA test should be performed in patients with a nonreactive CSF VDRL test and suspected neurosyphilis; CSF FTA test is very sensitive and is not as specific, so a nonreactive CSF FTA test is thought to exclude virtually all probability of neurosyphilis.[90]

The treatment of choice for neurosyphilis in HIV+ patients is IV aqueous crystalline penicillin G, 18 to 24 million units daily, administered as 3 million to 4 million units every 4 hours or by continuous infusion for 10 to 14 days, or intramuscular (IM) procaine penicillin, 2.4 million units once daily plus probenecid 500 mg orally 4 times a day for 10 to 14 days. HIV+ patients who are allergic to sulfa-containing medications should not be given probenecid because of potential allergic reaction.[71] Because neurosyphilis treatment regimens are of shorter duration than those used in late-latent syphilis, 2.4 million units of IM benzathine penicillin once per week for up to 3 weeks after completion of neurosyphilis treatment can be considered to provide a comparable duration of therapy.[71] Ceftriaxone may be an alternative for patients with penicillin allergy.[71] The response to antibiotic treatment is reported to differ in HIV+ persons, particularly if they have severe immunosuppression or are not treated with ART, because they are more likely to fail conventional treatment of neurosyphilis.[87,91,92]

There is no consensus that antibiotic treatment of neurosyphilis produces a persistent improvement in cognition in persons with GP (note that most of the patients studied were HIV negative).[93] Further, although neurosyphilis remains associated with psychiatric and behavioral symptoms even in HIV-negative patients,[94] there is no consensus or RCT describing how to best manage these symptoms. Sanchez and colleagues[95] published a case series describing treatment of neurosyphilis with mood stabilizers and atypical antipsychotic drugs; however, these agents need to be used with caution in HIV+ patients receiving concurrent treatment with ART.

HERPES SIMPLEX VIRUS 1 ENCEPHALITIS

Herpes simplex virus 1 (HSV-1) encephalitis (HSVE) is the most common encephalitis in the HIV-negative population and can also occur in HIV+ patients. It is hypothesized that HSV-1 enters the brain via the olfactory nerves and spreads into the limbic system, frontal lobe, and temporal lobe.[96] Infected neurons and other cells can undergo cytolysis, causing hemorrhagic destruction of brain tissue. Particularly vulnerable areas include the fronto-orbital region, temporal lobes, hippocampus, cingulate gyrus, and insular cortex.[96]

The most common clinical presentation of HSVE includes fever, headache, seizures, and altered level of consciousness, and culminates in stupor or coma.[96] However, patients with HSVE can have a presentation dominated by behavioral symptoms, such as irritability; confusion; psychomotor retardation; anosmia; auditory, gustatory, or olfactory hallucinations; delusions; paranoia; or aggression. It is common for patients with HSVE to be mistakenly referred to a psychiatric unit.[97,98]

The diagnosis of HSVE is confirmed by brain MRI with/without contrast showing characteristic contrast-enhancing lesions in the frontal and/or temporal areas, and/or by a positive HSV-1 PCR or increased levels of HSV-1 antibodies in CSF.[99] Occasionally the CSF studies are negative, and a repeat CSF examination or a brain biopsy is required to make the diagnosis. Treatment is IV acyclovir (60 mg/kg/d, given in 3 divided doses) for 21 days.[100] A repeat CSF examination should be performed at the end of therapy to ensure that the virus has cleared. The use of continued outpatient treatment with oral valacyclovir is common but has not been shown to improve outcomes.[101] survivors of HSVE often have behavioral sequelae,[102] such as aphasia, memory deficits, visuospatial deficits, executive dysfunction, or Klüver-Bucy syndrome (hypersexuality, hyperoral behavior, and hyperphagia).

There are no RCTs of treatment of the neurobehavioral sequelae of HSVE in HIV+ patients, but case reports describe the management of post-HSVE neurobehavioral deficits with antipsychotics and mood stabilizers.[103]

PROGRESSIVE MULTIFOCAL LEUKOENCEPHALOPATHY

The John Cunningham virus (JCV), a polyoma virus, is the cause of progressive multifocal leukoencephalopathy (PML), a serious and often fatal CNS demyelinating disease. The JCV is a ubiquitous virus transmitted by casual contact. Worldwide, more than 50% of adults are JCV infected (JCV+).[104] Once established, JCV takes up residency in a latent form in the kidneys, and, possibly, in the brain.[105] Under conditions of immunosuppression, including HIV infection, JCV can reactivate and cause PML. HIV+ patients are doubly at risk, because JCV replication can also be increased by the HIV tat protein.[106]

Before ART, most patients with AIDS/PML presented with an absolute CD4+ cell count fewer than 100 cells/μL. However, unlike some other CNS OIs, PML can occasionally occur in HIV+ patients with absolute CD4+ cell counts more than 200 cells/μL,[107] in HIV+ patients who receive adequate ART, and in patients recently started on ART who experience immune reconstitution inflammatory syndrome uncovering an occult JCV infection.[108] However, the number of PML cases has declined overall in ART-treated populations.

The clinical presentation of PML can include cognitive decline, aphasia, acalculia, right-left confusion, agnosia, cortical blindness, akinetic mutism, emotional lability (pseudobulbar affect), apraxia, dysarthria, involuntary movements, catatonia, diplopia, or seizures.[109–113] Other common features include visual field cuts, monoparesis or hemiparesis, gait disturbance, oculomotor palsy, sensory loss, tremors, incoordination, and ataxia.[110] Signs and symptoms are usually referable to the locations of the demyelinating lesions. Fever, headache, and stiff neck are rarely seen in uncomplicated AIDS/PML.

The most common neuroimaging findings are 1 or more space-occupying white matter lesions that are nonenhancing, hyperintense on T2 and fluid-attenuated inversion recovery, hypointense on T1, and spare the cortical U fibers. Virtually any brain area can be involved. Only 5% to 10% of cases have some degree of contrast enhancement.

A possible diagnosis of AIDS/PML should be considered in an HIV+ patient with 1 or more CNS signs/symptoms, MRI that shows at least 1 characteristic brain lesion, and no other CNS diseases that might explain the signs and symptoms. Historically, a diagnosis of definitive PML required a brain biopsy or autopsy showing demyelination, bizarre astrocytes, and enlarged oligodendroglial nuclei, along with histopathologic or electron microscopy demonstration of JCV.[114] However, in 2013, this was expanded to include patients without a tissue diagnosis who had characteristic presentation, MRI, and a positive CSF JCV PCR.[114]

The routine CSF examination in AIDS/PML is nonspecific, with mild or no pleocytosis, increased total protein level, and normal glucose level, but is essential to exclude diagnoses that mimic the appearance of PML, such as other viral infections.

One potential problem in confirming the diagnosis of AIDS/PML is that the sensitivity of the CSF JCV PCR test, especially in ART-treated patients, is as low as 58%.[115] In addition, JCV has occasionally been detected in the CSF of immune-suppressed persons, and in clinically and radiologically normal persons, without PML. For this reason, both clinical and laboratory features are necessary to establish a diagnosis of PML.[114]

There is no specific drug that treats JCV infection. Multiple agents have been studied in RCT without success, including topotecan,[116] cytarabine,[117,118] cidofovir,[119] and mefloquine.[120] The use of mirtazapine[121] and other 5HT2a receptor blockers (olanzapine, ziprasidone, mirtazapine, cyproheptadine, and risperidone) have been suggested because JCV may use the serotonergic 5HT2a receptor to enter glial cells in culture systems, but no RCTs have been conducted. ART has improved the course of AIDS PML, decreasing the mortality, improving the neuroimaging features, improving survival, and decreasing CSF JCV viral load,[122–124] and should be optimized in all patients with AIDS/PML.[71]

Patients who survive AIDS PML are likely to have serious residual deficits. There are no RCTs that explore the appropriate medical treatment of behavioral abnormalities in AIDS/PML. Individual case reports have described the treatment of specific neuropsychiatric symptoms (eg, pseudobulbar affect, agitation, movement disorders) in patients with PML with conventional psychotropic medications (**Box 3**).[111,125]

ADVERSE EFFECTS OF MEDICATIONS USED TO TREAT HUMAN IMMUNODEFICIENCY VIRUS 1 AND ASSOCIATED CONDITIONS
Antiretroviral Therapy Toxicity

The ART drug efavirenz has been reported to cause CNS toxicity,[126,127] manifested by neuropsychiatric symptoms and histopathologic changes. Up to 60% of efavirenz-treated HIV+ patients experience the symptoms of mood disorders (mania or depression), suicidal thoughts, dizziness, confusion, lethargy, impaired concentration, hostile thoughts, aggression, psychosis, sleep disturbances (vivid dreams and insomnia), anxiety, catatonia, and hallucinations. This psychotropic effect is so well known that in some areas efavirenz is smoked as a recreational drug. The risk of suicide in HIV+ persons treated with efavirenz is also higher than in persons treated with other ARTs, particularly if there is a history of psychiatric disorder or substance abuse.[128] Behavioral disorders have been linked to increased serum levels of efavirenz associated with genetic variations in drug metabolism. Efavirenz has also been linked to CNS mitochondrial[129] and neuronal toxicity.[130]

Box 3
Behavioral disorders associated with HIV/AIDS treatment

I. Antiretroviral drugs

II. Drugs used to treat OI

III. Antipsychotic and dopamine-blocking drugs

Neuropsychiatric symptoms from efavirenz typically occur within the first few weeks of treatment. Patients who continue to take the drug may accommodate to these adverse effects but this may require up to 200 days of efavirenz use.

Individual cases of psychosis (with or without accompanying movement disorders) have been reported with other ARTs, including abacavir,[122] and zidovudine.[131]

Delirium has been reported as an idiosyncratic reaction to ART, catatonia has been reported in patients taking combination ART,[122] and acute dystonia has been reported with lamivudine.[132] Various ART drugs, such as zidovudine, abacavir, and efavirenz, have been reported to trigger depressive episodes in susceptible persons.[133] Note that a larger study indicated that ART might improve depression in HIV+ persons.[134]

Drugs Used to Treat Opportunistic Infections

Ganciclovir is an antiviral drug used to treat cytomegalovirus infections in patients with AIDS. Psychosis, confusion, visual and auditory hallucinations, aphasia, incontinence, and delirium have been reported.[116] These syndromes typically remit within 5 days after the drug is stopped. Ganciclovir is excreted by the kidneys, so persons with impaired renal function may be at higher risk for this complication; reducing the dose may prevent this problem. Valacyclovir and acyclovir have also been associated with psychosis, especially in patients with renal insufficiency.[117]

Sulfadiazine, a drug used extensively for the prophylaxis and treatment of TE in patients with AIDS, has also been associated with psychoses, hallucinations, and tremor.[118]

Antipsychotic and Dopamine-blocking Drugs

HIV has a predilection for the basal ganglia and is associated with disorders affecting the dopaminergic (DA) systems.[119] Particularly in the pre-ART era, patients with HAND were noted to manifest parkinsonian features, including psychomotor and motor slowing, tremor, increased tone, cogwheeling, hypomimia, and hypophonia.[123] However, most of these patients did not have a resting tremor and did not respond well to typical Parkinson drugs. The DA system is compromised in HIV, as shown by decreased levels of DA in the CNS of HIV+ patients.[124,135] Case reports indicate that HIV+ patients have developed parkinsonism and other extrapyramidal disorders when treated with DA-blocking drugs.[136]

SUMMARY

Patients with HIV/AIDS remain susceptible to significant and potentially life-threatening behavioral abnormalities even in the era of ART. These problems can be attributed to preexisting mental disorder, underlying infection, or adverse medication effects, so their physicians should consider whether new behavioral changes reflect a new and unwanted brain infection or other serious process. The management of HIV+ patients remains challenging because many commonly used psychiatric medications have unwanted adverse effects or potentially dangerous drug interactions. However, the development of psychiatric disease in the context of brain infection indicates the need to further explore the role of infectious agents in the pathogenesis of mental illness.

REFERENCES

1. Marks G, Gardner LI, Craw J, et al. The spectrum of engagement in HIV care: do more than 19% of HIV-infected persons in the US have undetectable viral load? Clin Infect Dis 2011;53(11):1168–9 [author's reply: 1169–70].

2. Tsao JC, Dobalian A, Moreau C, et al. Stability of anxiety and depression in a national sample of adults with human immunodeficiency virus. J Nerv Ment Dis 2004;192(2):111–8.

3. Rosenberg SD, Goodman LA, Osher FC, et al. Prevalence of HIV, hepatitis B, and hepatitis C in people with severe mental illness. Am J Public Health 2001; 91(1):31–7.

4. Meade CS, Kershaw TS, Hansen NB, et al. Long-term correlates of childhood abuse among adults with severe mental illness: adult victimization, substance abuse, and HIV sexual risk behavior. AIDS Behav 2009;13(2):207–16.

5. Alciati A, Fusi A, D'Arminio Monforte A, et al. New-onset delusions and hallucinations in patients infected with HIV. J Psychiatry Neurosci 2001;26(3):229–34.

6. Harris MJ, Jeste DV, Gleghorn A, et al. New-onset psychosis in HIV-infected patients. J Clin Psychiatry 1991;52(9):369–76.

7. Bing EG, Burnam MA, Longshore D, et al. Psychiatric disorders and drug use among human immunodeficiency virus-infected adults in the United States. Arch Gen Psychiatry 2001;58(8):721–8.

8. Cassol E, Misra V, Morgello S, et al. Altered monoamine and acylcarnitine metabolites in HIV-positive and HIV-negative subjects with depression. J Acquir Immune Defic Syndr 2015;69(1):18–28.

9. Gonzalez JS, Batchelder AW, Psaros C, et al. Depression and HIV/AIDS treatment nonadherence: a review and meta-analysis. J Acquir Immune Defic Syndr 2011;58(2):181–7.

10. Currier M, Nemeroff C. Inflammation and mood disorders: proinflammatory cytokines and the pathogenesis of depression. Antiinflamm Antiallergy Agents Med Chem 2010;9:212–20.

11. Beck AT, Steer RA, Ball R, et al. Comparison of Beck Depression Inventories-IA and -II in psychiatric outpatients. J Pers Assess 1996;67(3):588–97.

12. Radloff LS. The CES-D scale: a self report depression scale for research in the general population. Appl Psychol Meas 1977;1:385–401.

13. Steer RA, Cavalieri TA, Leonard DM, et al. Use of the Beck Depression Inventory for primary care to screen for major depression disorders. Gen Hosp Psychiatry 1999;21(2):106–11.

14. LeRoith D. Endocrinology and metabolism clinics of North America. HIV and endocrine disorders. Foreword. Endocrinol Metab Clin North Am 2014;43(3): xiii–xixv.

15. Hill L, Lee KC. Pharmacotherapy considerations in patients with HIV and psychiatric disorders: focus on antidepressants and antipsychotics. Ann Pharmacother 2013;47(1):75–89.

16. Brogan K, Lux J. Management of common psychiatric conditions in the HIV-positive population. Curr HIV/AIDS Rep 2009;6(2):108–15.

17. Rabkin JG, McElhiney MC, Rabkin R, et al. Modafinil treatment for fatigue in HIV/AIDS: a randomized placebo-controlled study. J Clin Psychiatry 2010;71(6): 707–15.

18. Schifitto G, Zhang J, Evans SR, et al. A multicenter trial of selegiline transdermal system for HIV-associated cognitive impairment. Neurology 2007;69(13): 1314–21.

19. Mendez MF. Mania in neurologic disorders. Curr Psychiatry Rep 2000;2(5): 440–5.

20. Nakimuli-Mpungu E, Musisi S, Kiwuwa Mpungu S, et al. Early-onset versus late-onset HIV-related secondary mania in Uganda. Psychosomatics 2008;49(6): 530–4.

21. Acharjee S, Branton WG, Vivithanaporn P, et al. HIV-1 Nef expression in microglia disrupts dopaminergic and immune functions with associated mania-like behaviors. Brain Behav Immun 2014;40:74–84.
22. Siddiqi O, Birbeck GL. Safe treatment of seizures in the setting of HIV/AIDS. Curr Treat Options Neurol 2013;15(4):529–43.
23. Birbeck GL, French JA, Perucca E, et al. Antiepileptic drug selection for people with HIV/AIDS: evidence-based guidelines from the ILAE and AAN. Epilepsia 2012;53(1):207–14.
24. Devarbhavi H, Andrade RJ. Drug-induced liver injury due to antimicrobials, central nervous system agents, and nonsteroidal anti-inflammatory drugs. Semin Liver Dis 2014;34(2):145–61.
25. Okulicz JF, Grandits GA, French JA, et al. The impact of enzyme-inducing antiepileptic drugs on antiretroviral drug levels: a case-control study. Epilepsy Res 2013;103(2–3):245–53.
26. Sewell DD, Jeste DV, McAdams LA, et al. Neuroleptic treatment of HIV-associated psychosis. HNRC group. Neuropsychopharmacology 1994;10(4):223–9.
27. Hernandez JL, Palacios-Araus L, Echevarria S, et al. Neuroleptic malignant syndrome in the acquired immunodeficiency syndrome. Postgrad Med J 1997; 73(866):779–84.
28. Dolder CR, Patterson TL, Jeste DV. HIV, psychosis and aging: past, present and future. AIDS 2004;18(Suppl 1):S35–42.
29. Spiegel DR, Weller AL, Pennell K, et al. The successful treatment of mania due to acquired immunodeficiency syndrome using ziprasidone: a case series. J Neuropsychiatry Clin Neurosci 2010;22(1):111–4.
30. Vergara-Rodriguez P, Vibhakar S, Watts J. Metabolic syndrome and associated cardiovascular risk factors in the treatment of persons with human immunodeficiency virus and severe mental illness. Pharmacol Ther 2009;124(3):269–78.
31. Penzak SR, Hon YY, Lawhorn WD, et al. Influence of ritonavir on olanzapine pharmacokinetics in healthy volunteers. J Clin Psychopharmacol 2002;22(4): 366–70.
32. Panos SE, Del Re AC, Thames AD, et al. The impact of neurobehavioral features on medication adherence in HIV: evidence from longitudinal models. AIDS Care 2014;26(1):79–86.
33. McIntosh RC, Rosselli M, Uddin LQ, et al. Neuropathological sequelae of human immunodeficiency virus and apathy: a review of neuropsychological and neuroimaging studies. Neurosci Biobehav Rev 2015;55:147–64.
34. Marin RS, Biedrzycki RC, Firinciogullari S. Reliability and validity of the apathy evaluation scale. Psychiatry Res 1991;38(2):143–62.
35. Cummings JL, Mega M, Gray K, et al. The Neuropsychiatric Inventory: comprehensive assessment of psychopathology in dementia. Neurology 1994;44(12): 2308–14.
36. Malloy P, Grace J. A review of rating scales for measuring behavior change due to frontal systems damage. Cogn Behav Neurol 2005;18(1):18–27.
37. Devos D, Moreau C, Maltete D, et al. Rivastigmine in apathetic but dementia and depression-free patients with Parkinson's disease: a double-blind, placebo-controlled, randomised clinical trial. J Neurol Neurosurg Psychiatry 2014; 85(6):668–74.
38. Prommer E. Methylphenidate: established and expanding roles in symptom management. Am J Hosp Palliat Care 2012;29(6):483–90.
39. Hatherill S, Flisher A. Delirium in children with HIV/AIDS. J Child Neurol 2009; 24(7):879–83.

40. Uldall KK, Harris VL, Lalonde B. Outcomes associated with delirium in acutely hospitalized acquired immune deficiency syndrome patients. Compr Psychiatry 2000;41(2):88–91.
41. Sno HN, Storosum JG, Swinkels JA. HIV infection: psychiatric findings in The Netherlands. Br J Psychiatry 1989;155:814–7.
42. Breitbart W, Marotta R, Platt MM, et al. A double-blind trial of haloperidol, chlorpromazine, and lorazepam in the treatment of delirium in hospitalized AIDS patients. Am J Psychiatry 1996;153(2):231–7.
43. Celesia BM, Nigro L, Pinzone MR, et al. High prevalence of undiagnosed anxiety symptoms among HIV-positive individuals on cART: a cross-sectional study. Eur Rev Med Pharmacol Sci 2013;17(15):2040–6.
44. Shacham E, Morgan JC, Onen NF, et al. Screening anxiety in the HIV clinic. AIDS Behav 2012;16(8):2407–13.
45. Kelly B, Raphael B, Judd F, et al. Posttraumatic stress disorder in response to HIV infection. Gen Hosp Psychiatry 1998;20(6):345–52.
46. Smith MY, Egert J, Winkel G, et al. The impact of PTSD on pain experience in persons with HIV/AIDS. Pain 2002;98(1–2):9–17.
47. Safren SA, Gershuny BS, Hendriksen E. Symptoms of posttraumatic stress and death anxiety in persons with HIV and medication adherence difficulties. AIDS Patient Care STDS 2003;17(12):657–64.
48. Tucker JS, Burnam MA, Sherbourne CD, et al. Substance use and mental health correlates of nonadherence to antiretroviral medications in a sample of patients with human immunodeficiency virus infection. Am J Med 2003;114(7):573–80.
49. Thames AD, Hinkin CH, Byrd DA, et al. Effects of stereotype threat, perceived discrimination, and examiner race on neuropsychological performance: simple as black and white? J Int Neuropsychol Soc 2013;19(5):583–93.
50. Thames AD, Panos SE, Arentoft A, et al. Mild test anxiety influences neurocognitive performance among African Americans and European Americans: identifying interfering and facilitating sources. Cultur Divers Ethnic Minor Psychol 2015;21(1):105–13.
51. Capron DW, Cougle JR, Ribeiro JD, et al. An interactive model of anxiety sensitivity relevant to suicide attempt history and future suicidal ideation. J Psychiatr Res 2012;46(2):174–80.
52. Capron DW, Fitch K, Medley A, et al. Role of anxiety sensitivity subfactors in suicidal ideation and suicide attempt history. Depress Anxiety 2012;29(3):195–201.
53. Zinbarg RE, Brown TA, Barlow DH, et al. Anxiety sensitivity, panic, and depressed mood: a reanalysis teasing apart the contributions of the two levels in the hierarchial structure of the Anxiety Sensitivity Index. J Abnorm Psychol 2001;110(3):372–7.
54. Ammassari A, Trotta MP, Murri R, et al. Correlates and predictors of adherence to highly active antiretroviral therapy: overview of published literature. J Acquir Immune Defic Syndr 2002;31(Suppl 3):S123–7.
55. Parker J. Psychotropic prescribing in HIV. South Afr J HIV Med 2009;10(3):44–7.
56. Hsu AJ, Carson KA, Yung R, et al. Severe prolonged sedation associated with coadministration of protease inhibitors and intravenous midazolam during bronchoscopy. Pharmacotherapy 2012;32(6):538–45.
57. Clay PG, Adams MM. Pseudo-Parkinson disease secondary to ritonavir-buspirone interaction. Ann Pharmacother 2003;37(2):202–5.
58. Heaton RK, Marcotte TD, Mindt MR, et al. The impact of HIV-associated neuropsychological impairment on everyday functioning. J Int Neuropsychol Soc 2004;10(3):317–31.

59. Reger M, Welsh R, Razani J, et al. A meta-analysis of the neuropsychological sequelae of HIV infection. J Int Neuropsychol Soc 2002;8(3):410–24.

60. Heaton RK, Franklin DR, Ellis RJ, et al. HIV-associated neurocognitive disorders before and during the era of combination antiretroviral therapy: differences in rates, nature, and predictors. J Neurovirol 2011;17(1):3–16.

61. Beguelin C, Vazquez M, Bertschi M, et al. Viral escape in the CNS with multidrug-resistant HIV-1. J Int AIDS Soc 2014;17(4 Suppl 3):19745.

62. McArthur JC, McDermott MP, McClernon D, et al. Attenuated central nervous system infection in advanced HIV/AIDS with combination antiretroviral therapy. Arch Neurol 2004;61(11):1687–96.

63. Sidtis JJ, Gatsonis C, Price RW, et al. Zidovudine treatment of the AIDS dementia complex: results of a placebo-controlled trial. AIDS Clinical Trials Group. Ann Neurol 1993;33(4):343–9.

64. Letendre S, Marquie-Beck J, Capparelli E, et al. Validation of the CNS Penetration-Effectiveness rank for quantifying antiretroviral penetration into the central nervous system. Arch Neurol 2008;65(1):65–70.

65. Nightingale S, Winston A, Letendre S, et al. Controversies in HIV-associated neurocognitive disorders. Lancet Neurol 2014;13(11):1139–51.

66. Perkins D, Evans DL. HIV-related major depression: response to zidovudine treatment. Psychosomatics 1991;32(4):451–4.

67. Hinkin CH, Castellon SA, Hardy DJ, et al. Methylphenidate improves HIV-1-associated cognitive slowing. J Neuropsychiatry Clin Neurosci 2001;13(2): 248–54.

68. Fernandez F, Levy JK, Samley HR, et al. Effects of methylphenidate in HIV-related depression: a comparative trial with desipramine. Int J Psychiatry Med 1995;25(1):53–67.

69. Breitbart W, Rosenfeld B, Kaim M, et al. A randomized, double-blind, placebo-controlled trial of psychostimulants for the treatment of fatigue in ambulatory patients with human immunodeficiency virus disease. Arch Intern Med 2001; 161(3):411–20.

70. Johannessen DJ, Wilson LG. Mania with cryptococcal meningitis in two AIDS patients. J Clin Psychiatry 1988;49(5):200–1.

71. Panel on Opportunistic Infections in HIV-infected Adults and Adolescents. Guidelines for prevention and treatment of opportunistic infections in HIV-infected adults and adolescents. 2015. Available at: http://aidsinfo.nih.gov/contentfiles/lvguidelines/adult_oi.pdf. Accessed July 15, 2015.

72. Spiegel DR, Bayne CE, Wilcox L, et al. A case of mania due to cryptococcal meningitis, successfully treated with adjunctive olanzapine, in a patient with acquired immunodeficiency syndrome. Gen Hosp Psychiatry 2011;33(3): 301.e3–6.

73. Levine AJ, Hinkin CH, Ando K, et al. An exploratory study of long-term neurocognitive outcomes following recovery from opportunistic brain infections in HIV+ adults. J Clin Exp Neuropsychol 2008;30(7):836–43.

74. Ho YC, Sun HY, Chen MY, et al. Clinical presentation and outcome of toxoplasmic encephalitis in patients with human immunodeficiency virus type 1 infection. J Microbiol Immunol Infect 2008;41(5):386–92.

75. Donnet A, Harle JR, Cherif AA, et al. Acute psychiatric pathology disclosing subcortical lesion in neuro-AIDS. Encephale 1991;17(2):79–81 [in French].

76. Ilniczky S, Debreczeni R, Kovacs T, et al. Aids-related toxoplasma-encephalitis presenting with acute psychotic episode. Ideggyogy Sz 2006;59(7–8):289–93 [in Hungarian].

77. Alla P, de Jaureguiberry JP, Galzin M, et al. Hemiballism with manic access caused by toxoplasmic abscess in AIDS. Ann Med Interne (Paris) 1997; 148(7):507–9 [in French].

78. Ozkaya G, Kurne A, Unal S, et al. Aphasic status epilepticus with periodic lateralized epileptiform discharges in a bilingual patient as a presenting sign of AIDS-toxoplasmosis complex. Epilepsy Behav 2006;9(1):193–6.

79. Hirose G. Parkinsonism in a patient with AIDS. Intern Med 2000;39(12): 1006–7.

80. Linazasoro G. Movement disorders with cerebral toxoplasmosis and AIDS. Mov Disord 1994;9(2):244–5.

81. Monroe JM, Buckley PF, Miller BJ. Meta-analysis of anti-*Toxoplasma gondii* IgM antibodies in acute psychosis. Schizophr Bull 2015;41(4):989–98.

82. Mikita K, Maeda T, Ono T, et al. The utility of cerebrospinal fluid for the molecular diagnosis of toxoplasmic encephalitis. Diagn Microbiol Infect Dis 2013;75(2): 155–9.

83. Halonen SK, Weiss LM. Toxoplasmosis. Handb Clin Neurol 2013;114:125–45.

84. Berger JR, Dean D. Neurosyphilis. Handb Clin Neurol 2014;121:1461–72.

85. Hutto B. Syphilis in clinical psychiatry: a review. Psychosomatics 2001;42(6): 453–60.

86. Hicks CB, Benson PM, Lupton GP, et al. Seronegative secondary syphilis in a patient infected with the human immunodeficiency virus (HIV) with Kaposi sarcoma. A diagnostic dilemma. Ann Intern Med 1987;107(4):492–5.

87. Lukehart SA, Hook EW 3rd, Baker-Zander SA, et al. Invasion of the central nervous system by *Treponema pallidum*: implications for diagnosis and treatment. Ann Intern Med 1988;109(11):855–62.

88. McArthur JC, Sipos E, Cornblath DR, et al. Identification of mononuclear cells in CSF of patients with HIV infection. Neurology 1989;39(1):66–70.

89. Wong T, Fonseca K, Chernesky MA, et al. Canadian public health laboratory network laboratory guidelines for the diagnosis of neurosyphilis in Canada. Can J Infect Dis Med Microbiol 2015;26(Suppl A):18A–22A.

90. Jaffe HW, Larsen SA, Peters M, et al. Tests for treponemal antibody in CSF. Arch Intern Med 1978;138(2):252–5.

91. Johns DR, Tierney M, Felsenstein D. Alteration in the natural history of neurosyphilis by concurrent infection with the human immunodeficiency virus. N Engl J Med 1987;316(25):1569–72.

92. Katz DA, Berger JR. Neurosyphilis in acquired immunodeficiency syndrome. Arch Neurol 1989;46(8):895–8.

93. Moulton CD, Koychev I. The effect of penicillin therapy on cognitive outcomes in neurosyphilis: a systematic review of the literature. Gen Hosp Psychiatry 2015; 37(1):49–52.

94. Lin LR, Zhang HL, Huang SJ, et al. Psychiatric manifestations as primary symptom of neurosyphilis among HIV-negative patients. J Neuropsychiatry Clin Neurosci 2014;26(3):233–40.

95. Sanchez FM, Zisselman MH. Treatment of psychiatric symptoms associated with neurosyphilis. Psychosomatics 2007;48(5):440–5.

96. Steiner I, Benninger F. Update on herpes virus infections of the nervous system. Curr Neurol Neurosci Rep 2013;13(12):414.

97. Steadman P. Herpes simplex mimicking functional psychosis. Biol Psychiatry 1992;32(2):211–2.

98. Boyapati R, Papadopoulos G, Olver J, et al. An unusual presentation of herpes simplex virus encephalitis. Case Rep Med 2012;2012:241710.

99. Steiner I, Schmutzhard E, Sellner J, et al. EFNS-ENS guidelines for the use of PCR technology for the diagnosis of infections of the nervous system. Eur J Neurol 2012;19(10):1278–91.

100. Widener RW, Whitley RJ. Herpes simplex virus. Handb Clin Neurol 2014;123: 251–63.

101. Gnann JW Jr, Skoldenberg B, Hart J, et al. Herpes simplex encephalitis: lack of clinical benefit of long-term valacyclovir therapy. Clin Infect Dis 2015;61(5): 683–91.

102. Dagsdottir HM, Sigurethardottir B, Gottfreethsson M, et al. Herpes simplex encephalitis in Iceland 1987-2011. Springerplus 2014;3:524.

103. Vasconcelos-Moreno MP, Dargel AA, Goi PD, et al. Improvement of behavioural and manic-like symptoms secondary to herpes simplex virus encephalitis with mood stabilizers: a case report. Int J Neuropsychopharmacol 2011;14(5): 718–20.

104. Padgett BL, Walker DL. Prevalence of antibodies in human sera against JC virus, an isolate from a case of progressive multifocal leukoencephalopathy. J Infect Dis 1973;127(4):467–70.

105. White MK, Khalili K. Pathogenesis of progressive multifocal leukoencephalopathy–revisited. J Infect Dis 2011;203(5):578–86.

106. Wright CA, Nance JA, Johnson EM. Effects of Tat proteins and Tat mutants of different human immunodeficiency virus type 1 clades on glial JC virus early and late gene transcription. J Gen Virol 2013;94(Pt 3):514–23.

107. Berger JR, Pall L, Lanska D, et al. Progressive multifocal leukoencephalopathy in patients with HIV infection. J Neurovirol 1998;4(1):59–68.

108. Corti M, Villafane M, Trione N, et al. Progressive multifocal leukoencephalopathy presenting as IRIS in an AIDS patient. A case report and literature review. Neuroradiol J 2013;26(2):151–4.

109. Sudhakar P, Bachman DM, Mark AS, et al. Progressive multifocal leukoencephalopathy: recent advances and a neuro-ophthalmological review. J Neuroophthalmol 2015;35(3):296–305.

110. Berger JR. The clinical features of PML. Cleve Clin J Med 2011;78(Suppl 2): S8–12.

111. King RR, Reiss JP. Treatment of pseudobulbar affect with citalopram in a patient with progressive multifocal leukoencephalopthy. J Clin Neurosci 2012;19(1): 185–6.

112. Naito K, Ueno H, Sekine M, et al. Akinetic mutism caused by HIV-associated progressive multifocal leukoencephalopathy was successfully treated with mefloquine: a serial multimodal MRI Study. Intern Med 2012;51(2):205–9.

113. Saito H, Sakai H, Fujihara K, et al. Progressive multifocal leukoencephalopathy in a patient with acquired immunodeficiency syndrome (AIDS) manifesting Gerstmann's syndrome. Tohoku J Exp Med 1998;186(3):169–79.

114. Berger JR, Aksamit AJ, Clifford DB, et al. PML diagnostic criteria: consensus statement from the AAN Neuroinfectious Disease Section. Neurology 2013; 80(15):1430–8.

115. Marzocchetti A, Di Giambenedetto S, Cingolani A, et al. Reduced rate of diagnostic positive detection of JC virus DNA in cerebrospinal fluid in cases of suspected progressive multifocal leukoencephalopathy in the era of potent antiretroviral therapy. J Clin Microbiol 2005;43(8):4175–7.

116. Southworth MR, Dunlap SH. Psychotic symptoms and confusion associated with intravenous ganciclovir in a heart transplant recipient. Pharmacotherapy 2000; 20(4):479–83.

117. Asahi T, Tsutsui M, Wakasugi M, et al. Valacyclovir neurotoxicity: clinical experience and review of the literature. Eur J Neurol 2009;16(4):457–60.
118. Reboli AC, Mandler HD. Encephalopathy and psychoses associated with sulfadiazine in two patients with AIDS and CNS toxoplasmosis. Clin Infect Dis 1992; 15(3):556–7.
119. Kieburtz KD, Epstein LG, Gelbard HA, et al. Excitotoxicity and dopaminergic dysfunction in the acquired immunodeficiency syndrome dementia complex. Therapeutic implications. Arch Neurol 1991;48(12):1281–4.
120. Clifford DB, Nath A, Cinque P, et al. A study of mefloquine treatment for progressive multifocal leukoencephalopathy: results and exploration of predictors of PML outcomes. J Neurovirol 2013;19(4):351–8.
121. Lanzafame M, Ferrari S, Lattuada E, et al. Mirtazapine in an HIV-1 infected patient with progressive multifocal leukoencephalopathy. Infez Med 2009;17(1): 35–7.
122. Foster R, Olajide D, Everall IP. Antiretroviral therapy-induced psychosis: case report and brief review of the literature. HIV Med 2003;4(2):139–44.
123. Rosso AL, Mattos JP, Correa RB, et al. Parkinsonism and AIDS: a clinical comparative study before and after HAART. Arq Neuropsiquiatr 2009;67(3B): 827–30.
124. Kumar AM, Fernandez JB, Singer EJ, et al. Human immunodeficiency virus type 1 in the central nervous system leads to decreased dopamine in different regions of postmortem human brains. J Neurovirol 2009;15(3):257–74.
125. Cotton PJ, Le B. Progressive multifocal leukoencephalopathy and palliative care: a report of three cases and review of the literature. Palliat Med 2013; 27(3):286–8.
126. Jena A, Sachdeva RK, Sharma A, et al. Adverse drug reactions to nonnucleoside reverse transcriptase inhibitor-based antiretroviral regimen: a 24-week prospective study. J Int Assoc Physicians AIDS Care (Chic) 2009; 8(5):318–22.
127. Rihs TA, Begley K, Smith DE, et al. Efavirenz and chronic neuropsychiatric symptoms: a cross-sectional case control study. HIV Med 2006;7(8):544–8.
128. Mollan KR, Smurzynski M, Eron JJ, et al. Association between efavirenz as initial therapy for HIV-1 infection and increased risk for suicidal ideation or attempted or completed suicide: an analysis of trial data. Ann Intern Med 2014;161(1): 1–10.
129. Funes HA, Blas-Garcia A, Esplugues JV, et al. Efavirenz alters mitochondrial respiratory function in cultured neuron and glial cell lines. J Antimicrob Chemother 2015;70(8):2249–54.
130. Tovar-y-Romo LB, Bumpus NN, Pomerantz D, et al. Dendritic spine injury induced by the 8-hydroxy metabolite of efavirenz. J Pharmacol Exp Ther 2012;343(3):696–703.
131. Kermani E, Drob S, Alpert M. Organic brain syndrome in three cases of acquired immune deficiency syndrome. Compr Psychiatry 1984;25(3):294–7.
132. Song X, Hu Z, Zhang H. Acute dystonia induced by lamivudine. Clin Neuropharmacol 2005;28(4):193–4.
133. Kaestner F, Anneken K, Mostert C, et al. Depression associated with antiretroviral drug therapy in HIV: case report and overview. Int J STD AIDS 2012;23(6): e14–9.
134. Judd FK, Cockram AM, Komiti A, et al. Depressive symptoms reduced in individuals with HIV/AIDS treated with highly active antiretroviral therapy: a longitudinal study. Aust N Z J Psychiatry 2000;34(6):1015–21.

135. Kumar AM, Ownby RL, Waldrop-Valverde D, et al. Human immunodeficiency virus infection in the CNS and decreased dopamine availability: relationship with neuropsychological performance. J Neurovirol 2011;17(1):26–40.

136. Hollander H, Golden J, Mendelson T, et al. Extrapyramidal symptoms in AIDS patients given low-dose metoclopramide or chlorpromazine. Lancet 1985; 2(8465):1186.

Traumatic Brain Injury and Behavior: A Practical Approach

Jeanie McGee, DHEd, Nadejda Alekseeva, MD, Oleg Chernyshev, MD,
Alireza Minagar, MD*

KEYWORDS

- Traumatic brain injury • Psychosis • Suicide • Behavioral abnormalities • Seizures
- Mania • Depression • Sleep-wake disorder

KEY POINTS

- Traumatic brain injury (TBI) comprises a heterogenous array of disorders that stem from an initial trauma to the head and in many patients leads to death or significant morbidity and disability. Presently an estimated 1.4 million cases of TBI occur annually in the United States.
- TBI is associated with a broad spectrum of neurologic and psychiatric abnormalities that directly affect the patient's behavior. Cognitive decline (particularly memory loss), epilepsy, and mood disorders are among the most common complications of TBI.
- Frontal lobes are prone to injury in the course of TBI, and damage to these areas and their neuroanatomic connections to other cortical and subcortical regions may cause frontal lobe syndromes and executive dysfunction syndromes.
- A wide array of sleep-wake disorders including insomnia, excessive daytime sleepiness, posttraumatic hypersomnia, circadian rhythm sleep wake disorders, narcolepsy, sleep-related breathing disorder, REM sleep behavior disorder, non-REM parasomnias (sleepwalking, sleep terrors), periodic limb movements in sleep, and rhythmic movement disorders may occur in patients with TBI.

INTRODUCTION

Traumatic brain injury (TBI) is a significant cause of morbidity and mortality in adult and pediatric populations. Rather than being a congenital or neurodegenerative injury to the brain, TBI results from the application of external mechanical force to the head and leads to transient or permanent damage. The negative outcomes of TBI include, but are not restricted to, cognitive decline, neurologic and physical deficits, and impairment of psychosocial activities and function. Clinically, TBI may present with decreased or altered mental status. Rather than being a simple event, TBI is a complex

Department of Neurology, Louisiana State University Health Sciences Center - Shreveport, 1501 Kings Highway, Shreveport, LA 71130, USA
* Corresponding author.
E-mail address: aminag@lsuhsc.edu

Neurol Clin 34 (2016) 55–68
http://dx.doi.org/10.1016/j.ncl.2015.08.004   **neurologic.theclinics.com**
0733-8619/16/$ – see front matter © 2016 Elsevier Inc. All rights reserved.

neuroanatomic, neuropathologic, and biochemical process that affects several areas of the human brain through the original impact and injury and via secondary events, such as ischemia, seizure, and infection. TBI interrupts the physiologic activity of the brain. In addition, TBI is not a solitary disorder with a clear-cut set of clinical manifestations. Indeed, the term TBI is a multifaceted and heterogeneous group of disorders, which adversely affects a wide range of neuropsychiatric functions of the patient. Neuropsychiatric disorders, and particularly cognitive decline, are common following TBI and reflect the depth and width of the injury induced by the initial impact to the head. As an injury, TBI stems from penetrating, blunt, or acceleration-deceleration forces.

Based on a comprehensive report by the Centers for Disease Control and Prevention to the United States Congress in 2010, an estimated 2.5 million emergency room visits resulted from TBI, which included isolate TBIs and TBIs associated with other injuries.[1] TBIs affect civilians and military individuals. TBIs are categorized as mild, moderate, and severe based on the victim's clinical manifestations and the associated outcomes. Most civilian cases of TBI are mild. Grossly, TBI is divided into penetrating and nonpenetrating. Most cases of TBI are mild; nonpenetrating; and result from falls, motor vehicle accidents, violence and assault, and sport and recreational activities.[1]

Epidemiologic data indicate that annually in the United States, more than 2 million cases of TBI occur and a significant number of them occur in the elderly population.[2] A significant number of patients with TBI require hospital admission and treatment. Every year an appraised 300,000 sports-associated TBI cases occur in the United States.

Clinically, TBI is associated with a wide gamut of neurologic and psychiatric disorders that include, but are not limited to, amnesia, cognitive decline, seizures, attention and concentration deficits, depression, manic behavior, psychosis, hostile and violent behavior, and personality alterations. Civilian TBIs most often stem from falls, motor vehicle accidents, getting hit in the head by a moving or standing object, and being attacked. Military TBIs mainly are cause by blasts and shock waves from explosives. In both populations, TBI can be blunt or penetrating. Because TBI includes a heterogeneous group of disorders, therapy and rehabilitative efforts should be designed based on the type of injury and the patient's specific needs.

COGNITIVE DECLINE FOLLOWING TRAUMATIC BRAIN INJURY

TBI sets off an array of primary and secondary insults to the human brain that, in turn, affect the neurophysiologic activity of the cerebral cortex, subcortical structures, and neuroanatomic pathways, which serve cognition. All or any of these areas are potentially affected by TBI, which most often translates into cognitive impairment. Cognitive decline, a broad-term that covers many aspects of human cognition, is observed more often following moderate to severe TBIs and is less frequently associated with mild TBI cases. Cognitive decline, particularly memory loss, is a common and well-recognized complication of TBIs. Impairment of cognitive capabilities directly and adversely affects the patient's intellectual creativity and productivity and causes disability. Other troubling cognitive issues include attention deficit; difficulty with concentration and multitasking; impairments of language use and visual perception; and difficulty with abstract reasoning, thought process, problem-solving, insight, and judgment. These impairments, indeed, pose significant and insurmountable barriers to patients' paths toward having a normal independent life, securing a job, and establishing social adaptation.[3]

All forms of TBI affect and impair the patient's attention. For example, during the posttraumatic amnestic period that acutely occurs following mild TBI, the patient shows difficulty with awareness of the surrounding events, attention, and concentration. Furthermore, executive function of attention also may be impaired and result in the patient's inability to perform lower-level attentional processes because of a lack of coordination.

Memory impairment and difficulty with learning are among the salient clinical features of TBI. Many patients with TBI suffer from retrograde amnesia and posttraumatic amnesia, which indicate the memory dysfunction is initiated during the acute stage of TBI and may continue beyond this stage.[4,5] Long-term memory is frequently classified as declarative (explicit) memory and procedural (implicit) memory. By definition, explicit memory, which refers to "knowing what," points to memories that can be consciously and purposefully recalled and declared. The declarative memory is further subcategorized into episodic memory and sematic memory. Episodic memory is about personal events, whereas semantic memory covers common knowledge and basic facts about the world, such as the capital of countries. The concepts and ideas within this portion of memory do not stem from personal experience. Procedural (implicit) memory or knowing how to do things refers to unconscious memory skills to certain things, such as riding a bike or how to make a bowtie. This type of memory is formed by repetition of any activity to the point that it is "automatic." Abnormality of the episodic memory is an outstanding characteristic of TBI and its harshness usually parallels the severity of the TBI.[4] Impairments of executive functioning related to memory are often noted in TBI. Working memory, which consists of temporary information storage and manipulation; strategic memory involving active information organization; source memory related to conceptual episodic memory; prospective memory, such as task performance recall; and metamemory, which relates to the patient's self-awareness of memory recollection, are all vulnerable to impairment resulting from TBI.[6]

Frontal lobes, and more specifically the prefrontal cortex, with their complex neuroanatomic pathways and connections to other cortical and subcortical structures, serve to establish long-term memory and executive functions, and their injury during TBI leads to serious behavioral abnormalities. Damage to these areas during the course of TBI is associated with, but not limited to, increased distractibility, forgetfulness, difficulty with focusing one's attention and concentration on a mental task, impairment of working memory and retrieval, dysexecutive syndromes, and disinhibited behavior. The various categories of frontal executive functions include executive cognition, activation-regulating function, behavioral self-regulation and inhibition, and metacognitive processes. Patients suffering TBI may develop executive function impairments in the areas of planning and completing goals, initiating and inhibiting responses, developing various response alternatives, mental flexibility, problem-solving and conceptual reasoning, decision-making, working memory, memory and attention processes, emotional response regulation and self-monitoring, and appropriate functioning in social situations.[6]

TRAUMATIC BRAIN INJURY AND DEMENTIA

Dementia, as a serious and devastating event, may stem from TBIs, and several epidemiologic assessments indicate that suffering from TBI in early to mid-life is associated with an elevated danger of dementia in late life.[7,8] A recent systemic review of risk of dementia and chronic cognitive decline by Godbolt and colleagues[9] reported a lack of conclusive evidence supporting elevated risk of dementia following mild TBI.

However, frequent and repeated mild TBIs for many years, a condition commonly seen in professional boxers, is associated with a high risk of chronic traumatic encephalopathy (CTE).[10] CTE carries its own clinical and neuropathologic characteristics.

CTE is a neurodegenerative disease resulting from head trauma as observed in professional boxers, wrestlers, football players, and hockey players, and in military veterans. Clinical characteristics of CTE most often include, but are not limited to, headache and/or head pain, mood disorders, motor dysfunction, attention and memory difficulties, and dementia. It is currently believed that about 50% of all head injuries among professional athletes can be categorized as CTE.[11]

A significant issue is that dementia may occur in the context of multiple and repeated blows to the patient's head. Indeed, repeat minor rotational blows to the head translate into collective brain damage known as "dementia pugilistica." Dementia pugilistic is often observed in professional boxers, and it particularly occurs if the boxers initiated boxing in their teenage years, boxed for longer than 10 years, collected more than 150 competitions, and were known to take punches.[12,13]

Presently, it remains unknown whether dementia in TBI survivors is pathophysiologically similar to Alzheimer disease, CTE, or some other entity. Such information is critical for developing preventive and treatment strategies for a common cause of acquired dementia. The epidemiologic data linking TBI and dementia, existing clinical and pathologic data, and areas where future research is needed are discussed elsewhere in this issue.

An interesting and significant research topic in TBI and cognition is the role of apolipoprotein E as a prognostic factor in the development of dementia following TBI. A recent systemic assessment and review by Lawrence and colleagues[14] concluded that APOEε4 adversely affected recovery from TBI, and this was noticeable in dementia and other cognitive impairments in patients with severe TBIs.

TRAUMATIC BRAIN INJURY AND EPILEPSY

Seizures and epilepsy are well recognized complications of TBI and are categorized as immediate if they happen within the first 24 hours, early if they happen between 24 hours and 7 days, and late if they happen after 7 days. In a significant number of patients with TBI, the risk of post-TBI seizures is greatest in the first 12 months following the initial impact, and it declines after that. Haltiner and colleagues[15] reported that a cumulative incidence of recurrent seizures in this group of patients was up to 86% by almost 2 years. A recent review on this subject by Pitkanen and Immonen[16] reports that post-TBI epilepsy constitutes 10% to 20% of patients with symptomatic epilepsy and 5% of all epilepsy.

Perhaps a significant factor in the development of post-TBI epilepsy is the severity and harshness of the head trauma. Other potential risk factors for development of post-TBI seizures include age older than 65 years, cerebral contusion with subdural hematoma or intracerebral bleeding, and development of early post-TBI seizures (within 1 week from TBI).[17,18]

Lastly, one must realize that posttraumatic epilepsy, by itself, results or is associated with several behavioral abnormalities, such as depression, aggressive behavior, memory loss, and omnipresent feeling of losing control.

A major issue related to post-TBI seizures is the prophylactic use of antiepileptic drugs (AEDs). For patients with mild TBI, use of AEDs is not recommended unless the patient seizes. In patients with severe TBI, prophylactic use of phenytoin defends against early post-TBI seizures (7 days). Because there is no concrete evidence to support preventive efficacy of AEDs after 7 days and their capability to influence the risk of development of post-TBI epilepsy, chronic use of these medications to avoid late post-TBI seizures is not suggested.[19] In general, therapy of post-TBI seizures is virtually the same for epilepsy.

TRAUMATIC BRAIN INJURY AND MOOD DISORDERS

Since 1904, researchers have associated TBI with subsequent mood disorders, with mania and depression being common manifestations following TBI.[20] Mood disorders are believed to be the most common psychiatric diagnosis made in post-TBI patients, second only to anxiety disorders.[21] Depression is noted in around 6% to 77% of patients with TBI and is suspected to be associated with the disruption of neurons containing biogenic amines as their neuronal signals travel through frontal subcortical white mater or basal ganglia.[20,22] A recent prospective study found that patients with a history of depression before TBI were more than five times more likely to develop post-TBI depressive disorders following injury, and the odds of developing depression increased with each subsequent month following initial TBI.[21] Post-TBI depression manifests in 25% to 50% of patients within the first year following injury and in 26% to 64% over their lifetime.[20] Post-TBI depressive mood disorders may present clinically as a general depressed mood, fatigue or loss of energy, or anhedonia and are noted to be most clinically significant at 6 and 12 months post-TBI before treatment of symptomology.[21]

As with depression resulting from other etiologies, patients suffering from post-TBI depression can be treated with antidepressants, and electroconvulsive therapy has been proven highly effective in this patient population.[20] Other effective treatments include such approaches as cognitive behavioral therapy (CBT), which may decrease depressive symptoms, anger, and anxiety. CBT also assists in improving the patient's self-esteem, which may result in increased psychosocial functioning. Additional treatments include such approaches as the use of psychotherapy groups and other support groups or therapy that focuses on education, interpersonal skills development, and ongoing social support.[22]

Manic tendencies occur less frequently following TBI than depressive moods with estimates of prevalence in less than 10% of patients with TBI.[20] A recent prospective study reported even lower prevalence rates of 1.7% to 9% of post-TBI bipolar and related disorders, including mania and hypomania.[22] Changes in mood resulting in mania in post-TBI patients may present clinically as insomnia, aggression or agitation, irritability, or uncharacteristic violent tendencies and most commonly manifests following TBI involving the right hemisphere affecting the limbic system.[20] When post-TBI behavioral changes occur, they are most often associated with head injuries involving the right ventral frontal or basotemporal regions.[22]

TRAUMATIC BRAIN INJURY AND PSYCHOSIS

Although the published research varies considerably regarding the severity of TBI that most often results in psychosis, most researchers agree that in severe cases of TBI, patients may develop psychotic symptoms similar to those noted in patients diagnosed with schizophrenia. The current Diagnostic and Statistical Manual-IV diagnosis assigned to patients experiencing psychosis following TBI is termed "psychotic disorder due to traumatic brain injury" (PDTBI).[23] Recent studies of post-TBI psychosis report rates ranging from less than 1% to 15% of patients with TBI developing these symptoms.[20] Prevalence rates of post-TBI psychosis of 20% have been reported among patients considered to have chronic TBI.[24] A recently published meta-analysis examining the relationship between TBI and psychosis revealed a significant association between TBI and psychosis, specifically schizophrenia, indicating an increased risk of developing schizophrenia following TBI that is two times greater than the risk of schizophrenia in the normal population.[25] Other published research suggests that post-TBI psychosis may occur even more frequently, at a rate up to three times higher than in the non-TBI population.[26] However, researchers have concluded that in some cases TBI is the primary cause of psychosis, whereas in other cases post-TBI psychosis can development as a result of TBI-related seizure onset. Furthermore, the risk for developing post-TBI psychosis has been determined to be directly related to the severity of the injury, with psychosis onset being more likely in patients with severe TBI.[27]

Among the most commonly noted psychotic symptoms are illogical thinking and beliefs, delusions, and hallucinations. Furthermore, regression, inappropriate emotional expressions, such as laughter or grimacing, and agitation may be noted in these patients.[20] A comprehensive review of patients specifically diagnosed with PDTBI determined that the most common symptoms of psychosis presenting in this group included delusions (most often, persecutory delusions) and hallucinations, with negative symptomology being rare.[23]

Post-TBI psychosis is most likely to manifest when the brain injury involves the frontal and temporal lobes.[27] A publication by Fuji and Ahmed[23] noted electroencephalogram abnormalities in more than 70% of patients diagnosed with PDTBI, with more than half of the abnormalities localized to the temporal lobe. However, research has shown that post-TBI psychosis may result from injuries sustained to either the left or right hemispheres, and treatment approaches are most effective when the hemisphere of injury is considered. For example, anticonvulsants are commonly most effective in treating post-TBI psychoses in left-temporal injuries.[20] However, patients diagnosed with PDTBI have shown improvement when treated with a variety of medications, including anticonvulsants, lithium, and antidepressants.[23]

TRAUMATIC BRAIN INJURY AND SUBSTANCE ABUSE

There is a substantial amount of published literature indicating an association between TBI and subsequent increases in drug and alcohol use, especially in individuals with substance abuse history before the injury. However, the cause of such increases is not always clear and may be from drug use for pain or other injury-related complications or may be a direct result of proximal neurobiologic sequelae.[28] On the contrary, some researchers have reported declines in post-TBI substance abuse in patients with prior use ranging from 4% to 66%.[29] Correlations between TBI and substance abuse are noted to occur at the onset of TBI, with more than 30% of patients suffering a brain injury reportedly being under the influence of illegal drugs at the time of the injury, making an accurate interpretation of the relationship between the two variables postinjury complicated.[30] Epidemiologic studies have noted a high incidence of reported alcohol and drug use, and high levels on laboratory testing, at the time of initial brain injury.[28] Still, other studies suggest that the presence of comorbid substance abuse and mental illness places patients at a higher risk of TBI, and post-TBI increased substance abuse.[31]

Systematic reviews of TBI as a risk factor for substance abuse have indicated differences in patient clinical status post-TBI depending on the type of substance used. Therefore, it is difficult to ascertain whether the long-term effects of post-TBI substance abuse have negative implications in terms of patient outcomes.[29] Furthermore, these differences could contribute significantly to the patient's response to treatment, making both pre- and post-TBI substance abuse histories integral to effective treatment following TBI.[31] Additionally, TBI location may directly influence a patient's use of drugs and/or alcohol postinjury, because patients sustaining frontal lobe TBI may have impairments in terms of their ability to predict potential outcomes of substance abuse.[28] Thus, it sometimes becomes difficult for clinicians to determine the most effective treatments for post-TBI substance abuse because of unclear etiology.

TRAUMATIC BRAIN INJURY AND SUICIDE

Years of research have shown that patients with TBI are at an increased risk of taking their own lives, with one study reporting that around 17% of patients who had suffered TBI reported at least one suicide attempt.[32] Recent studies examining suicide rates among patients with TBI report frequencies of suicide attempts up to 4.5 times that of individuals without TBI, and more than 8% higher frequency in attempted suicide among patients with TBI who also suffer alcohol abuse.[33] Most often suicidal ideation, attempts, and completion results from anxiety and depression that occurs following the injury, and is frequently combined with other specific predisposing variables.[34,35] Various research studies have determined that such factors as post-TBI aggression, feelings of hopelessness, number of head injuries sustained, severity of TBI, symptoms of posttraumatic stress disorder, and demographics including younger age and male gender are significantly correlated with the risk of suicide in patients with TBI.[32–36]

TRAUMATIC BRAIN INJURY AND SLEEP-WAKE DISORDERS

Sleep-wake abnormalities after TBI are very common, ranging from 30% to 70% of patients who suffer head injury.[37,38] The precise prevalence of posttraumatic sleep disorders is not well known, especially in the pediatric and elderly populations.[39] The reported spectrum of post-TBI sleep-wake disorders is broad and consists of insomnia as a symptom and disorder (20%–60%)[37,39–42]; excessive daytime sleepiness (14%–57%)[37,43–48]; posttraumatic hypersomnia (11%–30%)[38,46,49]; circadian rhythm sleep-wake disorders (13%)[50]; narcolepsy (6%)[38]; sleep-related breathing disorder (23%–25%)[38,51,52]; rapid eye movement (REM) sleep behavior disorder; non-REM parasomnias (sleepwalking, sleep terrors); periodic limb movements in sleep (7%)[38]; rhythmic movement disorders (3.3%); and Kleine-Levin syndrome.[53] In the pediatric population, from 10% to 38% of children with TBI have sleep disturbances, specifically in the acute period following injury.[54–58] There is a lack of research in the area of geriatric TBI.[58] Thus, the prevalence of post-TBI sleep-wake disorders in the geriatric population is not well-established.

PATHOPHYSIOLOGY

There are two subtypes of head injury, closed and open (perforating). TBI can lead to the development of diffused or localized cerebral lesions and increased intracranial pressure, specifically during the acute phase. Diffuse axonal injury can result from acceleration/deceleration forces. A coup-contrecoup TBI mechanism is responsible for localized cerebral lesions. The severity of head injury is classified as mild, moderate, or severe. Sleep disorders may be present in patients with TBI regardless of severity of the TBI.[59] Cerebral structural lesions, either diffuse or focal, can affect function of sleep-promoting and wake-promoting anatomic centers. Posttraumatic hypersomnia is associated with diffuse and/or focal lesions, affecting wake-promoting structures in the brainstem reticular formation, posterior hypothalamus, and the periventricular structures surrounding the third ventricle.[60–62]

Decreased levels of hypocretin 1 concentrations (a marker of narcolepsy type 1) may contribute to the development of excessive daytime sleepiness after TBI.[46,63,64] Interestingly, the hypocretin 1 concentrations tend to return to normal by 6 months after injury,[46] which may provide an explanation for resolution and improvement of posttraumatic sleepiness. Reduced secretion of melatonin has been identified in the acute[65,66] and chronic phases[67] of TBI. TBI can compromise the suprachiasmatic nucleus or its outputs and disturb circadian rhythmicity causing concomitant hypersomnia and insomnia.[52] A 41% loss of histaminergic wake-promoting neurons in the tuberomammillary nucleus was found during postmortem brain autopsies in patients after TBI in a persistent coma. Insomnia could result from the coup-contrecoup brain trauma with consequent damage to the inferior frontal and anterior temporal regions, including basal forebrain, a sleep-promoting area.[52,60]

The exact mechanism of sleep-disordered breathing in TBI is unknown. Sleep-related breathing disorders are possibly caused by focal and or diffuse cerebral and spinal cord injuries affecting central respiratory control and/or upper airway collapsability, and may be precipitated by coexisting multiorgan injuries, specifically compromising the upper airway.[60,62,68,69]

The glymphatic system is a recently discovered cerebral macroscopic waste clearance system, using a unique system of glial aquaporin-4 water channels, to promote efficient elimination of soluble proteins and metabolites from central nervous system, and facilitation of brain-wide distribution of several compounds (glucose, lipids, amino acids, growth factors) and neuromodulators (adenosine), responsible for "sleep pressure" generation and maintenance. The glymphatic system functions mostly during sleep and is in inactive mode during wakefulness.[70] Recent research demonstrated the evidence of glymphatic system malfunction in TBI, which may be a significant contributing factor in the development of posttraumatic sleep-wake disturbances.[71]

CLINICAL PRESENTATION AND TREATMENT

The results of available research projects are diverse because of an absence of uniform measures and inconsistencies in methodologic tools. Delayed sleep-wake phase disorder (10%) and irregular sleep-wake rhythm disorder (3%) are the primary manifestations of posttraumatic circadian rhythm sleep-wake disorders.[72] Chronotherapy and chronobiotics, such as melatonin, can be used for treatment of chronic sleep-wake disturbance after TBI.[73,74]

Sleep-related breathing disorders, primarily obstructive sleep apnea, have been noted in TBI populations undergoing evaluations for excessive daytime sleepiness.[51] Sleep-related breathing disorders resulting from TBI are treated with continuous positive airway pressure therapy or bilevel positive airway pressure therapy. In some cases, adaptive servoventilation is used to control central sleep apnea or complex sleep apnea. Lifestyle modifications, such as weight loss, and positional therapy are used in selected cases. Other available individualized treatment options include oral mandibular advancement appliances; tongue-retaining devices; and surgical procedures, including maxilla-mandibular advancement, uvulopalatopharyngoplasty, genio-glossus advancement, and tonsillectomy.

Posttraumatic Hypersomnia

Posttraumatic hypersomnia commonly occurs after TBI. It may be present in patients recovering from posttraumatic coma or in those who had mild closed head injury (concussion) without associated loss of consciousness. The diagnosis can be established if hypersomnia (with or without cataplexy) persists for 3 months after TBI with a mean sleep onset latency of less than 8 minutes and less than one sleep onset REM period is found on Multiple Sleep Latency Test.[75] Common complaints of patients with post-TBI hypersomnolence are related to daytime sleepiness and include difficulty with concentration, memory impairment, fatigue, depressive mood, speech difficulty, headaches, restless sleep, night terrors, night sweats, nightmares, seizures during sleep, heavy snoring, and leg and/or body jerks.[52]

Posttraumatic Narcolepsy

Posttraumatic narcolepsy has been reported in several cases.[44,76] This diagnosis is established if hypersomnia (with or without cataplexy) persists for 3 months after TBI with a mean sleep onset latency of less than 8 minutes and two or more sleep onset REM periods are found on Multiple Sleep Latency Test.[75] Narcolepsy may have preceded the TBI, or the head trauma may have triggered clinically silent, premorbid narcolepsy.[44,76] It is proposed that head injury can affect the hypothalamic system and alter transiently or permanently hypocretin neuronal function, leading to decreased cerebrospinal fluid hypocretin levels.[77] Stimulant therapy (modafinil, amphetamine, methylphenidate, amantadine, armodafinil) can be a treatment of choice in posttraumatic hypersomnia and narcolepsy, and in recurrent hypersomnia (Kleine-Levin syndrome).[60,78] Strategic napping and conventional stimulants, such as caffeine, are used in mild cases of posttraumatic narcolepsy. The role of sodium oxybate for posttraumatic narcolepsy is not clear. More randomized controlled studies are needed.

Posttraumatic insomnia is common and is presented as a symptom or as an insomnia disorder (sleep onset or and sleep maintenance insomnia).[37,40,41] In one recent study, 29% of patients with mild to severe TBI met the diagnostic criteria for insomnia disorder, and 21% presented with insomnia as a symptom. Most studies of posttraumatic insomnia rely on subjective questionnaires or sleep diaries. In this same study, mild TBI was associated with more insomnia complaints when compared with severe TBI.[79–81] Given that chronic persistent insomnia affects about 30% of the adult population, it is not clear in patients with TBI if insomnia represents as a pre-existing condition exacerbated by head injury and comorbidities. Insomnia-promoting comorbid factors include pain, depression, anxiety, environmental disturbances, and sedating medications.[82,83] The identification of factors contributing to insomnia is critical for initiation of appropriate behavioral and/or pharmacologic therapy. Posttraumatic insomnia is treated with pharmacologic and/or nonpharmacologic approaches. Benzodiazepines are commonly used in insomnia patients with underlying anxiety. The nonbenzodiazepine-benzodiazepine receptor agonists (eszopiclone, zolpidem, zaleplon) are used in posttraumatic sleep onset and sleep maintenance insomnia, most often resulting in therapeutic success. CBT for post-TBI insomnia, which includes stimulus control, cognitive restructuring, sleep restriction, sleep hygiene education, and fatigue management, can improve sleep quality, total wake time, sleep efficiency, and daytime fatigue.[84]

Parasomnias, including sleep-walking and sleep terrors, were reported in TBI and REM sleep behavior disorder, which presents with abnormal dream enactment, injurious behavior commonly associated with REM sleep without atonia.[85] Parasomnias are usually treated with nonpharmacologic behavioral techniques (mental imagery, relaxation techniques, anticipatory awakenings) and pharmacologic agents (eg, benzodiazepine (clonazepam), and tricyclic antidepressants). Lifestyle modifications and avoidance of triggering factors for parasomnia (hypnotics, especially zolpidem, alcohol use, stress) should be used. Safe sleeping environment (locking doors, removing sharp objects and weapons/guns from the house, sleeping on the floor) should be encouraged in case of sleep-walking and dream-enactment behaviors. For REM sleep behavior disorder (RBD) management a low dose of melatonin and/ or clonazepam may be used to control this condition and the implementation of safety measures. The periodic limb movements in sleep,[38,51] rhythmic movement disorders,[50] and Kleine-Levin syndrome (a condition consisting of recurrent hypersomnia, cognitive disturbances, compulsive behavior, and hypersexuality)[53] have also been reported in patients with TBI, although the prevalence and curative therapies are not well-established. Current management is focused on guideline-based symptomatic therapy. Posttraumatic periodic limb movement disorder can be treated with dopamine agonist medications (ropinirole or pramipexole). The patient's iron storage level should be reviewed and treated with ferritin less than 75 ng/mL. Lifestyle modifications and avoidance of periodic limb movement disorder triggers (nicotine, alcohol, selective serotonin reuptake inhibitors, caffeine) before bedtime is recommended. Rhythmic movement disorder is treated with low-dose clonazepam and appropriate safety measures in the bedroom.[75]

SUMMARY

TBI is a complex neurologic and neuropathologic process that may affect the patient's behavior permanently. Gaining familiarity with the behavioral disorders outlined in this article and understanding how to identify and treat them plays a significant role in the management of patients with TBI.

REFERENCES

1. United States Department of Health and Human Services. Traumatic brain injury. 2012. Available at: http://www.hhs.gov/asl/testify/2012/03/t20120319a.html.
2. Papa L, Mendes ME, Braga CF. Mild traumatic brain injury among the geriatric population. Curr Transl Geriatr Exp Gerontol Rep 2012;1(3):135–42.
3. McAllister TW. Neurobehavioral sequelae of traumatic brain injury: evaluation and management. World Psychiatry 2008;7(1):3–10.
4. Levin HS, Hanten G, Zhang L, et al. Selective impairment of inhibition after TBI in children. J Clin Exp Neuropsychol 2004;26(5):589–97.
5. Vakil E. The effect of moderate to severe traumatic brain injury (TBI) on different aspects of memory: a selective review. J Clin Exp Neuropsychol 2005;27(8): 977–1021.
6. Rapoport MJ, McCullagh S, Shammi P, et al. Cognitive impairment associated with major depression following mild and moderate traumatic brain injury. J Neuropsychiatry Clin Neurosci 2005;17(1):61–5.
7. Broglio SP, Eckner JT, Paulson HL, et al. Cognitive decline and aging: the role of concussive and subconcussive impacts. Exerc Sport Sci Rev 2012;40(3):138–44.
8. Moretti L, Cristofori I, Weaver SM, et al. Cognitive decline in older adults with a history of traumatic brain injury. Lancet Neurol 2012;11(12):1103–12.
9. Godbolt AK, Cancelliere C, Hincapié CA, et al. Systematic review of the risk of dementia and chronic cognitive impairment after mild traumatic brain injury: results of the International Collaboration on Mild Traumatic Brain Injury Prognosis. Arch Phys Med Rehabil 2014;95(3 Suppl):S245–56.
10. Zhang L, Ravdin LD, Relkin N, et al. Increased diffusion in the brain of professional boxers: a preclinical sign of traumatic brain injury? AJNR Am J Neuroradiol 2003;24(1):52–7.

11. Maroon JC, Winkelman R, Bost J, et al. Correction: chronic traumatic encephalopathy in contact sports: a systematic review of all reported pathological cases. PLoS One 2015;10(6):e0130507.
12. Erlanger DM, Kutner KC, Barth JT, et al. Neuropsychology of sports-related head injury: dementia pugilistica to post concussion syndrome. Clin Neuropsychol 1999;13(2):193–209.
13. Roberts GW, Allsop D, Bruton C. The occult aftermath of boxing. J Neurol Neurosurg Psychiatry 1990;53(5):373–814.
14. Lawrence DW, Comper P, Hutchison MG, et al. The role of apolipoprotein E episilon (ε)-4 allele on outcome following traumatic brain injury: A systematic review. Brain Inj 2015;29(9):1018–31.
15. Haltiner AM, Temkin NR, Dikmen SS. Risk of seizure recurrence after the first late posttraumatic seizure. Arch Phys Med Rehabil 1997;78(8):835–40.
16. Pitkänen A, Immonen R. Epilepsy related to traumatic brain injury. Neurotherapeutics 2014;11(2):286–96.
17. Annegers JF, Coan SP. The risks of epilepsy after traumatic brain injury. Seizure 2000;9(7):453–7.
18. Temkin NR. Risk factors for posttraumatic seizures in adults. Epilepsia 2003; 44(Suppl 10):18–20.
19. Beghi E. Overview of studies to prevent posttraumatic epilepsy. Epilepsia 2003; 44(Suppl 10):21–6.
20. Rao V, Lyketsos C. Neuropsychiatric sequelae of traumatic brain injury. Psychosomatics 2000;41(2):95–103.
21. Gould KR, Ponsford JL, Johnston L, et al. The nature, frequency and course of psychiatric disorders in the first year after traumatic brain injury: a prospective study. Psychol Med 2011;41:2099–109.
22. Jorge RE, Arciniegas DB. Mood Disorders after TBI. Psychiatr Clin North Am 2014;37(1):13–29.
23. Fujii D, Ahmed I. Characteristics of psychotic disorder due to traumatic brain injury: an analysis of case studies in the literature. J Neuropsychiatry Clin Neurosci 2002;14(2):130–40.
24. Masel BE, DeWitt DS. Traumatic brain injury: a disease process, not an event. J Neurotrauma 2010;27:1529–40.
25. Molloy C, Conroy RM, Cotter DR, et al. Is traumatic brain injury a risk factor for schizophrenia? A meta-analysis of case-controlled population-based studies. Schizophr Bull 2011;37:1104–10.
26. Kim E. Does traumatic brain injury predispose individuals to develop schizophrenia? Curr Opin Psychiatry 2008;21:286–9.
27. Keshavan MS, Kaneko Y. Secondary psychoses: an update. World Psychiatry 2013;12:4–15.
28. Bjork JM, Grant SJ. Does traumatic brain injury increase risk for substance abuse? J Neurotrauma 2009;26:1077–82.
29. Graham DP, Cardon AL. An update on substance use and treatment following traumatic brain injury. Ann N Y Acad Sci 2008;1141:148–62.
30. O'Phelan K, McArthur DL, Chang CWJ, et al. The impact of substance abuse on mortality in patients with severe head injury. J Trauma 2008;65(3):674–7.
31. Corrigan JD, Deutschle JJ. The presence and impact of traumatic brain injury among clients in treatment for co-occurring mental illness and substance abuse. Brain Inj 2008;22(3):223–31.
32. Wasserman L, Shaw T, Vu M, et al. An overview of traumatic brain injury and suicide. Brain Inj 2008;22(11):811–9.

33. Wortzel HS, Arciniegas DB. A forensic neuropsychiatric approach to traumatic brain injury, aggression, and suicide. J Am Acad Psychiatry Law 2013;41: 274–86.

34. Reeves RR, Laizer JT. Traumatic brain injury and suicide. J Psychosoc Nurs Ment Health Serv 2012;50(3):32–8.

35. Simpson GK, Tate RL, Whitting DL, et al. Suicide prevention after traumatic brain injury: a randomized controlled trial of a program for the psychological treatment of hopelessness. J Head Trauma Rehabil 2011;26(4):290–300.

36. Bryan CJ, Clemens TA. Repetitive traumatic brain injury, psychological symptoms, and suicide risk in a clinical sample of deployed military personnel. JAMA Psychiatry 2013;70(7):686–91.

37. Mathias JL, Alvaro PK. Prevalence of sleep disturbances, disorders, and problems following traumatic brain injury: a meta-analysis. Sleep Med 2012;13:898–905.

38. Castriotta RJ, Wilde MC, Lai JM, et al. Prevalence and consequences of sleep disorders in traumatic brain injury. J Clin Sleep Med 2007;3:349–56.

39. Ouellet MC, Beaulieu-Bonneau S, Morin CM. Sleep-wake disturbances after traumatic brain injury. Lancet Neurol 2015;14:746–57.

40. Ouellet MC, Savard J, Morin CM. Insomnia following traumatic brain injury: a review. Neurorehabil Neural Repair 2004;18(4):187–98.

41. Wiseman-Hakes C, Colantonio A, Gargaro J. Sleep and wake disorders following traumatic brain injury: a systematic review of the literature. Crit Rev Phys Rehabil Med 2009;21:317–74.

42. Bryan CJ. Repetitive traumatic brain injury (or concussion) increases severity of sleep disturbance among deployed military personnel. Sleep 2013;36:941–6.

43. Kempf J, Werth E, Kaiser PR, et al. Sleep-wake disturbances 3 years after traumatic brain injury. J Neurol Neurosurg Psychiatry 2010;81:1402–5.

44. Verma A, Anand V, Verma NP. Sleep disorders in chronic traumatic brain injury. J Clin Sleep Med 2007;3:357–62.

45. Imbach LL, Valko PO, Li T, et al. Increased sleep need and daytime sleepiness 6 months after traumatic brain injury: a prospective controlled clinical trial. Brain 2015;138:726–35.

46. Baumann CR, Werth E, Stocker R, et al. Sleep-wake disturbances 6 months after traumatic brain injury: a prospective study. Brain 2007;130:1873–83.

47. Parcell DL, Ponsford JL, Rajaratnam SM, et al. Self-reported changes to nighttime sleep after traumatic brain injury. Arch Phys Med Rehabil 2006;87:278–85.

48. Watson NF, Dikmen S, Machamer J, et al. Hypersomnia following traumatic brain injury. J Clin Sleep Med 2007;3:363–8.

49. Masel BE, Scheibel RS, Kimbark T, et al. Excessive daytime sleepiness in adults with brain injuries. Arch Phys Med Rehabil 2001;82:1526–32.

50. Gardani M, Morfiri E, Thomson A, et al. Evaluation of sleep disorders in patients with severe traumatic brain injury during rehabilitation. Arch Phys Med Rehabil 2015. http://dx.doi.org/10.1016/j.apmr.2015.05.006.

51. Castriotta RJ, Atanasov S, Wilde MC, et al. Treatment of sleep disorders after traumatic brain injury. J Clin Sleep Med 2009;5(2):137–44.

52. Viola-Saltzman M, Watson N. Traumatic brain injury and sleep disorders. Neurol Clin 2012;30(4):1299–312.

53. Arnulf I, Zeitzer JM, File J, et al. Kleine-Levin syndrome: a systematic review of 186 cases in the literature. Brain 2005;128(Pt 12):2763–76.

54. Blinman TA, Houseknecht E, Snyder C, et al. Postconcussive symptoms in hospitalized pediatric patients after mild traumatic brain injury. J Pediatr Surg 2009;44(6):1223–8.

55. Hawley CA, Ward AB, Magnay AR, et al. Children's brain injury: a postal follow-up of 525 children from one health region in the UK. Brain Inj 2002;16(11):969–85.
56. Kraus J, Hsu P, Schaffer K, et al. Preinjury factors and 3-month outcomes following emergency department diagnosis of mild traumatic brain injury. J Head Trauma Rehabil 2009;24(5):344–54.
57. Gagner C, Landry-Roy C, Laine F, et al. Sleep-wake disturbances and fatigue following pediatric traumatic brain injury: a systematic review of the literature. J Neurotrauma 2015;32:1–14.
58. Breed ST, Flanagan SR, Watson KR. The relationship between age and the self-report of health symptoms in persons with traumatic brain injury. Arch Phys Med Rehabil 2004;85(Suppl 2):S61–7.
59. Katz DI, Cohen SI, Alexander MP. Mild traumatic brain injury. Handb Clin Neurol 2015;127:131–56.
60. Valko PO, Gavrilov YV, Yamamoto M, et al. Damage to histaminergic tuberomammillary neurons and other hypothalamic neurons with traumatic brain injury. Ann Neurol 2015;77:177–82.
61. Skopin MD, Kabadi SV, Viechweg SS, et al. Chronic decrease in wakefulness and disruption of sleep-wake behavior after experimental traumatic brain injury. J Neurotrauma 2014;32:289–96.
62. Willie JT, Lim MM, Bennett RE, et al. Controlled cortical impact traumatic brain injury acutely disrupts wakefulness and extracellular orexin dynamics as determined by intracerebral microdialysis in mice. J Neurotrauma 2012; 29:1908–21.
63. Baumann CR, Bassetti CL, Valko PO, et al. Loss of hypocretin (orexin) neurons with traumatic brain injury. Ann Neurol 2009;66:555–9.
64. Baumann CR, Stocker R, Imhof HG, et al. Hypocretin-1 (orexin A) deficiency in acute traumatic brain injury. Neurology 2005;65:147–9.
65. Paparrigopoulos T, Melissaki A, Tsekou H, et al. Melatonin secretion after head injury: a pilot study. Brain Inj 2006;20:873–8.
66. Seifman MA, Gomes K, Nguyen PN, et al. Measurement of serum melatonin in intensive care unit patients: changes in traumatic brain injury, trauma, and medical conditions. Front Neurol 2014;5:237.
67. Shekleton JA, Parcell DL, Redman JR, et al. Sleep disturbance and melatonin levels following traumatic brain injury. Neurology 2010;74:1732–8.
68. Leduc BE, Dagher JH, Mayer P, et al. Estimated prevalence of obstructive sleep apnea-hypopnea syndrome after cervical cord injury. Arch Phys Med Rehabil 2007;88(3):333–7.
69. Kryger MH, Roth T, Dement WC, et al. Other neurological disorders. In: Principles and practice of sleep medicine. 50th edition. Elsevier Saunders; 2011. p. 1064–74.
70. Jessen NA, Finmann Munk AS, Lundgaard I, et al. The glymphatic system: a beginner's guide. Neurochem Res 2015. http://dx.doi.org/10.1007/s11064-015-1581-6.
71. Plog BA, Dashnaw ML, Hitomi E, et al. Biomarkers of traumatic injury are transported from brain to blood via the glymphatic system. J Neurosci 2015;35(2):518–26.
72. Ayalon L, Borodkin K, Dishon L, et al. Circadian rhythm sleep disorders following mild traumatic brain injury. Neurology 2007;68(14):1136–40.
73. Kemp S, Biswas R, Neumann V, et al. The value of melatonin for sleep disorders occurring post-head injury: a pilot RCT. Brain Inj 2004;18:911–9.
74. De La Rue-Evans L, Nesbitt K, Oka RK. Sleep hygiene program implementation in patients with traumatic brain injury. Rehabil Nurs 2013;38:2–10.

75. American Academy of Sleep Medicine. The international classification of sleep disorders. 3rd edition. Darien (IL): American Academy of Sleep Medicine; 2014.
76. Ebrahim IO, Peacock KW, Williams AJ. Posttraumatic narcolepsy—two case reports and a mini review. J Clin Sleep Med 2005;1:153–6.
77. Ripley B, Overeem S, Fujiki N, et al. CSF hypocretin/orexin levels in narcolepsy and other neurologic conditions. Neurology 2001;57:2253–8.
78. Menn SJ, Yang R, Lankford A. Armodafinil for the treatment of excessive sleepiness associated with mild or moderate closed traumatic brain injury: a 12-week, randomized, double-blind study followed by a 12-month open-label extension. J Clin Sleep Med 2014;10:1181–91.
79. Ouellet MC, Beaulieu-Bonneau S, Morin CM. Insomnia in patients with traumatic brain injury: frequency, characteristics, and risk factors. J Head Trauma Rehabil 2006;21:199–212.
80. Mahmood O, Rapport LJ, Hanks RA, et al. Neuropsychological performance and sleep disturbance following traumatic brain injury. J Head Trauma Rehabil 2004; 19:378–90.
81. Parcell DL, Ponsford JL, Redman JR, et al. Poor sleep quality and changes in objectively recorded sleep after traumatic brain injury: a preliminary study. Arch Phys Med Rehabil 2008;89:843–50.
82. Fichtenberg NL, Millis SR, Mann NR, et al. Factors associated with insomnia among post-acute traumatic brain injury survivors. Brain Inj 2000;14:659–67.
83. Thaxton L, Myers MA. Sleep disturbances and their management in patients with brain injury. J Head Trauma Rehabil 2002;17:335–48.
84. Ouellet MC, Morin CM. Efficacy of cognitive-behavioral therapy for insomnia associated with traumatic brain injury: a single-case experimental design. Arch Phys Med Rehabil 2007;88:1581–92.
85. Schenck CH, Boyd JL, Mahowald MW. A parasomnia overlap disorder involving sleepwalking, sleep terrors, and REM sleep behavior disorder in 33 polysomnographically confirmed cases. Sleep 1997;20(11):972–81.

Alzheimer's Disease

Prototype of Cognitive Deterioration, Valuable Lessons to Understand Human Cognition

Maryam Noroozian, MD

KEYWORDS

- Alzheimer's disease • Dementia • Cognition • Cognitive domains • Aging
- Mild cognitive impairment • Neuropsychology

KEY POINTS

- With the aging of the population and limitation of access to complex diagnosis tools for Alzheimer's disease, now is the proper time to emphasize for neurologists how important it is to become more familiar with neuropsychological evaluation because of its crucial role in early detection of cognitive decline in the elderly population.
- The ever-increasing growth of this method in research, as an available, inexpensive, and noninvasive diagnostic approach, which can be administered even by non–specialist-trained examiners, makes this knowledge more necessary than ever.
- Such knowledge has a basic role in planning national programs in primary health care systems for prevention and early detection of Alzheimer's disease as a debilitating disorder.
- This is more crucial in developing countries, which have to deal with higher rates of dementia prevalence along with cardiovascular risk factors, lack of public knowledge about dementia, and limited social support.

INTRODUCTION

With the aging of the population, more neuroscientists, neurologists, psychiatrists, and psychologists focus their research on age-related medical disorders in general, and more specifically dementia. Alzheimer's disease (AD) is the most common cause of severe memory loss and cognitive deterioration in the elderly; the main goal of research on cognitive aging has been to find treatments for AD and other dementias. However, apart from the disease process, it is also crucial to understand the normal

Disclosure: The author has nothing to disclose.
Conflict of Interest: None.
Memory and Behavioral Neurology Division, Department of Psychiatry, Roozbeh Hospital, Tehran University of Medical Sciences, 606 South Kargar Avenue, Tehran 1333795914, Iran
E-mail address: mnoroozi@tums.ac.ir

process of cognitive decline with age: age is the greatest predisposing factor for a spectrum of neurodegenerative disorders. Thus, understanding what the brain goes through in the normal process of aging helps not only to improve the quality of life for the general population but may also ultimately help unravel pathologic changes that at present seem unrelated.[1] AD is one of the most prevalent conditions in the elderly and the most common cause of memory impairment in old age.[2] Nearly 40 years ago, dementia, and particularly AD, was first emphasized as a major public health problem.[3] According to the World Health Organization (WHO), in the year 2011, 35.6 million people were affected by dementia.[4] This number is destined to increase rapidly. The aging of the population affects both the incidence and the prevalence of this syndrome,[5,6] thus, it has been estimated that, by the year 2050, 115.4 million people will be affected.[4] In Western industrial nations, AD is the most common form of dementia[7]: approximately 60% to 80% of dementia cases in these countries are AD[8]; thus, AD is the fourth cause of death (after cardiovascular disorders, cancer, and cerebral hemorrhage). Over the past 30 years, neuropsychological assessment has played one of the central roles in characterizing the dementia associated with AD. As well as being available, noninvasive, and inexpensive, it has helped identify the most significant cognitive and behavioral symptoms; it has also contributed greatly to the staging and tracking of the disease.[9–13] At present, no curative treatments exist for AD. However, several promising strategies are being developed that may delay or even prevent the progression of AD.[14] It is now known that decades before the onset of cognitive symptoms, such as episodic memory loss, AD-related neurologic changes begin to accumulate.[15,16] Thus, intervention well before the onset of observable symptoms could provide a promising opportunity to slow the progression of the disease or minimize the damage, particularly if targeted at individuals with the greatest risk of developing AD.[17] This article describes the neuropsychological profile of AD and its contrast with cognitive changes that occur in normal aging and in mild cognitive impairment (MCI) over the course of time.

The Spectrum of Alzheimer's disease as a Prototype of Cognitive Disorder

The first case of the disease was described by Alois Alzheimer's in November 4, 1906, in his lecture at the 37th Conference of South-West German Psychiatrists in Tübingen and the condition was later called AD by Emil Kraepelin.[18,19] This first case (Aguste D) was a 51-year-old woman with progressive cognitive and behavioral impairment in middle age; however, in general, AD affects the elderly. The first clinical signs in most patients with AD are shown during the seventh decade. Early-onset cases are often familial; in many of these patients mutations have been discovered. In contrast, late-onset cases are sporadic, and their cause is still unknown. In both the sporadic and familial forms of AD there is a remarkably selective defect in declarative memory, which is discussed later.[1] Recent research, which has increasingly focused on earlier stages of AD, has made clear that cognitive and behavioral symptoms of the illness can be preceded by biological markers by years.[9] AD disorder is usually initially selective for limbic regions that subserve episodic memory, which in turn brings about circumscribed memory deficit in the early stages of the disease.[20–22] Over time, with the progress of the disorder to other neocortical regions,[23–26] further cognitive symptoms emerge and the full dementia syndrome manifests itself. The established research diagnostic criteria for AD dementia has served well since 1984; however, these recent discoveries have prompted its revision.[27] In addition to defining the dementia of AD,[28] the new criteria also incorporate a fuller spectrum of cognitive aging, and include an intermediate stage of MCI that precedes the full-blown dementia.[29] A third, even earlier, stage of preclinical AD has also been identified.[30]

The Structure and Function of the Brain Change with Age

Fig. 1[30] presents the different pathways in the brain aging process (from normal to MCI and AD). The quality of life in most people is not seriously compromised by age-related cognitive changes. However, in a subset of elderly people, cognitive decline reaches a pathologic level. Age-related declines in mental abilities are highly variable with regard to rate, severity, and type of cognitive capacity. First, there are considerable differences in the rate and severity of cognitive decline among individuals. Some rare individuals retain their cognitive functions throughout life, whereas others experience decline in mental agility: for some, the decline is gradual, for some rapid[31] **(Fig. 2)**.[1,32] There are well-known instances of the former group: in his late 80s, Titian was still painting masterpieces, and they say Sophocles wrote *Oedipus at Colonus* in his 92nd year.[1] The infrequency of cases with completely preserved function suggests that this retention of cognitive function may be suggestive of special properties in the life experiences or genes of the individual. Accordingly, great interest has been shown in studying these rare individuals, who retain nearly intact cognition well into their tenth or even eleventh decade. These centenarians might provide insight regarding environmental or genetic factors that protect against normal cognitive decline with age, or potentially even prevent the pathologic progression to dementia.[1] Typically, personalities and interests are retained in those individuals who age normally; personality traits and interests include their levels of initiative, motivation, sociability, sensitivity to others, sympathy, affect, and behavior.[32]

Second, averaged data gathered from many individuals show that although some cognitive capacities decline significantly with age, others are largely spared[33] **(Box 1, Fig. 3)**.[1,34]

Alterations that occur with age in memory, motor activity, mood, sleep pattern, appetite, and neuroendocrine function result from alterations in the structure and function of the brain. The volume of the brain mildly shrinks in the elderly, a loss in brain weight is observable, and the ventricles are enlarged. These cellular changes lead

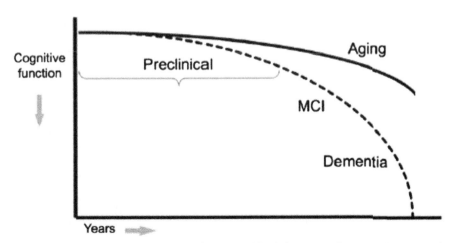

Fig. 1. Model of the clinical trajectory of aging and (AD). (*From* Sperling RA, Aisen PS, Beckett LA, et al. Toward defining the preclinical stages of Alzheimer's disease: recommendations from the National Institute on Aging-Alzheimer's Association workgroups on diagnostic guidelines for Alzheimer's disease. Alzheimer's Dement 2011;7(3):280–92; with permission.)

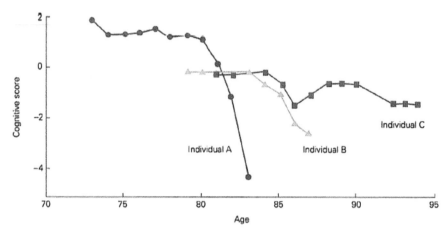

Fig. 2. Cognitive scores of 3 people who were given a battery of cognitive tests annually for decades. Person A declined rapidly. Persons B and C showed similar cognitive performances into their 80s but then diverged. (*Adapted from* Rubin EH, Storandt M, Miller JP, et al. A prospective study of cognitive function and onset of dementia in cognitively healthy elders. Arch Neurol 1998;55:395–401; with permission; and Kandel ER. The principles of neural science, 5th edition. New York: McGraw-Hill Education, 2013; with permission.)

to alterations in the integrity of the neural circuits through which mental activities are mediated. Age-related cognitive decline is thought to be greatly contributed to by loss of synapses along with impairment in functioning of retained synapses. MCI is a constellation of changes at the lesser end of the pathologic range. MCI is characterized by memory impairments that the individual might find alarming but that are not serious enough to affect day-to-day life. Because of its subtlety, MCI is difficult to diagnose; neurologists have been convinced by longitudinal studies that it is a real condition and needs additional attention. Approximately 15% of individuals diagnosed with MCI develop AD within a few years of diagnosis, and another 50% eventually succumb to AD. In contrast, some individuals with MCI remain at a stable plateau for decades. At present, intense interest exists with regard to learning how to distinguish individuals with MCI who will progress to AD from those who will age normally (**Box 2**).[1]

Box 1
Aging brain

- Working and long-term memories, visuospatial abilities, and verbal fluency usually decline with old age. In contrast, there is minimal decline in measures of vocabulary, information, and comprehension in normal individuals well into their 80s.

- From college age onward, brain weight decreases 0.2% per year on average; this number is about 0.5% per year in the 70s.

- Widespread changes are detectable in white matter, which are especially notable in the prefrontal and temporal cortex. Considering the localization of encoding and storing memory functions in the frontal-striatal systems and the temporal lobes, it is possible that notable alterations in white matter may underlie age-related decline in executive functions and reduction in the ability to focus attention as a major cause of cognitive decline.

Adapted from Kandel ER. The principles of neural science, 5th edition. New York: McGraw-Hill Education, 2013; with permission.

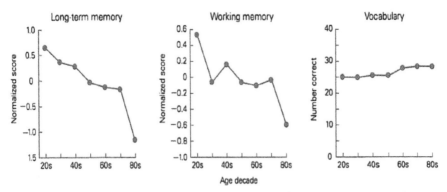

Fig. 3. Average scores on several cognitive tests administered to a large number of people. Long-term declarative memory and working memory decline throughout life, and more so in advanced age. In contrast, knowledge of vocabulary is maintained. (*Adapted from* Park DC, Smith AD, Lautenschlager G, et al. Mediators of long-term memory performance across the life span. Psychol Aging 1996;11:621–37; with permission; and Kandel ER. The principles of neural science, 5th edition. New York: McGraw-Hill Education, 2013; with permission.)

LEARNING AND MEMORY

In most patients with dementia, memory problems are evident early in the course of their disease.[35] Therefore, understanding memory is vital to explaining the neuropsychology of dementia. Learning and memory are crucial for people and animals to fully function and survive independently (**Box 3**).[1]

The nature and function of learning and memory can be investigated by observing the imperfections and errors in remembering. During the past several decades, significant progress has been made in the analysis and understanding of learning and memory. There are several fundamentally different types of memory, each of which has its own distinctive cognitive properties and is mediated by a specific brain region; thus, specific regions of the brain are more crucial for some types of storage. Memory can be classified along 2 dimensions: (1) the time course of storage, (2) the nature of the information stored (**Box 4**).

MEMORY TYPES AND TIME COURSE OF STORAGE: SHORT-TERM VERSUS LONG-TERM MEMORY

Historically, memory has been categorized into three temporal stages.[36]

Box 2
Mentalizing

- The concept of mentalizing is defined as the ability to infer other people's mental states.
- Using functional MRI (fMRI), a recent study has confirmed the results of previous studies indicating that mentalizing capacity decreases in older adults.[34]
- There was also an association between this decline and decreases in blood oxygen level–dependent response in the dorsomedial prefrontal cortex (PFC).
- Thus, the possibility is raised that PFC might be important for mentalizing, becoming less active with advancing age.

Box 3
Learning and memory

- Learning refers to a change in behavior that results from acquiring knowledge about the world.

- Memory is the ability of the brain to store information for later retrieval and is the capacity by which that knowledge is encoded, stored, and retained to be later retrieved. Thus, memory is the necessary prerequisite that makes learning possible.[35]

- Memory can be deconstructed into discrete encoding, storage consolidation, and retrieval processes.

Immediate Memory

Immediate memory comprises the amount of information a subject can keep in conscious awareness without having to actively memorize the information. Normal human beings can retain 7 digits in active memory span. Perhaps by coincidence, a local telephone number is also 7 digits. Most normal people can hear a telephone number, walk across the room, and dial the number without having actively memorized it. Implementing supraspan numbers (numbers of more than 7 digits) requires active memory processing, similar to unnatural tasks, such as reverse digit span. This first temporal stage corresponds with Baddeley's[37] concept of working memory. Attention disorders affecting digit span and focal lesions of the superior frontal neocortex affecting Brodmann areas 8 and 9 may extensively affect immediate memory.[38] Many patients with aphasia secondary to left frontal lesions manifest impaired immediate memory. Individuals normally forget the items in immediate memory as soon as their attention switches to another topic unless they try actively to memorize them.

Recent Memory

The second stage of memory, which clinicians call short-term or recent memory, comprises the ability to register and recall items, such as words or events, after a delay of minutes or hours. This type of memory has such synonyms as declarative and episodic memory.[39,40] The function of the hippocampus and parahippocampal areas of the medial temporal lobe is required by this second stage of memory for both storage and retrieval. The function of the amygdala, a structure adjacent to the medial temporal cortex, is not crucial for episodic memory, but seems essential for recalling

---

Box 4
The so-called 7 sins of memory

- Seven basic sins comprise the misdeeds of memory: transience, absentmindedness, blocking, misattribution, suggestibility, bias, and persistence.

- The first 3 denote different types of forgetting, the next 3 involve different types of distortions, and the seventh sin refers to disturbing recollections that are not easy to forget.

- Cognitive, social, and clinical psychology and cognitive neuroscience studies indicate that the 7 sins may only seem to reflect flaws in system design; instead, it is argued that the flaws are by-products of features of memory, which are otherwise adaptive.

Adapted from Schacter DL. The seven sins of memory: insights from psychology and cognitive neuroscience. Am Psychol 1999;54(3):182; with permission.

the emotional contexts of, and the reactions associated with, specific events and such reactions as fear or pleasure associated with those events. The familiar bedside test of asking the patient to recall 3 unrelated memory items at 5-minute intervals assesses episodic (short-term) memory; asking the patient about this morning's breakfast or the result of yesterday's football match is similar.

Long-term Memory

Remote memory refers to storage of long-known information such as a person's first-grade teacher, where a person grew up, or the names of grandparents. The factual knowledge that is consciously recalled is known in current parlance as semantic memory.[41]

To test semantic memory, the patient is asked to recall a famous figure or event, such as presidents or wars; also, the patient's knowledge of semantic information is assessed, such as the definitions of words and the differences between words. Semantic memory is different from personal long-term memory; the latter can be replenished continuously through daily life events.

NEURAL BASIS OF MEMORY: HISTORICAL EVIDENCE

In the mid-1950s, important new evidence began to emerge about the neural basis of long-term memory from studies performed on patients in whom bilateral removal of the hippocampus and neighboring regions in the medial temporal lobe was performed as treatment of epilepsy. The first and most thoroughly studied case was a patient called H.M. He is a historic case because his deficit for the first time linked clearly memory and the medial temporal lobe, including the hippocampus.[1]

After the surgery, H.M.'s seizures were managed more effectively, but he had developed a distressing memory deficit (or amnesia). H.M.'s deficit was highly specific. His working memory was still normal, for seconds or minutes, which indicated that the medial temporal lobe is not necessarily related to transient memory. Also, he had long-term memory for events that had occurred before the operation. He remembered his name, his previous job, and his childhood; however, he did not have robust recollection of memories in the years just before the surgery. In addition, he retained a command of language, including his vocabulary, which indicated that semantic memory was preserved. H.M. dramatically lacked the ability to move new information from working memory into long-term memory. He did not have the ability to retain information about people, places, or objects that he had just come across for lengthy periods. H.M. was able to repeat a new telephone number only immediately for seconds to minutes because his working memory was intact. If he was even briefly distracted, he forgot the number. H.M. could not recognize people whom he met after the surgery, even if he met them repeatedly. The physiologic findings are consistent with clinical observations: lesions in the right hippocampus cause problems with spatial orientation, whereas lesions of the left hippocampus affect verbal memory. Another critical observation regarding H.M. was that all types of long-term memory were not impaired. Despite H.M. and other patients with damage to the medial temporal lobe showing profound memory deficits, they were as able as healthy subjects to form and retain certain types of enduring memories. Such patients retained simple reflexive learning, including habituation, sensitization, classical conditioning, and operant conditioning.

The results from the observations of amnesic patients with damage to the medial temporal lobe, such as H.M., are suggestive that old memories are not stored in the medial temporal lobe itself. They are stored in various other cortical regions. Squire and Zola-Morgan,[42] and others, suggest that the medial temporal region may play only a temporary role in the consolidation of memories, but, after a sufficiently long period, because memories can be retrieved directly from cortical regions, the medial temporal region is no longer needed. Their finding is consistent with the observation that remote memories are more readily recalled by amnesic patients compared with memories from the period just before they became amnestic. The activation of neocortical representations that were present during encoding is thought to be facilitated by medial temporal lobe activity (**Box 5**).

LONG-TERM MEMORY: EXPLICIT VERSUS IMPLICIT MEMORY

Considering whether or not conscious awareness is required for recalling a memory, two types of long-term memory are differentiated.[1] **Fig. 4** shows the classification of all types of human memory and the anatomic substrates.

Implicit Memory

Also known as nondeclarative or procedural memory, this type is an unconscious form of memory that underlies the task performance; it typically manifests in an automatic manner that requires little conscious processing from the individual. Different forms of implicit memory give rise to priming, skill learning, habit memory, and conditioning.

Explicit Memory

The other type comprises the conscious retrieval of previous experiences as well as conscious recall of factual knowledge about people, places, and things. This type is also referred to as declarative memory. Explicit memory is highly flexible; various pieces of information are registered in accordance with their associated circumstances, which also influence their retrieval. However, implicit memory is closely related to the conditions under which the learning originally took place.

DECLARATIVE (EXPLICIT) VERSUS NONDECLARATIVE (IMPLICIT) MEMORY

Memory is not a monolithic entity but comprises several separate entities that function in association with different brain systems. The main distinction is between the capacity for conscious recalling of facts and events (declarative memory) and a heterogeneous collection of capacities for nonconscious learning (nondeclarative memory), which are expressed through performance and cannot access any conscious memory material.[1,39] Declarative and nondeclarative memory systems need to be distinguished not only in terms of anatomy but also in terms of operating characteristics, the kind of information processed, and the purpose served by each system.[43]

Box 5
Memory localization

- The function of the hippocampus and parahippocampal areas of the medial temporal lobe is required for both storage and retrieval parts of recent memory.

- The function of the amygdala seems to be essential for recalling the emotional contexts of the reactions, such as fear or pleasure, associated with specific events.

- Once a memory is well deposited in the neocortex, it can be retrieved without the hippocampal system being engaged. Thus the effects of medial temporal damage do not affect remote memory.[36]

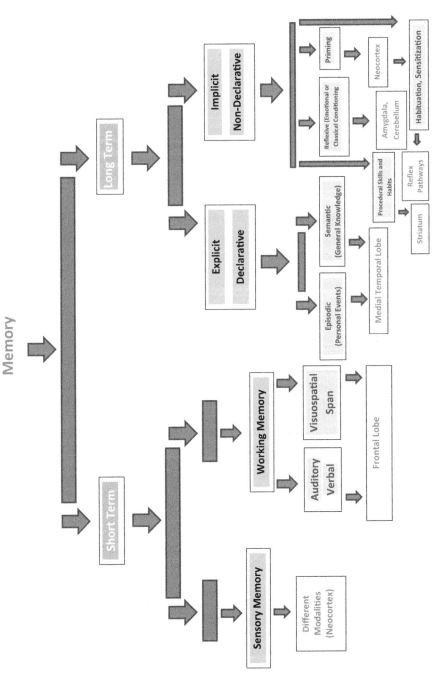

Fig. 4. Memory classification and the main localization of its subcomponents.

EXPLICIT MEMORY: EPISODIC VERSUS SEMANTIC MEMORY

The idea of a distinction between explicit memory (the memory of personal experiences or autobiographical memory) and semantic memory (memory for facts) was first developed by the Canadian psychologist Endel Tulving.[44]

Episodic Memory

Episodic memory serves to recall that a person saw the first snow of winter yesterday or that several months ago heard Beethoven's Hammerklavier.[1]

Semantic Memory

Semantic memory is used to learn the meanings of new words or concepts.

In both episodic and semantic memory, the medial temporal lobe plays a critical role; this is evident in patients like H.M., who have difficulties in forming new conscious memories of their personal experiences or the meanings of new concepts and their retention.

EXPLICIT MEMORY PROCESSING INVOLVES AT LEAST 4 DISTINCT OPERATIONS

Two additional important things need to be considered about explicit memory.[1] First, there exists no single long-term store for explicit memories in the brain. Instead, every item of knowledge is stored in a widely distributed manner among many brain regions and can be independently accessed (by visual, verbal, or other sensory clues). Second, at least 4 related but distinct types of processing mediate explicit memory: encoding, storage, consolidation, and retrieval.[45]

Encoding

Through this process, new information is attended and linked to existing information in memory. Determining how well the learned material will be remembered almost entirely depends on the depth of this process. The incoming information needs to be encoded thoroughly in order for a memory to persist and be well remembered; this is called deep encoding. This process is performed by attending to the new item of information and associating it with knowledge that is already well established in memory. Furthermore, memory encoding is stronger when there is high motivation for remembering. Different neurodegenerative conditions can affect functioning of memory in different ways. Patients with frontosubcortical atrophy have problems with encoding and initial learning; retention is left fairly intact. In addition, there exists normal recognition memory.[46,47] In contrast, in patients with AD, normal immediate recall may be shown, but they may have difficulty retaining information over brief minutes-long delays; recognition tends to be poor in such patients as well. Functional MRI (fMRI) scans show that, when people engage in deep encoding (eg, attending to the meaning of information by judging whether a word is concrete or abstract), there is greater activity in the medial temporal lobe compared with when they engage in shallow encoding (eg, judging whether a word is registered in upper-case or lower-case letters). During deep encoding, there is enhancement in activity in parts of the left prefrontal cortex (PFC), which suggests that, for encoding episodic memory, frontal lobe and medial temporal lobe processing are involved. Moreover, it has been shown that, at the time of encoding, when subjects are studying words that they were later able to recall, there is enhanced activity in several regions of the left PFC. In comparison, there is greater activity in the right PFC during encoding of pictures that were later recalled compared with pictures that could not be recalled (Box 6).

Box 6
Memory and encoding[45]

- Explicit memory processing involves at least four distinct operations: encoding, storage, consolidation, and retrieval.
- fMRI scans show that activity in the medial temporal lobe is greater when patients engage in deep encoding (eg, attending to the meaning of information by judging whether a word is concrete or abstract) than when they engage in shallow encoding (eg, judging whether a word is presented in upper or lower-case letters).
- Activity in parts of the left PFC is also enhanced during deep encoding, suggesting that frontal lobe and medial temporal lobe processing contribute to encoding episodic memory.
- Functional imaging of the brain in healthy humans shows increasing activity in the right hippocampus when spatial information is recalled and in the left hippocampus when words, objects, or people are recalled.

Storage

This operation comprises the neural mechanisms and sites by which memory is retained over time. Remarkably, long-term storage seems to have an almost unlimited capacity; long-term storage has known limits with regard to the amount of information it can store. In contrast, working memory storage is very limited; at any given time, it is thought that human working memory can hold only a certain number of pieces of information.

Consolidation

Consolidation is the process that renders the information that is stored temporarily and is still labile more stable. In this process genes are expressed and proteins synthesized that bring about structural changes at the synaptic level.

Retrieval

Retrieval is the process by which stored information is recalled. In this process, different kinds of information that are stored in different sites are brought back to mind. Retrieval of memory closely resembles perception: it is a constructive process and can therefore be distorted, much as perception may be subject to illusions.[45] Individuals can be reminded of how they initially encoded an experience through a retrieval cue.

EPISODIC MEMORY

Episodic memory refers to the system though which particular experiences or episodes are remembered. These memories are context dependent and are associated with a particular time, place, and feeling. In evaluating memory in patients with AD using clinical neuropsychological tests, it is clear that recall and recognition performance are impaired in both the verbal and nonverbal domains.[48,49] Studies using postmortem examination,[23] structural imaging,[50] resting metabolism,[51] and functional imaging[52–55] have linked explicit memory deficits in AD to pathologic, structural, and functional abnormalities within the mesial temporal lobe (MTL). These findings are consistent with evidence that suggests MTL structures are crucial for new episodic memories to be formed[56] (**Box 7**).

When examiners assess episodic memory in the clinic, they should use enough information to exceed immediate memory span. They should also consider initial

---

Box 7
Episodic memory

- The earliest neurofibrillary alterations, which are part of the disease process of AD, usually occur in structures in the medial temporal lobe (eg, hippocampus and entorhinal cortex).[9,20]

- Hence, deficits in episodic memory, which are caused by medial temporal lobe atrophy and neuronal loss in the basal forebrain cholinergic system, characterize the early stages of AD.[57]

- The impact of this disorder is interruption of the neural network that is critical for episodic memory function. Thus, the clinical hallmark of AD is a deficit in the ability to learn and remember new information.

---

learning versus retention, and recall versus recognition separately. For bedside evaluation of memory, supraspan list learning tasks with delayed recall and recognition conditions (eg, California Verbal Learning Test-II [CVLT-II][58] and Rey Auditory Verbal Learning Test[59,60]) are more suitable. Patients with AD manifest a general episodic memory deficit: such patients cannot benefit from cueing or inherent structure; their ability to recognize is as defective as their free recall performance. Rather than accelerated forgetting or disrupted retrieval, patients with AD show impaired learning. In addition, regardless of the perceptual modality of the stimuli implemented in episodic memory tasks, patients with AD manifest impaired performance. The relative irrelevance of delayed recall trials and perceptual modality is an important finding considering that these factors strongly influence clinical memory testing (**Box 8**).

It has been shown, through a comparison of patients with AD with amnestic patients with Korsakoff syndrome (KS) and demented patients with Huntington disease (HD) that patients with AD recalled significantly fewer words over a 2-minute delay.[62] Although the subjects with KS and HD and the normal control subjects lost an average of 10% to 15% of the verbal information between the 15-second and 2-minute delay intervals, patients with AD lost an average of 75% of the material. Severe recall deficits of the patients with AD have been shown, through similar studies, compared with the patients with frontotemporal dementia (FTD) and progressive supranuclear palsy (PSP)[63] (**Box 9**).

Note that, in order to stage patients with AD across levels of severity, measures of episodic memory are not particularly useful, mainly because memory is much impaired early in the course of the disease. These findings support the observation that, in most patients with AD, memory is impaired preceding impairments in language and spatial function. There is substantial agreement that memory tests are significantly different among nondemented individuals who show mild memory deficits with a diagnosis of AD on follow-up, compared with those who also have memory problems but do not progress to AD within a few years.[64–68]

Box 8
Delayed recall task

- A study has assessed the effectiveness of using 3-word recall tasks (such as the task in the Mini–Mental State Examination [MMSE]) in order to assess recall performance. There was major variability among the subjects, and a significant share of normal subjects recalled zero or 1 word.[61]

- When simple recall performance is interpreted as an index of memory, the investigators noted that caution must be taken. For bedside evaluation of memory, supraspan list learning tasks with delayed recall and recognition conditions are more suitable.

> **Box 9**
> **Severity of delayed recall impairment in AD**
>
> - Patients with AD recalled significantly fewer words over a 2-minute delay.[62] Hence the patients with AD lost an average of 75% of the material.
> - In the Korsakov syndrome, Huntington dementia, and normal control subjects, the patients lost an average of 10% to 15% of the verbal information between the 15-second and 2-minute delay intervals, whereas patients with AD lost an average of 75% of the material.

SEMANTIC MEMORY

Semantic knowledge comprises general knowledge about the world: facts, concepts, and information about objects, as well as words and their meanings. Semantic knowledge is distinguished from episodic knowledge in that it is typically not linked to the context in which the information was first acquired.[1] All of the semantic knowledge that has been acquired over a lifetime is not stored in a single storage site. It is instead stored in a distributed manner among many brain regions, such as the neocortex, including the lateral and ventral temporal lobes, the visual association cortex for visual memories, and the temporal cortex for auditory memories. Thus, specific features (eg, form, color, or motion) are represented by various brain regions. Functional brain imaging research supports this view of multiple localizations of semantic memory.[69] Patients have been reported to have an impaired knowledge about living things, whereas their knowledge about inanimate objects was spared and vice versa. Hence, it seems that the brain organizes semantic knowledge according to conceptual primitives (eg, form and function). Some categories mainly depend on information about form (eg, living things), whereas others depend on knowledge of function (eg, inanimate things). Therefore, loss of memory for particular semantic categories can result from focal brain damage, whereas knowledge of others is left intact.[70] It is thought that the left lateral temporal cortex is where specific semantic knowledge of word meanings resides. Semantic memory plays an important role in several tests, as listed in **Table 1**.[17] Before the diagnosis of AD can be made, changes in semantic memory can be detected[71,72]: initially, patients cannot name low-frequency exemplars and later they go on to lose more common elements. It is concluded that, in AD, it is the impaired verbal fluency performance that is caused by loss of knowledge, rather than impaired initiation of retrieval.[72–74] Contrary to early-phase dementia, and AD in particular, semantic memory, and certain forms of implicit memory, are thought to be relatively spared in normal aging.[75,76] Another prominent influence of AD on mental status testing is a decrease in category fluency in the context of preserved letter fluency. In a study by Rascovsky and colleagues,[77] verbal fluency results from 32 patients, whose AD was confirmed by autopsy, were compared with those of 16 patients with autopsy-confirmed FTD. Those with AD were more impaired in terms of semantic fluency than letter fluency (in which, within a certain time limit [usually 1 minute] as many words as possible are to be recalled beginning with a particular letter), whereas the pattern of impairment was reversed in those with FTD. Semantic category fluency deficits in AD may be suggestive of the gradual progression of AD in the temporal association areas that serve semantic memory.[77,78] However, these tests do not usually serve to measure semantic memory. Thus, it could be argued that (purely) episodic memory processes should not be considered crucial for prediction, otherwise important information could be missed. Several studies suggest

Table 1
Cognitive domains and their assessment in an office visit

Domain and Subdomains	Instructions for the Patient
Orientation	• Person: state name; name the present family members • Place: name the county, state, town, hospital or clinic building, floor • Time: state the year, month, date, day, time of day
Attention	• Recite the days of the week or months of the year in forward then reverse order • Spell a word (eg, world) in forward then reverse order • Recite a string of numbers (presented at a rate of a number per second, starting with a short string and increasing string length by 1 number each time (eg, 2, 7...5, 8, 6...6, 9, 3, 4...) • An impaired attention span is usually apparent during history taking. It can be tested more formally by having the patient repeat a series of numbers or count backward[1]
Memory	
Immediate memory	• Repeat a list of words immediately, and again after 10 min • Digit span tests are widely used, with the forward digit span component used to assess immediate auditory memory
Recent memory	• At the beginning of the visit, tell the patient you will be hiding 3 objects in the room (eg, watch, pencil, and ruler). Then show the patient where you are hiding them, and ask the patient to try to remember the items and their locations. At the end of the visit, ask the patient to name the objects and to show (or tell) you where they are located • Ask the patient to memorize 3 to 5 unrelated words and, after 5-min intervals, prompt the patient to repeat them
Remote memory	• Ask the patient to say the patient's (own, spouse, first child's) birthday, the name of city where the person has done military service, name of the high school or college, an important social or political event in the past years (with regard to the patient's education and culture). All of the personal information needs to be confirmed by the informant caregiver
Working memory	• The backward span component evaluating working memory (ie, the capacity to juggle information mentally). Research has shown that, on average, people can keep 7 ± 2 items in their short-term memory • Recite a string of numbers using the method described earlier, but instructing the patient to recite the numbers in reverse order (eg, "If I say '7, 8, 3,' you would say '3, 8, 7'"). • Recite a string of numbers using the method described earlier, but instructing the patient to recite the numbers in numeric order, starting with the lowest number (eg, "If I say '7, 2, 5,' you would say '2, 5, 7'"). • Working memory is also assessed on the MMSE when the patient carries out serial 7s or spells "world" backward. Other bedside techniques include reciting the months of the year in reverse order
Language	
Naming	• Name several objects in the room, starting with high-frequency items (pen, pencil, watch, ruler, glasses) and moving to low-frequency items (glasses lens, watch clasp, tip of pencil)

(continued on next page)

Table 1 *(continued)*	
Domain and Subdomains	**Instructions for the Patient**
Fluency	• Recite as many words as possible in 1 min that start with a given letter (eg, C) or a given semantic category (eg, grocery store items)
Reading	• Read aloud simple sentences, words, or letters • Reading comprehension can be tested by having the patient follow written commands that were previously successfully executed as oral commands or by having the patient answer written yes-or-no questions. such as following a written command (eg, "Close your eyes")
Repetition	• Repetition of high-frequency and low-frequency word combinations (eg, no ifs, ands or buts)
Comprehension	• Comprehension of single words (give the patient simple commands, such as "Show me your chin," or have the patient say the word that a picture is illustrating), comprehension of complex syntax (eg, "Put your left hand on your right ear"), or follow a multistep verbal command (eg, "Touch your left ear with your right index finger then touch your nose") • Answer a complex question (eg, "If a lion and a tiger fight and the tiger eats the lion, which animal is still alive?")
Visuospatial	• Ask the patient to copy the predrawn shapes on a page, starting with simple shapes (eg, a square, pentagon) and progressing to more complex shapes (eg, a cube, intersecting pentagons), building shapes with triangles or blocks, drawing a clock, and eventually a Rey-Osterrieth complex figure task[368],[b]
Praxis	
	• In most of the classifications,[1],[255] there are 3 types of testing: (1) gesture ("Show me how you would throw a ball"), (2) imitation ("Watch how I point upward, then you do it"), and (3) use of an object ("Here is a spoon. Show me how you would use it")
Limb-kinetic praxis	With limb-kinetic apraxia the act is understood but motor execution is faulty. There is loss of hand and finger dexterity resulting from inability to connect or isolate individual movements[254] • Ask the patient to wave the patient's hands as a goodbye (symbolic), touch the patient's nose (nonsymbolic), transitive (ie, using tools and instruments; eg, a hammer or a hairbrush), and intransitive (ie, communicative gestures; eg, representational tasks such as waving goodbye and nonrepresentational tasks such as touching the nose and wiggle the fingers)
Ideomotor praxis	The ability to correctly form the necessary postures and movements to perform a task using a tool, which can be tested by: • Asking the patient to pretend by showing you how to scramble an egg with a fork (a transitive task) or by asking the patient to show you how to salute (a nontransitive task)
Ideational praxis	The ability to correctly temporally sequence independent actions/task components to perform a goal. Ideational apraxia is present when the idea of the act (the neural representation of the act, or engram) is disrupted. The patient does not know what to do • Ask the patient to verbalize, step by step, how to make a sandwich Error types include impairment in carrying out sequences of actions requiring the use of various objects in the correct order so as to achieve an intended purpose,[262] and loss of tool action knowledge

(continued on next page)

Table 1
(*continued*)

Domain and Subdomains	Instructions for the Patient
Constructional praxis[a]	• Draw a copy of crossed pentagons (as in MMSE) or copy a cube (as in the MoCA scale) or more complex task, such as the Rey-Osterrieth Complex Figure Test • Dressing praxis is a type of constructional praxis. Ask the patient to wear an inside-out jacket, and then button or zip it up
Calculation	• This can range from simple arithmetical (eg, "What is 9 plus 14?" "What is 28 minus 17?") to calculations involving money (eg, "How many nickels are there in 65 cents?"), to figuring out the change (eg, "If you bought something that cost $3.73 and you paid with a $5 bill, how much change should you receive back?"), to calculating more complex bills involving percentages (eg, "If you went to a restaurant and the bill came to $120, how much total money would you leave if you wanted to also include a 15% tip?")
Executive Functions	
Abstract thinking	• Identify the similarities between words (eg, "In what way are a banana and an orange alike?") • Ask the patient to explain about the concept of a familiar proverb or metaphor (check with the informant whether this item is routine for the patient in terms of culture and education) • Abstraction can be assessed by asking for the meaning of common proverbs as well as asking the patient to delineate the similarity (eg, "In the most general sense, how are a bicycle and a train similar?") and difference between 2 things (eg, "What is the difference between a lie and a mistake?"). Identify the similarities between words (eg, "In what way are a banana and an orange alike?"). • Abstract reasoning can be evaluated by asking patients to describe conceptual similarities or differences between word pairs (eg, dog–lion), give opposites (eg, healthy–sick), find analogies (eg, "Table is to leg as bicycle is to…?"),[60] or interpret proverbs (eg, "An old ox plows a straight row")
Sequencing and planning	• Imitate hand movements in a sequence demonstrated by the examiner • Continue a sequenced drawing that is started by the examiner (eg, XOXO; ramparts)
Reasoning/ problem solving	• Provide solutions to everyday problems (eg, "What should you do if you are in a movie theater and you smell smoke?")
Set switching	• Alternate between counting and reciting the alphabet (eg, "I want you to switch between counting in numeric order and reciting the alphabet, like this: 1-A-2-B-3… Now you try it") • Alternate between counting by 6s and reciting the days of the week (eg, "I want you to alternate between counting by 6s and reciting the days of the week in order, like this: 0, Sunday; 6, Monday; 12… Now you try it")
Specialized Mental Functions	
Visual Gnosis[b]	
Visual object agnosia	• Ask the patient to name the different segments of an object, name different parts of a schematic outline of an image or recognize each object in pictures of overlapping objects

(*continued on next page*)

Table 1 *(continued)*	
Domain and Subdomains	**Instructions for the Patient**
Prosopagnosia	• Show an image of a famous or familiar person (for the patient) and ask the patient to say the person's name
Simultanagnosia	• Describe a complex scene (eg, the Boston Cookie Theft picture) or identify a large object that is made up of smaller shapes (eg, an A made on a page with small As)
Color agnosia	• Ask the patient to name the color of such fruits as banana, carrot, lemon and so forth; name similar colors in terms of tonality or different shades of a color
Neglect	• Bisect a line drawn on a page • Draw a clock face on a page
General impression[253]	Note processing speed, psychomotor retardation Note the patient's mood, behavior, and frontal lobe signs Note the patient's movement disorders, eye movement, and pyramidal signs

Abbreviation: MoCA, Montreal Cognitive Assessment.

[a] Note that some overlaps exist between active cognitive domains in many of the mentioned tasks (eg, visuospatial, constructional praxis, and planning during the clock drawing task).

[b] These tasks are helpful for the diagnosis of posterior cerebral atrophy or the occipital variant of AD.

Adapted from Dickerson B, Atri A. Dementia: comprehensive principles and practice. Oxford University Press; 2014, with permission.

that, typically, normal elderly subjects perform better on the category fluency task than on the letter fluency task. The reverse pattern is seen in patients with AD: despite showing impairment in both types of performance, they perform better on letter fluency than on category fluency.[73,74,79] This performance pattern usually helps differentiate patients with AD and normal elderly controls, and shows the clear semantic memory problems of patients with AD compared with normal elderly controls. In addition, the qualitative performance of patients with AD on the category fluency task may help detect these patients: in addition to naming few correct exemplars in general, they typically name the most common elements (ie, broad category information is preserved) and produce few different subcategories, few items per subcategory, and relatively numerous category labels.[80–82] As mentioned before, to examine semantic memory, the most frequently and extensively used task is verbal fluency.[83] Hodges and Patterson[84] tried to explore how early in the course of AD, and how consistently, semantic memory problems occur. The patients with minimal AD showed impaired performance on various tests of semantic memory (eg, category fluency, naming, naming to verbal description, semantic feature questions) and on episodic memory (ie, delayed story recall). In patients with minimal AD, recognition memory was less impaired, which may be a better index of severity of the disease.[84] Hodges and Patterson[84] concluded that semantic memory is impaired very early in the course of AD, although patients with the same overall level of dementia showed considerable variability in the extent of semantic impairment. Other investigators who examined category fluency performance in patients with early AD have supported the findings regarding the early semantic memory impairment in AD.[74] Other studies[83,85] have confirmed that patients with early AD (mean Mini–Mental State Examination [MMSE] score: 23.7) are impaired in several tasks of semantic memory. They also showed the impaired performance on a category fluency test and several tests of semantic knowledge (eg, Boston Naming Test, Wechsler Adult Intelligence Scale-Revised [WAIS-R] subtests Vocabulary and Similarities). Another study[86] also found early semantic memory impairment and reported that very mild dementia was best detected by 3 tests assessing episodic memory, semantic memory, and visuospatial functioning (according to a stepwise discriminant analysis).

EPISODIC VERSUS SEMANTIC MEMORY IN ALZHEIMER'S DISEASE BIOMARKER RESEARCH

Aspects of memory functioning are used as part of tasks presented to participants in several fMRI studies. These studies frequently assess 2 general categories of memory performance: episodic memory (eg, discriminating between previously learned and novel stimuli) and semantic memory (recall of general facts and knowledge about the world that is not contextually specific; eg, making a categorical or attributional judgment to a presented item). Episodic memory impairment is a hallmark of AD,[87] and thus most fMRI studies of AD risk have used episodic memory tasks.[88] However, there may be challenges in the use of episodic memory tasks in fMRI studies that focus on prediction of MCI, AD, and risk factors for these conditions. Episodic memory is typically impaired not only in association with onset of MCI or AD[68,89–92] but also in normal aging.[93] Furthermore, episodic memory tasks might be fundamentally more difficult than semantic memory tasks, making individuals who are in the preliminary stages of cognitive decline exert greater effort and paradoxically display a greater blood oxygen level–dependent signal (a marker for metabolic activity) because of the greater cognitive challenge. In longitudinal studies that use episodic memory tasks, participants displaying a greater extent of activation are usually at the greatest risk of subsequent cognitive decline.[94–96]

IMPLICIT (NONDECLARATIVE) MEMORY

Implicit memory systems such as procedural memory (remembering how to perform a skilled motor act) are less likely to be affected by amnestic or dementing illnesses. Although patients with AD consistently manifest impaired explicit (episodic or declarative) memory, they show intact implicit (priming or procedural) memory.[75] The ability to play a musical instrument has been shown to be unforgettable in some musicians with AD.[97] The dissociation between impaired and intact memory capacities seems to reflect the distinction between neural systems that are injured or spared in the early stages of AD. Nonconscious influence of past experiences on subsequent performance affects implicit memory. The hippocampus seems to be required for the recognition or recall of items. As discussed earlier, large areas of the neocortex specialized for specific cognitive functions, such as auditory or visual analysis, are involved as sites for storage of memories. Once items are processed in the neocortex and stored for a long period of time, they can be recalled even in the presence of hippocampal damage, as is the case with remote or semantic memories. Following hippocampal damage, a retrograde period of memory loss may extend back from minutes to years, and the patient cannot form new anterograde memories.[98,99]

WORKING MEMORY

Miller and colleagues[100] coined the term working memory and used it in 1960 in their classic book *Plans and the Structure of Behavior*; it was used in 1968 by Atkinson and

Shiffrin[101] in an influential article and afterward adopted as the title for a multicompo-nent model by Baddeley and Hitch.[102] Working memory refers to the system or sys-tems that are thought to be essential for keeping things in mind while such complex tasks as reasoning, comprehension, and learning are being performed. The term working memory evolved from the earlier concept of short-term memory. These two terms are sometimes still used interchangeably (**Box 10**).

It has been proposed by Baddeley and Hitch[102] that working memory could be cate-gorized into 3 subsystems. (1) the first subsystem is concerned with verbal and acous-tic information (the phonological loop);. (2) the second subsystem is the visuospatial sketchpad providing its visual equivalent; whereas both are dependent on (3) the third attentionally limited control system, called the central executive. Baddeley[103,104] later discussed the modification of his first model in a comprehensive article and has added a fourth component: the episodic buffer (**Fig. 5**).[103]

The Central Executive

The central executive is the most complex component of working memory. As pre-sented in the original model, it was assumed to be capable of attentional focus (eg, during dual tasks performed on 2 different modalities: one verbal, involving recalling digit sequences, and the other requiring visuospatial tracking), storage, and decision making.

The Phonological Loop

The phonological loop is the verbal subsystem that functions when people attempt to keep phonological information (speech, sign, lip reading, music, environmental sounds) in conscious awareness; for instance, when people mentally rehearse a phone number that they have just obtained from an operator. The verbal subsystem consists of 2 components that are interactive: a reservoir that stores phonological in-formation and a rehearsal mechanism that keeps the stored information active for as long as it is needed.

Visuospatial Sketchpad

The visuospatial sketchpad is related to the characteristics of such variables as visual (information about the shape and color), spatial (the location of objects in space), and haptic domains (the kinesthetic and tactile information).

Box 10
Short-term memory versus working memory

- Short-term memory is the simple temporary storage of information, whereas working memory is a functional system that implies concomitant storage and manipulation.[103]

- working memory is a common substrate to patients' difficulty with multitasking.

- The forward digit span component of digit span tests is used to assess immediate auditory memory, and the backward span component evaluates working memory (ie, the capacity to mentally juggle information).

- Research has shown that, on average, people can keep 7 ± 2 items in their short-term memory.

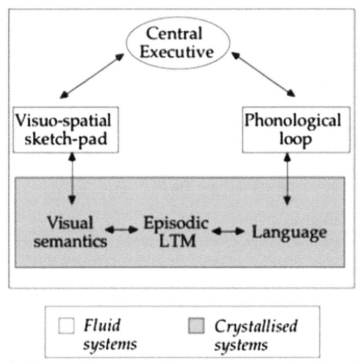

Fig. 5. A modification of the original model to take into account the evidence of links between working memory and long-term memory (LTM). (*From* Baddeley A. Working memory: theories, models, and controversies. Annu Rev Psychol 2012;63:1–29; with permission.)

The Episodic Buffer

The episodic buffer is assumed to hold integrated episodes or chunks of information in a multidimensional code. It acts as a buffer store, not only between the components of working memory but it also links working memory to perception and long-term memory. The episodic buffer does this through its capability to hold multidimensional representations; however, like most buffer stores, its capacity is limited.

In brief, this model presents a processing system in which a limited-capacity, language-based or visually based, immediate memory buffer holds the information that is the immediate focus of attention, while this information is manipulated by a central executive.[9,103,105] Activated long-term memory influences working memory in many ways. For example, when a telephone number is spoken in a person's native language, memory for it is substantially better than when a number is spoken in a foreign language. This difference reflects the influence of long-term phonological knowledge on short-term verbal memory. Furthermore, the capacity to remember and repeat a string of irrelevant words is about 5 items, but if the words comprise a meaningful sentence, the capacity expands to 15 words, which reflects a contribution from grammar and meaning, both of which depend on different aspects of long-term memory. Hence, neuroimaging studies of short-term or working memory tasks have also been shown to activate areas related to long-term memory. The mental manipulation deficit that patients with AD manifest may also express itself in working memory tests.[9] Studies indicate that the working memory deficit in patients with AD is mild to begin with; this deficit primarily disrupts the central executive and relatively spares immediate memory.[106,107] Working memory assessment has been used in the development and validation of a dual-task performance measure in order to detect AD in early stages.[108] It is only in later stages of AD that all aspects of the working memory system become compromised.[107,109] Mildly demented patients with AD often manifest impairment in complex attention tasks that depend on the efficient allocation of attention (eg, dual-processing tasks) or that require efficient disengagement from tasks and shifting of attention.[110,111] In contrast, the ability to focus and sustain attention is usually not affected until later stages of the disease, which is evident when mildly demented patients with AD perform essentially normally on tests of immediate attention span compared with supraspan tests.[112]

MEMORY IN ALZHEIMER'S DISEASE

Kramer and colleagues[113] showed that, when conducting a dementia evaluation, delayed episodic memory needs to be examined as well and not just immediate memory. They established that hippocampal volume best predicts delayed recall, even after controlling for levels of initial acquisition. Numerous studies have found that patients with AD have greater memory impairments than other diagnostic cohorts.[114–117] Despite diffuse cognitive changes being typical in AD, particularly in the middle and later stages, this condition is associated with 2 particularly distinct findings on mental status testing: rapid forgetting on tasks of episodic memory and decreased category fluency compared with lexical fluency. Rapid forgetting is reflective of impairment in consolidating new information into long-term memory. Thus, even though patients with AD can show relatively intact immediate recall, much of the information is lost after even the briefest of delays.[113,118] With regard to memory function, patients with AD might partially or entirely forget important conversations, life events, dates, appointments, and obligations; misplace or lose belongings (and have difficulty retracing their steps; they may even put things in unusual places); be highly repetitive with questions and statements; and increasingly need to rely on external memory aids and others for tasks they used to perform efficiently and independently. In the moderate to severe stages of AD, severe memory loss is brought about by progression of memory dysfunction; also, there is difficulty with new learning in a way that only highly learned or overlearned material is retained, and new information is lost rapidly, including semantic knowledge and current and historical events (generally with a retrograde gradient). However, patients in the moderate stages of AD may still be able to remember details of events from decades ago. In severe dementia, no new learning occurs and no memory is formed; only patchy memory fragments remain. Patients increasingly lose not only personal and autobiographical information but also elementary semantic knowledge about the world.[32] Although this general progression is characteristic, it is important to keep in mind that individuals with AD often have both patchiness and fluctuations in cognition, function, and behavior. They do experience islands of relative stability in some mental or daily functions and, occasionally, otherwise low function and confusion is interspersed with moments of clarity. In contrast, patients with normal cognitive aging might occasionally have difficulty recalling a name, appointment, or details of a conversation, but this piece of information is not entirely lost and can typically be remembered later. This phenomenon is like when a name or piece of information is not readily within reach, but ultimately, if the person waits long enough, it comes back around and is retrieved. Cognitively healthy individuals may also occasionally misplace items; however, with time, they usually are able to remember and retrace their steps. By definition, daily functioning is not consistently adversely affected by this type of memory change. Numerous studies have shown that patients with AD manifest impairment in episodic memory tests that use a variety of cognitive procedures (eg, free recall, recognition, paired-associate learning) across virtually all modalities (eg, auditory, visual, olfactory). Evidence from many of these studies suggests that the episodic memory deficit of patients with AD, in general, results from ineffective consolidation or storage of new information.[9] Early studies that described the episodic memory deficit in AD used word list learning tasks, such as those from the Consortium to Establish a Registry for Alzheimer's Disease (CERAD)[119] and the CVLT.[120] These studies consistently showed that patients with AD rapidly forget information over time and are equally impaired (relative to age-matched controls) in recognition and free recall components of the tasks. This performance pattern is consistent with impaired consolidation rather than ineffective retrieval of new information.[120] Indices of rapid forgetting have important clinical utility in detecting AD in an early stage and making differential diagnoses. It was shown by Welsh and colleagues[119] that patients with very early AD could be differentiated from healthy elderly controls, using the amount of information recalled after a 10-minute delay on the CERAD word list learning task, with better than 90% accuracy. In this regard, this measure was superior to other measures derived from this task, including immediate recall on each of the 3 learning trials, recognition memory score, and the number of intrusion errors produced throughout the test. Other studies have shown that mildly demented patients with AD can be differentiated from healthy elderly controls using measures of rapid forgetting with 85% to 90% accuracy.[10,119,121–123] An additional mechanism that contributes to episodic memory impairment in AD includes an increased sensitivity to interference caused by defects in the inhibitory processes that in the natural state help people to exclude intruding phenomena while trying to register something in the memory. In other words, the brain in AD is more susceptible to these intruding phenomena and cannot resist them, which leads to the production of intrusion errors[120,124,125] and defective use of semantic information to bolster encoding.[126,127] Several prospective longitudinal studies of cognitive function in nondemented older adults have shown that a subtle decline in episodic memory can be registered before the emergence of the obvious cognitive and behavioral changes that are required for a clinical diagnosis of AD.[128–132] Some of these studies suggest that, several years before the development of the dementia syndrome, memory performance may be poor, but stable, and then rapidly decline in the period immediately before the diagnosis of AD dementia. Two studies[131,133] have shown that episodic memory was mildly impaired 6 years before the onset of dementia, but changed little over the next 3 years. Chen and colleagues[134] showed that, in individuals who were either asymptomatic in the first place or met the criteria for MCI at enrollment to the study, a significant and steady decline occurred in episodic memory on delayed recall conditions of word list and story memory tests.[134,135] Moreover, normal elderly individuals typically have difficulties with free recall conditions,[136,137] but they show normal benefit from (semantic) cueing and intrinsically structured material.[138–140] Compared with younger subjects, they show less efficiency in their recognition performance; however, this difference is negligible compared with the impairment they show on free recall tasks.[141] Taken together, more studies suggest that, to predict the imminent onset of dementia in an elderly individual, registering an abrupt decline in memory might serve better than poor but stable memory ability.[9] Recall performance of patients with AD is not improved by semantic cueing, possibly because of deficient semantic encoding.[89,142,143] Patients with AD are suggested to have a specific deficit in the ability to evaluate semantic relations. They are no longer able to discriminate between 2 related concepts, because they have lost the attribute knowledge that distinguishes these.[83] No relative better performance can be seen in patients with AD on verbal recognition tasks compared with recall tasks.[143–148] Greene and colleagues[149] found that patients with AD seem incapable of learning because of deficient encoding rather than because of impaired retrieval, because their free recall performance is as weak as their recognition performance; they are expected to be equally impaired on visual and verbal recognition trials. Furthermore, patients with AD show poor performance on the recognition of pseudowords.[150] In a study, they seemed not to be able to constrain irrelevant associations.[151] Many false-positive errors were shown by patients with AD because of their inability to discriminate between different semantic relations in the material that was presented to them: they were sensitive to category membership of words but, within a given category, they could not discriminate between different semantic attributes of words.[152] Contrary to early-phase dementia, AD in particular, semantic memory (in particular, but also certain forms of implicit memory) is alleged to be relatively spared in normal aging.[75,76] Another aspect of semantic memory deficit in AD is the patients' consistent deficiency on verbal fluency, compared with normal elderly controls.[79,80,83–85]

PRECLINICAL ALZHEIMER'S DISEASE

The period of cognitive decline that precedes the onset of AD is referred to as the preclinical phase of dementia.[153] At present, preclinical AD is a heatedly debated topic in dementia research. Two of the best studies in determining the characteristics of this phase and its practical implications were done by Elias and colleagues[154] and Linn and colleagues,[155] who worked on the Framingham cohort. With the advancement of research with respect to prognostic methods and therapeutic interventions, early detection of AD will be increasingly important.[129,155] Therefore, it is important for the timeline and the earliest evidence of cognitive decline that signals the preclinical phase of AD to be determined, and for the specific neuropsychological tests that have clinical applications for predicting this disorder to be identified. Deficits on the following tests may indicate the development of AD,[17] several years before the diagnosis: verbal and visuospatial episodic memory[155–159]; abstract reasoning[129,160]; new learning[161]; verbal abilities, including category and letter fluency[130,159,162]; and visuospatial and executive functioning.[129,159] Relations between measures of attention (eg, digit span forward and backward) have been seen in some studies[163] but not in others.[158,164] Moreover, delayed story recall,[154,165] similarities in WAIS-R,[154,166] verbal paired-associate learning,[155,166] delayed free recall and recognition of words,[133,155,157,165,167] recall of tactile memory, immediate visual memory,[168] and Digit Symbol in WAIS-R[166] have been shown to be valuable tests. There is also impairment in semantic memory in a very early stage: in patients with minimal AD[84] MMSE[169] is more than 23. Thus, it could be argued that, compared with (purely) episodic memory, semantic memory performance might be a better early marker for AD; episodic memory performance is left relatively intact by semantic processing capacities, as in free recall of lists of words that are inherently unstructured. A finding that supports this suggestion is that there is impairment in free recall conditions of normal elderly controls. However, in contrast with the performance of patients with AD, elderly controls show normal performance on tasks sensitive to semantic processing capacities.

Weingartner and colleagues[71] investigated semantic memory in patients with preclinical AD (using a category fluency task, 2 years before the diagnosis) and concluded that one of the early cognitive symptoms of AD is alterations in the extent to which uncommon exemplars of semantic networks are available.

PRINCIPLES OF COGNITIVE ASSESSMENT

Frequently, cranial nerves, reflexes, eye movements, and sensorimotor function seem to be intact in patients with neurodegenerative disease, particularly in the early stages.

Thus, to formally assess the cognitive, psychiatric, and behavioral abnormalities that define many dementing disorders, clinicians are in need of more effective neuropsychological tools. The regional variability in neuropsychological testing protocols and in the relative influence of various portions of the dementia evaluation on determining the clinical diagnosis has been recognized as a limiting factor in more effectively characterizing and treating AD.

Cognitive function is assessed by various scales, which are subject to educational and cultural bias. All of these scales have been designed to measure different cognitive domains, including memory, language, visuospatial functions, calculation, abstract thinking, planning, and other executive functions. Validation studies with proper methodological design are necessary to measure the cutoff point in any population in terms of culture adaptation and educational impact before any diagnostic decision.

Crum and colleagues[170] examined the distribution of MMSE scores in 18,056 adult participants. As measured by the MMSE scores, cognitive performance varied in accordance with both age and education level (**Box 11**).

The study of Crum and colleagues[170] emphasizes that, to interpret the MMSE scores, age and education need to be taken into account. However, it is important to bear in mind that the MMSE was primarily designed to quantify the severity of dementia and not to make differential diagnoses.

FUNCTIONAL STATUS

To diagnosis dementia, it is necessary to detect impairment in both cognition and everyday functioning. Functional status refers to the capacity to perform effectively such activities of daily living as food preparation, management of medication, driving,

---

Box 11
Mini Mental State Examination (MMSE)

- Perhaps the most widely used cognitive rating scale is the MMSE. Although this scale is extremely useful, it is weighted significantly toward aspects of memory and attention. The language tasks are fairly insensitive; there is limited assessment of visuospatial ability, and executive performance is not tested.

- There is an inverse relationship between age and MMSE scores and a positive relationship between years of education and MMSE scores.

- The impact of age: the median MMSE score of those participants aged 18 to 24 years was 29, whereas the median score for individuals more than 80 years of age was 25 in the study by Crum and colleagues.[170]

- The impact of educational level: the median MMSE score for participants with at least 9 years of formal education was 29, whereas the median score for those with 0 to 4 years of education was 22.

- The strength of tests like the MMSE lies in that they provide researchers with composite scores that can be used as markers of disease severity over time.

- Healthy older adults perform in a fairly stable manner in MMSE, whereas, over time, MMSE scores of patients with AD decrease at an average rate of around 3 points per year.[171]

- The patients with dementia with Lewy bodies performed worse than patients with AD on attention and construction items, whereas patients with AD performed worse on the MMSE on temporal orientation items and memory items (delayed recall).[172]

- It needs to be taken into consideration that MMSE is not particularly sensitive indicator for manifestations in early stages of the disease.[173]

housekeeping, financial management, and shopping.[174,175] Memory and executive functioning bear the strongest relationship to functional abilities as components of the mental status examination.[176–179] Executive dysfunction often brings about impairments in planning, organization, and insight, all of which are likely to have an effect on people's ability to care for themselves.[176] Another study[174] determined that, among several elements of executive functioning (eg, working memory, generation, inhibition, planning, and sequencing), inhibition was the one most strongly related to impairments in instrumental activities of daily living in patients who were at risk of decline in cognition and function in future. Apart from executive dysfunction, apathy (a frontally mediated behavior) was also associated with impairment in instrumental activities of daily living.[179] Extensive research efforts have been directed toward developing strategies that could predict risk of developing AD before the appearance of observable symptoms. The efficacy, invasiveness, and ease of implementation of existing approaches vary for early detection of AD. Studies that investigate patients with preclinical AD (as the previous stage before MCI) generally recruit a large cohort of nondemented older subjects, who are subjected to a battery of neuropsychological tests at several times of measurement.[17] In the process of neuropsychological evaluation, it is important to precisely evaluate the level of education and schooling, culture, social status, and job exposures. To elaborate, in developing countries, patients are not familiar and comfortable with the setting of these types of assessments. Therefore, to reduce false-positive results, it is important to take into consideration consequences of such conditions; namely anxiety, reduced concentration, and their negative impact on the subjects' scores.[180]

Early to middle stage Alzheimer's dementia has the hallmark of a relatively preserved ability to immediately register new information but significant storage loss for the information when the patient is tested after an adequate delay that is not significantly amenable to cues or recognition by multiple-choice/forced-choice testing (**Box 12**).[32]

Box 12
Important consideration in delayed recall assessment

- It is important that patients are able to immediately register or encode the material, as well as having good hearing; this can be checked by asking the patient to repeat the presented items before the main test (at least once, and preferably twice, or more when a greater learning load is demanded).

- If the patient is not able to adequately register this material for any reason, then memory storage capacity cannot be reliably assessed.

- Once the patient has been mentally engaged with other tasks (ie, after a delay, ideally of at least 5 minutes) that do not require substantial learning and remembering of material that has the potential to interfere with this material/information, the patient should be asked to recall the specific information.

- Patients should not be allowed to rehearse the presented materials, a verbally presented word list or story, or to redraw a previously copied figure.

- When expressive language function can significantly interfere with verbal recall during memory testing, there are other alternatives to redrawing previously copied figures, which include testing recognition memory through presenting lists of words, patterns, or pictures, or hiding objects in particular locations in the examination room and asking the patient to remember and later show the locations.

Data from Dickerson B, Atri A. Dementia: comprehensive principles and practice. Chapter 16. Oxford University Press; 2014.

Note that standard cognitive testing sometimes does not verify the memory complaints of patients. Memorization in complex three-dimensional environments is required for acquisition of information in everyday life.[181] Among the hallmarks for the early clinical manifestations of dementia are impairment of episodic memory and spatial orientation.[182] To assess memory in specialized clinical settings, list learning paradigms such as the Auditory Verbal Learning Test[183] and the California Verbal Learning Test[184] are used. However, such assessments have been criticized for not representing naturalistic conditions and being irrelevant to everyday life.[185] Various cognitive domains that should be evaluated in the diagnostic process of dementia in clinical assessment are presented in **Table 1**.[32]

THE NEUROPATHOLOGIC BASIS OF ALZHEIMER'S CLINICAL PRESENTATION

The neuropathologic hallmarks of AD, namely neuritic plaques and neurofibrillary tangles, first appear in the entorhinal cortex and hippocampus,[24] and[186] subsequently spread to other MTL and neocortical sites. Some brain regions, including primary sensory and motor cortices, are relatively spared.[187] Within modality-specific neocortical areas, there is an increase in the scale of pathologic changes from primary to secondary to tertiary cortices.[188] Thus, the increase in pathologic changes in AD occurs in a hierarchical manner through the ventral visual pathway.[189] To learn the sequence of the symptoms it is vital to understand this pattern of disease progression. It has been revealed in patients with early-stage AD, through using fMRI that, compared with healthy age-matched neurologically normal control subjects, a dissociation exists in AD between impaired explicit memory encoding in MTL and fusiform regions and intact implicit encoding in earlier-stage occipital cortex.[189] During episodic memory encoding in AD, decreased MTL activation has been observed.[53,190–192]

Orientation

Patients with dementia show disorientation to place and time but not to person. With regard to spatial and temporal orientation, patients with AD have increased difficulty when they need to keep track of dates, the passage of time, and geographic relations and locations. Initially, this manifestation of disorientation might present as being disoriented only about the day and date, but, as AD progresses into the moderate and later stages, this confusion could progress to forgetting about the month, season, and year. In later stages, increasing confusion occurs about spatial location (eg, hospital or town) and patients can easily forget where they are or how they have arrived there. In normal cognitive aging, it is common not always to immediately remember the date (or even day of the week); however, in such cases the individual eventually remembers. It is also common to sometimes become distracted or become lost; to look for a car in the parking lot; become confused about a particular travel route; or have to ask for directions, need a map, or need a GPS (global positioning system). Although attention to some of these phenomena may have limited utility in detecting subtle signs of early dementia, they can still provide useful information for staging and tracking patients who are in the middle to late stages of dementia. Also, they may be beneficial in patients with mild dementia who have a greater disorientation, show impairment in forming new memories, or have a lack of insight and awareness into their cognitive problems. Also, through assessment of arousal and orientation, the clinician may be provided with an indication that an underlying medical complication that manifests as confusion and delirium is causing acute or subacute change or fluctuation in mental status.[32]

Attention

Attentional disturbances are frequently the first nonmemory impairments that develop in patients with AD. Therefore, an increasing number of investigations have attempted to identify the specific features of attention that are affected in the disease (for reviews, see Refs.[110,111,193,194]).

Although impairment in delayed recall may serve as an indicator of hippocampal dysfunction, immediate recall impairment may indicate problems in other brain regions involved in attention and organization.[113] The word attention is an umbrella term that refers to many different cognitive abilities, such as orientation to sensory stimuli, maintenance of the alert state, and orchestrating the computations needed for performing the complex tasks of daily life.[195] This last category also comprises the abilities to switch between tasks and to inhibit prepotent responses, also skills that are sometimes referred to as executive functions.[195,196] Although the core of AD is associated with memory impairments, evidence has accumulated over recent years that indicates early deficits in attention.[194,196–198] In early AD, hypometabolism is seen in some of the brain areas most important for attention. Moreover, attention is influenced by acetylcholine levels, which are decreased in AD.[199,200] These observations have led some researchers to propose that memory problems in AD may result in part from a cholinergic attention disruption.[201] The memory deficit in AD has been related chiefly to lesions of the hippocampus and medial temporal structures, whereas the attention deficits are thought to denote lesions of cortical association areas in the parietal and frontal lobes.[202–204] The pattern of attention impairments as observed in AD has been classified by Perry and Hodges[111] in terms of 3 broad subtypes.

Selective attention

Selective attention is the ability to focus on a single relevant stimulus or process while irrelevant stimuli are ignored. This ability includes ignoring perceptual distractors (ie, perceptual filtering) as well as the suppressing responses that conflict with the person's goals (ie, conflict resolution). Selective attention comprises various cognitive processes by which individuals are able to choose which stimuli to process and which to ignore. Thus, selective attention is fundamental for goal-directed behavior. Using the visual search task, selective attention in the visuospatial domain has been extensively studied.[103] In this task, reaction time increases with an increase in the number of distractors when the search is demanding with regard to attention. Possible deficits in selective attention were explored by Fernandez-Duque and Black[197] in patients with early AD, healthy elderly, and young adults under low memory demands; their study assessed perceptual filtering, conflict resolution, and set switching abilities. Neither evidence of impaired perceptual filtering nor evidence of impaired conflict resolution was found in early AD. In contrast, these patients did manifest a global cost in set switching, which was consistent with their not being able to maintain the goals of the task (mental set). These findings are important with regard to the impairment in executive attention, dual tasking, and working memory in AD.[197] However, it is not clear whether this deficit in the patients with AD is caused by their slowness in shifting attention from one item to another or to the processing of each item being ineffective.[44,104]

Divided attention

Divided attention is the ability to allocate attention to multiple stimuli or processes at the same time.[205] Neuropsychological studies of attentional systems in AD show that early in the course of the disease divided attention is affected,[202–204] whereas sustained attention remains preserved until later stages.[110,205] It has been observed that the histologic changes of AD are more pronounced in the parietal than in the frontal lobe during the early clinical stages of the disease. This observation points to the possibility that divided attention depends on the function of the posterior parietal attention site.[20,206,207] Another study has shown the role of frontal cortices as well as parietal dysfunction in the impairment of divided attention in probable AD.[203] To investigate the nature of the divided attention deficit in AD, most studies have used dual-task paradigms, in which tasks are performed both singly and in combination.[109,196,208–212] In these studies, relative to healthy elderly controls, patients with AD have consistently shown a disproportionate impairment in simultaneous performance of 2 tasks.[213,214] In patients with mild AD dual-task performance is also impaired.[213,215]

Sustained attention

Sustained attention is the ability to maintain attentional focus over time. Studies have shown that, although sustained attention is relatively well preserved early in AD, selective attention and divided attention were predominantly prone to disruption.[193] Patients with mild AD do not show impairments on a simple test of sustained attention that makes little demand on memory, such as digit span forward. However, such patients show selective impairments on more complex attentional tasks.[216] Given that AD is associated with impairments in both selective attention and divided attention, it is critical to understand how, in these patients, declines in the component processes of selective attention (eg, spatial attention, perceptual filtering, and inhibitory control) interact with the impairments in the executive processes that coordinate dual-task performance.[217] The functional neuroanatomy of attention is still much debated. Hypotheses range from models of attention monitored by a single central processor to network hypotheses.[1,218] Using PET study in the healthy elderly, a study has shown both sustained and divided attention to elicit activation of the right parietal (inferior lobule) and the right frontal (middle gyrus), whereas the anterior cingulate gyrus was activated only during sustained attention. In patients with AD, only medial frontal structures were activated. Compared with the healthy elderly, more cortical sites differed statistically in patients with AD during divided than during sustained attention. The activation patterns elicited by attention in this study supports the neuropsychological data suggesting that divided attention is more impaired than sustained attention in early AD.[219] Hence the evaluation of attention in general and divided attention specifically may provide important insight into the neural mechanisms of attention, and may aid early diagnosis and treatment of AD; therefore, studies on attention are important from both theoretic and clinical standpoints.[197]

DUAL-TASK DEFICIT IN ALZHEIMER'S DISEASE

Once these findings are taken together, it could be deduced that the dual-task deficit in AD is caused more by a specific inability to effectively coordinate processing across attentional networks[196,209] than by a general deficit in cognitive function or reduction in available attentional resources.[213] Furthermore, this impairment has been interpreted as a deficit in a specific dual-task coordination function of the central executive component of working memory.[102,220] This specific deficit in dual-task coordination in patients with AD suggests that being able to execute 2 competing tasks concomitantly may prove to be a particularly sensitive indicator of subtle changes in cognitive status. Dual-task impairments on selective attention tasks could be manifested in different ways with regard to behavior. First, dual-task conditions could bring about an overall increase in rate of error and/or response time, because coordinating and executing performance of the selective attention task become more difficult under dual-task conditions. Patients with AD also manifest impairment in rescaling the focus of attention, because, compared with healthy individuals, they benefit less from cues providing only imprecise information about the target location in the search display.[154] Maintaining a mental set is an ability related to working memory capacity; this ability may be compromised both in individuals experiencing healthy aging and those with AD. Furthermore, poor set switching performance in neuropsychological tasks can well predict the progression of the disease in patients at the preclinical stage.[64,221] The Trail Making Test, Part B, is one of these predicting tasks; letters and numbers are randomly distributed on a sheet of paper. The patient is asked to trace the items in an ascending manner and alternate between letter and number. In the case of healthy adults, performance in this task is related to performance in experimental set switching tasks.[153] There exists a consistency between these findings and the hypothesis that, even at very early stages of AD (including the prodromal stage called MCI), the ability to maintain mental set may be affected. As a group, patients with MCI may be impaired in response inhibition and set switching; however, a considerable number of patients seemingly show only deficits in episodic memory.[222] These latter meet the criteria for amnesic MCI (MCI-a).[129] Note that even the patients with MCI-a are a heterogeneous group, and patients reveal subtle deficits of attention in experimental designs. In one such study, researchers divided patients with MCI-a into 2 groups: those who had mostly hippocampal atrophy, and those who had mostly small vessel cerebrovascular disease (as registered by white matter hyperintensities on brain MRI).[155] Both groups were equally impaired with regard to episodic memory; however, subjects with small vessel disease showed more significant impairment in tasks that required them to maintain a mental set, such as working memory and continuous performance tasks. In a study by Festa and colleagues,[217] the findings are merely suggestive that a deficit in the ability to maintain a mental set is already detectable at very early stages in the disease. Their finding raises an important question: whether or not deficits in mental set maintenance could help predict who is at risk to progress from a preclinical stage to full-flown clinical manifestations. The difficulty in maintaining mental set also helps explain the deficit that exists in areas of higher cognition in AD. Dual-task studies have contended that it is not the increased perceived load by the patients that results in dual-task deficit in AD, but that it is caused by a deficit coordinating the two tasks.[209] Although task coordination is a concept in need of further development, one of its constituent parts might be the ability to maintain a mental set about task A while task B is being performed.[156] This concept forms a testable prediction: whether AD deficit in dual task is mediated, at least in part, by the inability to maintain set. In sum, the literature regarding early AD is suggestive of the existence of deficits in a variety of selective attention tasks; however, not much is known about the precise mechanisms underlying those deficits.

VISUOSPATIAL FUNCTION

Visuospatial function comprises the abilities to identify, integrate, and analyze space, and visual form, details, structure, and spatial relations in several (usually 2 or 3) dimensions.[32] Moreover, visuospatial skills include spatial navigation; perception of distance, depth, movement, and visual relations; visuospatial construction; and mental imagery. Assessment of visuospatial function is extremely useful and should thus be included in every mental status examination to detect organic brain disease.[35] Complex nonverbal cognitive functions are required for constructional abilities; these abilities also involve the integration of occipital, parietal, and frontal lobe functions.

Nevertheless, the parietal lobes are the principal cortical areas that are involved in visual-motor integration. According to the cognitive map theory[223] and similar studies,[224] representation of spatial locations are stored in the hippocampus. The hippocampus is also the critical structure for the memorization of verbal[225] and nonverbal lists of items.[226] It is not clear whether the learning of verbal material that occurs in spatial surroundings is different from classic word list learning. One of the crucial abilities for the preservation of autonomy in old age and AD is the ability to remember information and events while simultaneously moving in a complex environment.[227] At some point in the course of the disease, patients with AD often show deficits in visuospatial abilities.[158] Patients have also been reported to manifest visuospatial deficits early, even in preclinical stages.[159] Changes in visuospatial function are detectable on visuoconstructional tests and the tasks that require visuoperceptual abilities and visual orientation. This visuoperceptual deficit may partly arise from the loss of effective interaction between distinct and less damaged cortical information processing systems.[160] Studies have shown that, compared with controls in a visual search task, when patients with AD are asked to quickly identify targets from the aggregation of 2 or more features that are processed in different cortical regions (eg, color and shape), they have disproportionately greater response times than when they are asked to identify targets exclusively from a single feature.[228,229] In the course of normal aging, deficits are also observed in visual information processing and in selective and divided attention, but these deficits are intensified in individuals with AD.[230–233] In addition, visual motion detection has been shown to deteriorate in some individuals with MCI and more in patients with a diagnosis of AD dementia, which suggests that this symptom may serve as an independent marker to detect those who potentially have AD.[234]

Note that intact visuospatial functioning is essential for driving. Thus, given the safety implications, it is essential to question patients and their caregivers in detail regarding recent changes in driving ability.[157] With regard to visual and spatial relationships, patients with AD, even in the mild stages, can have difficulty understanding or interpreting visual images and spatial relationships, and navigating through space.[35] They may not be able to appreciate the big picture or notice objects that are right in front of them; they may also have difficulty judging distances, colors, and contrasts, and reading. Such problems can be a predominant and presenting sign of AD in some individuals (ie, patients with the visuospatial variant of AD). These problems can readily translate into substantial difficulties with work and particularly with driving.[9] Gross visuospatial dysfunction can be indicated by evidence of the patient's trouble navigating through space (eg, frequently bumping into things). Often, this early functional disability results in life-threatening complications caused by wandering and getting lost while driving.[78] Therefore, regardless of the degree of verbal memory impairment, as a symptomatic variant of MCI, this navigational impairment is a harbinger of AD-related cognitive decline.[235] However, it is important to bear in mind that the eyesight might be undergoing changes in individuals who are undergoing normal cognitive aging, as opposed to how their brain is integrating and interpreting visual images. For example, they may be shortsighted or have lost their visual clarity, because of cataracts, and have low visual acuity, caused by changes in the retina. In addition, compared with younger controls, older individuals react more slowly to peripheral stimuli; patients with AD show an even greater impairment. The increased incidence of car crashes in patients with AD dementia may be accounted for by these visual deficits.[159,161] There is an identical pattern of difficulty in associating visual scenes and locations in normal aging and AD; the difficulty becomes complicated in AD by the loss of navigational capacities that are verbally mediated.

Compared with normal controls, patients with mild AD present equal performances on simple copying tasks, such as drawing a clock or a triangle.[236,237] However, among mildly to moderately impaired patients, visuospatial impairments are commonly observed.[238,239] To assess visuospatial problems, patients can be asked to copy pre-drawn shapes on a page, starting with simple shapes (eg, a square or pentagon) and progressing to more complex shapes (eg, a cube or intersecting pentagons), to build shapes with triangles or blocks, and draw a clock. Also, visuospatial construction can be tested by asking the patient to imitate the construction of different interlocking finger patterns that the examiner has made. Another approach for assessment of visuospatial function[181] is checking navigation ability, which is impaired early in the course of AD.[182] Assessment of patients at various levels of severity,[240] as well as longitudinal data collected from the same patients,[239] indicates that, over time, performance on clock drawing to command becomes progressively worse, and that conceptual errors are particularly sensitive to the overall change in the severity of dementia. The sensitivity of clock drawing to command in patients with mild AD has led investigators to probe whether this task might also be sensitive to individuals in the prodromal phase of AD. However, several studies have indicated that clock drawing to command is not efficient for the identification of MCI cases.[241,242]

VISUAL GNOSIS

Agnosia, derived from agnosis, or nonknowledge (Greek: nosos meaning disease and gnosis meaning knowledge), is the loss of the ability to recognize objects, persons, sounds, shapes, or smells, without the specific sense being defective. Anosognosia is the lack of awareness of, or denial of, the existence of a deficit or handicap; this feature is seen often (but not necessarily), and early, in several dementias, particularly AD and behavioral variant of FTD (bvFTD).[32] Agnosia is a failure of recognition that cannot be explained by impaired primary sensation (tactile, visual, auditory) or cognitive impairment. It has been described as perception stripped of its meaning. Agnosia is different from anomia; the patient with agnosia not only fails to name an object but also cannot recognize it in a group or match it to a picture. In cases of tactile agnosia (astereognosis), touch threshold is normal but patients cannot recognize what they are touching. There exist comparable agnosias in the visual and auditory spheres. However, as the responsible lesions are usually bilateral, only rare cases of visual and auditory agnosias are seen. Simultanagnosia is the inability to recognize the meaning of a whole scene or object, despite its individual components being correctly recognized; individuals with this condition literally cannot see the forest because of the trees. To test simultanagnosia, the patient could be asked to identify on a page specific targets of various sizes, such as letters, numbers, or shapes; affected patients may be able to identify smaller individual targets but not bigger ones. Usually, language is processed in the left hemisphere and spatial information in the right hemisphere. Right hemispheric (particularly parietal) lesions impair spatial perception and manipulation. Patients with such lesions have difficulty reading maps or finding their way around (topographagnosia), or difficulty copying simple pictures or shapes or drawing simple objects such as a flower (constructional apraxia or apractagnosia).[1] It is important to assess anosognosia, and the patient's overall insight, in order to advise the caregivers about the best approaches to the patient's care and safety measures (like driving, handling guns, and cooking). To assess anosognosia, facts need to be compared with the patients' insights, perceptions, and understanding of their condition (deficits, disabilities, and behaviors, and their impact on others), current stations in life, and the reason for and context of the medical evaluation.

Posterior Cortical Atrophy: Occipital Variant of Alzheimer's Disease

Although rare, AD can initially show relatively circumscribed posterior cortical atrophy (PCA), and the dementia can be dominated by higher order visual dysfunction.[162] Patients with the clinical syndrome of PCA have relatively preserved memory functions, intact language, and preserved judgment and insight. However, such patients usually have prominent visual agnosia, constructional apraxia, and some or all of the features of Balint syndrome, which include optic ataxia, gaze apraxia, and simultanagnosia. Another key feature of this variant of AD is navigational impairment, which presents with disorders of spatial cognition, memory, and orientation[163,243–245]; this impairment is linked to the accumulation of AD neurologic disorder in peristriate cortices.[77] Components of Gerstmann syndrome may also be found in PCA, including acalculia, right-left disorientation, finger agnosia, and agraphia. Also, visual field defect, decreased visual attention, impaired color perception, or decreased contrast sensitivity may be present.[130] Usually, the clinical syndrome of PCA is associated with AD; however, this syndrome may also occur in association with neuropathologic changes of cortical Lewy body disease or Creutzfeldt-Jakob disease. Disproportionate atrophy and pathologic lesions are detected through neuropathologic examination in the occipital cortex and posterior parietal cortex.[163,246] Particular involvement of the dorsal visual stream has also been reported in studies using PET. In PCA caused by AD, neurofibrillary tangles and neuritic plaques in the posterior cortical regions are identical, with regard to their quality, to those in typical AD.[246] Using PET imaging with Pittsburgh compound-B ([11C]-PIB), an agent that binds to β-amyloid in the brain, it has recently been shown that pathologic features of AD in PCA have a disproportionately posterior cortical distribution.[247]

ARITHMETICAL ABILITY

Such common daily activities as handling money or consulting timetables,[248] apart from numerical and arithmetical processing (eg, comprehension of number meaning, simple calculation) are in need of executive control, set shifting, inhibition of interference, as well as temporary maintenance of information in short-term memory. In early stages of AD, patients show episodic memory deficits, along with functional impairment in everyday life activities including numerical activities.[46] In a recent study, patients with mild to moderate AD showed intact basic numerical skills (number comparison, transcoding, simple calculation), but performed very poorly in tasks such as checking the television program or calculating the money change.[47] There was a correlation between the patients' performance in these everyday numerical situations and their global cognitive status and measures of executive functioning. Early in AD, attentional and executive deficits present; these deficits manifest after impairments in episodic memory but before visuospatial and language disorders.[111] Among the first signs of AD, deficits in more abstract numerical processing (eg, dot counting, written complex calculation) have also been reported.[87,88,249] Daily-life financial abilities[32] may also be impaired in individuals with MCI. Patients with MCI typically have memory loss and show reduced performance on neuropsychological testing.[68,91] Also, mild deficits in episodic memory and executive functions, such as inhibition of interference and allocation of attention, have been described in MCI.[247] Activities of daily living, as tested by routine assessment, are usually found to be intact. However, slight impairments have been recently described in tasks related to high-order financial capacities, such as financial conceptual knowledge, bank statement management, and bill payment.[32] It has been shown that executive dysfunction may play a critical role in the functional change in MCI. To test arithmetical processing in routine neuropsychological assessment, well-structured test batteries are used in which, for example, knowledge of addition and multiplication facts ($2 + 3 = 6, 4 \times 3 = 12$) is tested by separate tasks. However, it is rare for people to be asked to solve series of addition or multiplication problems in real-life situations. Instead, it is typically required to shift between operations. A result acquired through routine laboratory testing may therefore not accurately reflect the individual's arithmetical ability in daily life. Moreover, it is assumed that arithmetical knowledge of addition and multiplication facts is stored in long-term memory in highly interrelated associative networks.[45,250,251] However, because attentional and executive deficits are shown early in AD,[111] patients may find difficulties with tasks that put high demand on these functions. With regard to MCI, minor executive deficits have also been reported.[247] A recent study on arithmetic by Zamarian and colleagues[248] showed that, in the mixed and the Stroop-like conditions, patients with MCI may manifest reduced performance. This finding may help in developing a diagnostic tool to differentiate mild AD or MCI from healthy aging. Zamarian and colleagues[248] showed that both patients with AD and MCI have intact arithmetical knowledge retrieval from long-term memory in the blocked condition. However, whenever a load was put on executive functions, patients with AD showed impairment, whereas patients with MCI successfully shifted between operations (mixed condition) but, if required to inhibit overlearned associations (Stroop-like condition), they had difficulties. These findings, in line with previous studies, signify the contribution of attentional and executive functions in arithmetic and are suggestive of the potential importance of assessing arithmetical processing not only in blocked presentations but also in mixed presentations. There is a high ecological value in the mixed condition because it mimics daily-life arithmetical activities (eg, checking the grocery bill). As shown by recent outcomes, patients with AD and MCI who are in the normal range in routine neuropsychological (blocked) arithmetical assessments might experience difficulties if extra requirements are demanded from nonnumerical resources, which means they may not process arithmetic efficiently in real daily-life situations.[248]

Praxis

Praxis denotes the performance of a learned motor act. In its broadest sense, apraxia refers to impaired learned skilled movements that cannot be explained by weakness, incoordination, abnormal tone, bradykinesia, movement disorder, dementia, aphasia, poor cooperation, sensory loss, lack of comprehension, or inattention.[1,252] Apraxia can be defined as the loss of the ability to execute purposeful, previously learned movements, despite the presence of the desire and the physical ability to perform such movements.[32] Apraxia is common in AD, and usually develops after the establishment of the impairments of memory and language. Apraxia also occurs in HD, corticobasal ganglionic degeneration, and occasionally in Parkinson disease. Failure to perform an act is not necessarily evidence of apraxia. In order for apraxia to be diagnosed, the act must be performed incorrectly, or components of the act must be performed imprecisely. There might be omissions in parts of the act, or the acts may be sequenced abnormally or incorrectly oriented in space. A complete assessment of apraxia should include these subcomponents: imitation of gestures, use of imagined objects, orobuccal movements, and a sequencing task such as the Luria 3-step command (fist, edge, palm) (see **Table 1**).[32,253]

Apraxias are traditionally classified as limb-kinetic, ideational, and ideomotor.

Limb-kinetic apraxia
With limb-kinetic apraxia the act is understood but there is fault in motor execution.- Hence, there is loss of hand and finger dexterity resulting from inability to connect or

isolate individual movements.[254] All types of movement are affected: symbolic, nonsymbolic, transitive (ie, using tools and instruments; eg, a hammer or a hairbrush), and intransitive (ie, communicative gestures; eg, representational tasks such as waving goodbye and nonrepresentational tasks such as touching the nose and wiggling the fingers). Movements of the mainly distal finger and hand are coarse and mutilated.[255] All cases that were pathologically confirmed have shown a degenerative process involving frontal and parietal cortices[256] or primary motor cortex.[257]

Ideomotor apraxia

In ideomotor apraxia, a disorder of goal-directed movements, there is impairment of pantomiming ability to use tool; hence, patients know what to do but not how to do it. Such patients are able to accurately describe using a hammer but might be unable to imitate its use and, if given a hammer, to use it correctly.[1] Transitive movements are more affected than intransitive. Voluntary automatic dissociation is present; therefore, that deficit is more apparent in clinical settings than in everyday life.[255] Ideomotor apraxia signifies a difficulty in producing gestures caused by an inability to translate the concept of a motor sequence into the corresponding motor action; this happens because of functional disconnection of the idea of the act and the motor components of its execution. Ideomotor praxis can be tested by evaluating the ability to correctly form the necessary postures and movements to perform a task using a tool (see **Table 1**).[32]

Anatomically diverse lesions mainly in left hemisphere typically involve parietal association areas and white matter bundles connecting frontal and parietal association areas.[196,255,258,259] Another classification for apraxia is described as ideomotor, dressing, and constructional apraxia.[258–260] One study performed on patients with AD and age-matched controls of apraxia showed that, on the tests of ideomotor and ideational apraxia, all types of movements were not affected to the same degree.[261] Limb transitive movements were especially susceptible, whereas limb intransitive, buccofacial, and axial movements were relatively intact. No significant difference existed between performance on verbal command and imitation; however, considerable improvement was observed with the use of objects.

Ideational (conceptual) apraxia

These patients do not know what to do. Content errors are readily evident. This terminology can be puzzling, not only because, among investigators, definitions of ideational and conceptual apraxia vary but also because some scholars are debating a distinction between the two.[255] Error types include impairment in carrying out sequences of actions that require the use of various objects in the correct order, in order to achieve a purpose,[262] and loss of tool action knowledge. This apraxia can be tested by asking the patient to verbalize, step by step, how to do a job (eg, make a sandwich).

Qualitatively, disorders of skilled movement in AD were similar to the apraxic syndromes caused by left parietal damage. This study suggested that apraxia in AD may reflect posterior left hemisphere cortical involvement and may be apparent even in patients who manifest good language functions. In an anterograde and neuropathologic study, Giannakopoulos and colleagues[263] investigated the neuroanatomic correlates of apraxia in 23 patients with clinically obvious AD. Their results suggest that ideomotor and dressing apraxias are associated with mild damage of the anterior cingulate cortex, whereas constructional apraxia is related to the disruption of cortical pathways that mediate visuospatial cognition in AD. However, this study included limitations: the neuropathologic analysis addresses only the left hemisphere whereas there is some evidence pointing to the role of the right hemisphere in dressing apraxia and drawing disability,[199,264,265] and in the impairment in the production of intransitive movements following verbal commands.[266] Moreover, depending on the neuropsychological tests selected, the definition of apraxia may vary in patients with AD. Although refined criteria exist for bvFTD, its differentiation from AD remains problematic at early clinical stages. Although apraxia is not considered as a supportive feature aiding the diagnosis of bvFTD, it is so considered for AD.[267] However, only a few studies have attempted to quantify praxis disturbances in mild disease stages; the specificity of these attempts remains indistinct for AD compared with bvFTD. In cortical dementias, breakdown in the praxis circuit is one of the early dysfunctions and results in perplexity, awkwardness, omission, substitution errors, toying behavior, and unrecognizable gestures in response to command.[268] Attentiveness to the organicity of these phenomena helps diagnosis to be made in early stages, which consequently helps in adopting appropriate therapeutic measures and slowing the progression of the disease. Cotelli and colleagues[268] conducted a study on 300 patients with dementia to test for ideational, ideomotor, limb-kinetic, buccopharyngeal, dressing apraxia, and constructional apraxia, and gait apraxias, in addition to recording rare apraxias if present. Patients with AD manifested apraxias in all the phases of the disease: ideational, ideomotor, dressing, and constructional apraxias in the early phases and buccopharyngeal and gait apraxia in the late phases. Late in the disease, patients with FTD showed buccopharyngeal and gait apraxias. Limb apraxias were seen in cortical basal ganglionic degeneration; diffuse Lewy body disease showed more agnosias and fewer apraxias. The most common apraxias were ideational and ideomotor.

Dressing apraxia
Dressing apraxia comprises a particular form of apraxia confined to the use of clothing and is often associated with focal lesions in the right parietal lobe.[264]

Constructional apraxia
Constructional apraxia signifies a visuospatial disorder that is characterized by impairment in the spatial organization that is required when fragments of objects are assembled to form a single entity. This impairment is thought to be related to parietal-occipital cortex disorder[194,264]; however, this view has been challenged.[199,269] Usually, apraxia develops in late stages of AD,[201] although reports have been made of patients with early constructional and ideomotor praxis disability.[195,196]

LANGUAGE DISORDERS

Aphasia is a disturbance of language, in which the patient shows an impaired production and/or comprehension of spoken language that cannot be explained by an impairment of the neural apparatus for hearing, vision, or vocalization.[1] Overall, language difficulties in AD often present as new problems with word finding, expression, comprehension, reading, writing, repetition, naming, and understanding the meaning of words. Patients may have difficulty following or joining a conversation; they may frequently have long pauses in the middle of a sentence, struggle with vocabulary, and use wrong or imprecise words (eg, call a watch a "hand clock," or frequently use "thing" instead of the correct word).[32] Over time, the patients' speech becomes increasingly inarticulate, it may lack information content, become simplified, agrammatic, and short. As the disease progresses, they also require frequent repetition and use of simple and short sentences in order to comprehend. Early on, this language problem can be confused with hearing problem. Older individuals experiencing normal cognitive aging frequently complain of the inability to retrieve the right word or name, which invariably comes back later. This difficulty is not sufficient to affect consistent, efficient, and successful communication.

Language Evaluation

To evaluate the patient's speech and language, gross signs of the motoric aspects of speech (eg, dysarthria; speech rhythm, prosody, and volume) as well as multiple aspects of language function need to be noted. These language functions can broadly be conceptualized as receptive language abilities (ie, the ability to process and understand written or spoken language) and expressive abilities (ie, the ability to express ideas in verbal or written language). It is important to make a distinction between whether a patient has a motor speech disorder (eg, dysarthria) or aphasia, which is a communicative disorder.[32] It might not be possible or appropriate to reach a perfect analysis of language function in a screening mental status examination format; however, a gross evaluation of expressive abilities can be attained. Close attention also should be paid to several features of the patient's spontaneous and conversational speech, including intonation, prosody, typical phrase length, the presence of grammatical terms, the presence and type of paraphasia, word-finding ability, and how well the patient seems to comprehend the content of what is being said. In addition, reading and writing also need to be assessed. Assessment of 6 basic elements of language can help identify clinical subtypes of aphasia: spontaneous speech, speech comprehension, naming, repetition, writing, and reading.[1]

Spontaneous Speech

Abnormality in the patient's spontaneous speech may be observed in several ways.[1]

Fluency

Fluency (ie, the quantity of speech produced over time) may be reduced. Fluency is an aspect of executive function, because it requires implementing organized search and retrieval strategies. Fluency can be assessed by asking the patient to generate words beginning with specified letters or belonging to certain semantic categories. Problems with semantic categories often suggest AD or Semantic Dementia (SD), whereas difficulty with letter prompts (phonemic cueing) suggests frontal and/or subcortical deficits.[77]

Semantic fluency

Semantic fluency is often evaluated using the category of animals.[270] Typically, nonverbal fluency tasks (eg, design fluency,[58] Ruff Figural Fluency Test[271]) present patients with boxes containing dots and the patients are then asked to generate as many novel designs as possible. The fluidity, speed, and ease with which patients expresses themselves in conversation are parameters that can be noted in order to assess fluency. If the patient has lengthy pauses or is hesitant in word finding or word substitutions, a nonfluent or dysnomic language disorder might be present (ie, if psychomotor processing is not also assumed to be generally affected to the same degree).

Verbal fluency

Verbal fluency is an aspect of language ability that conceptually is under both domains of executive and language function. Formal evaluation of verbal fluency is included on several of the standardized measures summarized later (eg, Saint Louis University Mental Status Examination [SLUMS],[272] Montreal Cognitive Assessment [MoCA],[243] Addenbrooke's Cognitive Examination Revised [ACE-R][273,274]). Typically, verbal fluency is assessed by asking patients to say as many words as they can think of that begin with a certain letter (letter or phonemic fluency task) or that belong to a certain semantic category (eg, animals, vegetables, tools; semantic category task). It is also informative to pay attention to the pattern of verbal fluency deficits. For example, in early AD, language dysfunction is often seen as a verbal fluency profile with worse performance on semantic tasks than letter fluency, which is likely to reflect temporal cortical dysfunction. In contrast, profiles of impaired word finding and naming (but improved naming when provided with hints or cues), and worse performance on letter fluency than semantic category fluency, are seen in early-stage patients with vascular cognitive impairment or other disorders that prominently affect frontoparietal language systems (eg, agrammatic or logopenic variants of primary progressive aphasia). If a patient's primary symptom is language difficulty, it is essential to perform a more detailed language assessment, which is usually performed by a specialist.

Prosody
Prosody (ie, the musical qualities of speech: pitch, accent, and rhythm) can also be impaired. Thus, dysprosody is an impairment of speech melody, inflection, and rhythm.

Paraphasia
Paraphasia is defined by substitution of incorrect words for correct ones.

Patients with literal (or phonemic) paraphasia use words that resemble the intended word phonetically but contain 1 or more substituted syllables (eg, "hosicle" instead of "hospital"). Patients with verbal (or semantic) paraphasia use words that are real but that are unintended (eg, "hotel" instead of "hospital"). In some patients, paraphasic mistakes occasionally contaminate speech; in others, they almost fully replace it. Even when paraphasia is absent, it may be difficult to grasp the content of aphasic speech. Logorrheic but empty speech, as well as hesitation before certain words, may be indicate a severely restricted vocabulary.

Paragrammatic
Paragrammatic speech preserves a facade of syntax despite profoundly restricted semantic content. By contrast, agrammatic (or telegrammatic) speech omits relational words (such as prepositions or conjunctions).

Speech Comprehension
Abnormalities of speech comprehension, whether mild, moderate, or even severe, cannot be revealed through casual conversation with the patient.[1] Particular testing is required. Clinicians should not depend on the patient's verbal responses to commands or questions in order to assess speech comprehension. A wrong answer could signify a paraphasic error rather than the patient's failure to comprehend. If the patients follow a command, whether simple or complex, it can be presumed that the command was understood. However, failure to follow a command could signify conditions other than impaired comprehension; for example, paralysis, apraxia, pain, or negativism. Asking yes-or-no questions is a more reliable method of testing speech comprehension. Even patients whose speech output is severely restricted can usually indicate affirmative or negative. Both the patient and the examiner must be aware of the correct answers. Another way to test speech comprehension is to ask the patient to point to objects or body parts. Similar to abnormal speech output, semantic and syntactic (relational) comprehension can be dissociated. Syntactic comprehension can be assessed by asking the patient to handle objects. For example, after the patient has identified a comb, a pen, and

a key, the patient could be asked to put the key on top of the comb or the comb between the key and the pen. The patient's comprehension can be assessed by asking a question with complex grammatical constructions in need of processing of the sentences or asking the patient to perform a multistep command, preferably across midline. It is important to bear in mind that during longer verbal statements challenge both language abilities and working memory are involved; thus, if a patient does not manage to perform such a task, further testing is needed to better define the nature of the deficit.

Naming

If patients have adequate vision, they can be challenged with confrontation naming (ie, being shown objects, body parts, colors, or pictures of actions). A range of anomalous responses indicate anomia (the loss of the ability to recall or recognize the names of things). Some patients show paraphasias. Some hesitate and struggle to find the correct word (tip-of-the-tongue phenomenon). Rather than naming an object, some patients describe it. For example, instead of saying "necktie," the patient says, "It's what you wear around your neck." Naming ability can briefly be assessed by asking the patient to name a few objects, starting with higher-frequency items and progressing to lower-frequency words (**Box 13**).

Repetition

One of the most important elements of language, which has an important role in differentiating types of dementia, is repetition. Evaluation of repetition is done by asking the patient to repeat sentences such as, "The cat always hid under the couch when dogs were in the room."[243] Patients may particularly have difficulty repeating syntactically complex sentences (eg, "If he were to come, I would go out"). Errors most often consist of paraphasic replacements.

Writing

In general, compared with reading, writing is more vulnerable to disruption; coordination of both central (spelling) and more peripheral (letter formation) components is involved in writing.[253] Testing of writing begins by having patients sign their names. More specific tests of writing include dictated sentences, words, or letters, as well

---

Box 13
Tip-of-the-tongue syndrome (TOTs)

- TOTs is a striking state of awareness; it is a common and dramatic word-finding failure, in which a person is temporarily unable to produce a well-learned word, despite being certain of knowing the word.

- Contradictory results are shown by the body of evidence for the nature of TOTs and its relationship with AD.

- For younger adults, episodes of TOTs occur about once a week and increase to about once a day for older adults.[275,276]

- TOTs is a phenomenon universally experienced by people of all languages and cultures; it is experienced by monolinguals and bilinguals, children, college-aged students, and older adults.[277]

- TOTs are also detectable in several neurologic conditions, including AD, anomic aphasia, and temporal lobe epilepsy (see Brown[278] and Schwartz and Brown[279]).

as spontaneous writing; for example, describing what is seen in a room (see **Table 1**).[32]

Reading

At first, the level of literacy should be assessed. The failure of comprehension is usually accompanied by an inability to read aloud; however, the reverse is not necessarily true. Reading ability is tested by having the patient read aloud simple sentences, words, or letters. Reading comprehension can be tested by having the patient follow written commands that were previously successfully executed as oral commands or by having the patient answer written yes-or-no questions (see **Table 1**).[32]

Dysgraphia

Several problems can be caused in daily living by neurologic damage and cognitive dysfunction, such as loss of memory, and difficulties of written and oral communication.[280,281] Reading and writing can be directly assessed; patients can be asked to read a paragraph and to write a whole sentence. To test repetition, medium to long phrases or sentences are used. Agraphia is an acquired impairment in writing. The term alexia signifies a loss of reading ability in a previously literate person. One of the best studies on dysgraphia was performed by Onofri and colleagues,[282] in whose comprehensive article the history of dysgraphia is also reviewed. As early as 1907, Alzheimer's[283] had observed in patients abnormal graphic gestures, which indicated that a unitary process does not constitute handwriting, but that a coordination of linguistic and visual-spatial abilities is required,[193] which reflects brain damage in different associative areas, such as parietal, temporal, occipital, and frontal regions,[284] in patients who are subsequently diagnosed with AD.[208] Lambert and colleagues[285] discussed a wide variety of agraphia syndromes, including a considerable number of patients with selective damage to one of the central or peripheral components, as well as patients who manifested multiple writing impairments. A positive correlation was registered between the severity of the dementia and spelling/writing measures. As observed in early AD,[284] agraphia or dysgraphia comprise a progressive disorganization and degeneration of the various components of handwriting[286]; these include the complexity of the structure of sentences,[287] the diversity and the accuracy of words used,[210] punctuation,[209] organization,[210] the production of grammatically incorrect sentences,[211,212] the length of the sentences,[211] the amount of written information,[212] the morphology of the letters[211] and spelling,[288] graphic and spatial layout of letters, and their arrangement in texts.[289] The possibility that agraphia/dysgraphia may be an early sign of degenerative dementia was examined by Fukui and Lee[290]; they reported on the simultaneous or subsequent emergence of nonfluent aphasia, ideomotor apraxia, executive dysfunction, and asymmetric akinetic rigid syndrome. Their observations indicate that degenerative processes engage the parietal-occipital-temporal regions, basal ganglia, and striatofrontal projections. Within the AD population, it has been observed that writing impairment is heterogeneous. Nevertheless, certain aspects of the writing process are more vulnerable than others and may be regarded as diagnostic signs.[291] The understanding of disease progression may be facilitated through the identification and staging patterns of writing impairments/deficits during different phases of AD; they may also provide conditions for the development of applicable interventions. The relationship between cognitive impairment and the performance of handwritten scripts was examined by Onofri and colleagues[282] by asking patients with AD to do some letter writing to a close relative. Agraphia or dysgraphia is often observed in early AD; therefore, it encompasses a progressive disorganization and degeneration of the various components of handwriting. The investigators showed that affected brain regions underlie functions in cognition, language, and motor domains, which are disturbed in AD. Dysgraphia manifests in the earlier as well as the later stages during the clinical course of AD[292–294]; it is associated with deficits in attention, motor, and memory functions that develop during progression of the disorder.[295] It has been suggested that, compared with anomia, dysgraphia is a more sensitive indicator for language deficits in AD.[296] In one study using Hangul (the Korean alphabet), PET imaging of glucose metabolism indicated that the hypometabolism in the right occipitotemporal lobe and left temporoparietal lobe was related to writing impairment.[297] Observations by other researchers[298–301] have shown that dysgraphia associated with deficits in semantic memory, seem to correspond with current notions concerning the progressive performance impairments of patients with AD within language and cognition domains from a staging perspective.[302,303] It has been concluded that the heterogeneous profiles of dysgraphia with primary signs of writing impairment in AD originate from changes in different regions of the brain networks that subserve writing and spelling performance.[285] There is evidence for altered parietal-motor connections in AD; therefore, the possibility of related motor deficits in dysgraphia ought to be taken into account.[304] It has also been found that, at an early stage of the disease, impairment occurs in the sensory-motor plasticity in the motor cortex of AD.[305] It can be inferred from such findings that assessment of dysgraphia could serve as an additional diagnostic tool, providing evidence of compromised functioning in motor, cognitive, and emotional domains.[306]

Alzheimer's Disease: Involvement of Language or Working Memory?

Impairments in working memory have dramatic consequences,[307] therefore it has been suggested that the language impairments in patients with AD result from reduced working memory capacity.[308] Other researchers have suggested that, in addition to having compromised working memory function, patients with AD have lost core linguistic knowledge.[309] In all cases, researchers have formed several assumptions about what linguistic working memory is. These assumptions centrally include the notion that damage can occur in the knowledge of language and working memory capacity independently.[310]

Language and Semantic Knowledge

On tests of object naming,[311,312] verbal fluency,[313] and semantic categorization,[314] mildly demented patients with AD often show impairment. There is evidence that these impairments reflect decline in the structure and content of semantic memory. As the neurologic disorder of AD impinges on the temporal, frontal, and parietal association cortices, in which knowledge for particular items or concepts are thought to be diffusely stored, the knowledge and associations between them may be disrupted.[84] Impairments in confrontation naming and verbal fluency are evident in mildly to moderately impaired patients with AD. It has been argued by some clinicians that these deficits result from a broader impairment in semantic memory.[315] Several studies that probed for knowledge of particular concepts across different modes of access and output (eg, fluency, confrontation naming, sorting, word-to-picture matching, and definition generation) have provided evidence for a deterioration of semantic memory in AD. These studies assume that loss of knowledge, and not impaired retrieval of intact knowledge, leads to consistency of performance across items.[142,316] For example, if the concept of a horse is lost with a patient, the patient should not be able to name a picture of a horse, generate "horse" on a verbal fluency test, sort horse into its proper category as a domestic animal, and so on.[9] Using a range of tasks that include category fluency,[316,317] category membership,[318] confrontation naming,[316] and similarity judgments,[317,319,320] semantic memory abnormalities in patients with AD have been documented. However, other studies that have used a variety of tasks, including recognition naming,[321] category-naming fluency, drawing fluency,[79] and category membership judgments,[318] have failed to reveal such category-specific differences. It has been suggested that inconsistent findings regarding category-specific semantic loss in patients with AD relate to the fact that, for category-specific judgments, some brain regions are more critical than others, and the presence of a deficit depends on the anatomic distribution of disease in the specific patients examined.[318] It is also assumed that loss of knowledge of the attributes and associations that define a particular semantic category reduces the ability of patients with AD to efficiently generate words from a small and highly related set of exemplars during tests of verbal fluency. Thus, patients with AD show more impairment on category fluency (eg, generating lists of animals) than letter fluency (eg, generating words beginning with a specific letter).[313,322,323] The fact that patients with AD are more impaired on the fluency task, which places greater demands on the integrity of semantic memory, is consistent with the assumption that their structure and organization of semantic memory has deteriorated, rather than having a general inability to retrieve or access semantic knowledge.[324,325] It is suggested by studies of semantic memory in patients with AD that some conceptual domains may be more impaired than others; in particular, that patients with AD have a specific impairment in the conceptual domain of living things. For example, in studies assessing confrontation naming[318,326] and picture recognition, patients with mild to moderate AD performed significantly worse in the category of living things than in the category of nonliving things.

VISUAL FUNCTION

Visual sensory functions are reported to be impaired in AD, including spatial contrast sensitivity,[327–330] color, stereopsis, temporal resolution,[331,332] and motion.[333,334] Visual attention[200,203] and higher visual functions such as reading, route finding, object localization, and recognition[335–339] can also be affected in AD. Through a better understanding of these vision-related deficits, diagnosis, interpretation of cognitive scores, and interventions could be aided to improve functional capacity in patients with AD.[340] On tests of static spatial contrast sensitivity, visual attention, shape from motion, color, visuospatial construction, and visual memory, patients with AD have been shown to perform significantly worse. AD affects several aspects of vision, which is compatible with the hypothesis that visual dysfunction in AD may contribute to declines in performance in other cognitive domains.[327]

EXECUTIVE FUNCTION

Executive functions generally mean higher-level cognitive functions that are involved in the control and regulation of lower-level cognitive processes and goal-directed, future-oriented behavior. Having been dubbed the most subtle and central realm of human activity, executive function is particularly important to assess because it is affected in most types of dementia.[341] The term executive function is an umbrella term denoting various complex cognitive processes and subprocesses. Most attempts to define executive function end up with a list of examples (such as decision making, task switching, planning, organization, fluency, abstract reasoning, solving novel problems, modifying behavior in the light of new information, generating strategies, or sequencing complex actions and skills such as mental flexibility and response inhibition) or that other useful umbrella term, working memory, which indicates that executive function is in no way a unitary concept.[342,343] Funahashi[344] summarized executive function as "a product of the coordinated operation of various processes to accomplish a particular goal in a flexible manner." It is the responsibility of executive control systems to achieve a specific goal through this flexible coordination of subprocesses. The neuropsychological literature is in agreement that successful performance on tests of executive function is critically dependent on the frontal cortex; the terms executive function and frontal lobe function are often used interchangeably. Moreover, PFC has been indicated to be critical for performing executive function tasks, through lesion studies and structural and functional neuroimaging studies.[345–348] However, it has recently been suggested that this view is simplistic; more recent theories point to the critical involvement of subcortical regions as well. Direct assessment of the neuronal basis of executive functions has been made possible through advances in neuroimaging. Perhaps unsurprisingly, these complex processes seem to be subsumed by distributed circuitry structures rather than discrete structures.[342] It is not necessary to evaluate specialized cognitive functions during all screening mental state examinations in the primary care setting. However, in certain primary care situations, some tests of specialized cognitive functions can be included and should often be included in screening by subspecialists. These tests include assessment of calculations, reasoning, problem solving, abstraction, agnosia, neglect, praxis, insight, and judgment. Some of these domains that include calculations are to be as complex as the patient's level of education or highest function allows.[32,349] The ability to generate verbal or nonverbal responses is another aspect of executive functioning. Verbal fluency is discussed earlier, but the executive component of these types of tasks is that they require the patient to generate novel responses in accordance with a set of rules (eg, to say or write words or create designs following a rule set). Executive function impairments are evident on these tasks in a reduction of ability or inability to generate responses, difficulties maintaining cognitive set (eg, when instructed to say as many "A" words as possible, a patient says a word beginning with another letter), and perseverative errors (ie, repeating previously stated responses). Impairments in executive functions that are responsible for the mental manipulation of information, concept formation, problem solving, and cue-directed behavior manifest early in the course of AD and are often evident in the MCI stage.[111,134] Initially, an alteration in executive function ability was not recognized among patients with AD, because early studies did not implement sensitive tests of executive function. Once sensitive tests of executive function began to be used to evaluate mildly impaired patients with AD, these impairments became apparent. For example, mildly impaired patients showed impairment on tasks that involved coordinating 2 concurrent tasks,[350] as well as tasks that required shifting between stimulus dimensions.[204] Mildly to moderately impaired patients also show executive function deficits.[351–353] Several studies have tried to determine whether impairment in executive function precedes significant deficits in spatial and language function or coexists with them. These studies have compared very mildly impaired patients with AD with controls on tasks assessing a range of cognitive domains. It was reported by Grady and colleagues[354] that deficits on tasks of memory and executive function preceded impairments in language. Lafleche and Albert[355] attempted to describe the specific aspect of executive function in which very mildly impaired patients with AD showed impairment. The investigators assessed a spectrum of executive abilities, including set shifting and self-monitoring (ie, the concurrent manipulation of information), cue-directed attention (eg, the ability to use cues to direct attention), and concept formation (eg, abstraction). The tasks that required set shifting and self-monitoring revealed the most significant deficit.

By contrast, patients did not show major impairment on tasks that assessed cue-directed attention and verbal concept formation. Similarly, no impairment was registered in performance on the tests of confrontation naming, figure copying, and sustained attention. These findings, taken together, suggest that very early in the course of the disease selected aspects of executive function are affected, particularly those involving set shifting and self-monitoring.

However, no consensus exists regarding whether during prodromal AD executive function deficits are prominent. The inconsistencies among studies are, at least partially, caused by the shortage of studies that have examined a wide variety of cognitive domains, and thus the types of associations that can be found are limited. Several studies have reported that, in the prodromal stage of AD, executive function abnormalities are shown.[64,134] Other studies have reported that people destined to develop AD are more likely to show declines in confrontation naming (eg, Ref.[356]). These discrepancies remain to be resolved. The brain abnormalities associated with executive function deficits that are seen among individuals destined to develop AD are also unclear. At least 2 potential neurobiological explanations have been put forth. During prodromal AD, findings from functional imaging indicate that dysfunction exists within a brain network that involves the dorsolateral PFC and the anterior cingulate.[357] An alternative possibility is that the disruption of the corticocortical connections that are seen in AD, and that are not specific to the frontal lobes,[358] may be responsible for executive dysfunction. In addition to difficulties with delayed memory recall, executive function deficits predict subsequent progression to AD dementia.[221] A well-controlled study has shown that very mildly demented patients with AD were significantly impaired relative to cognitively normal controls on tests that required set shifting, self-monitoring, or sequencing, but not on tests that required cue-directed attention or verbal problem solving. Thus, this study suggests that reduced ability to mentally manipulate information may be a particularly early feature of AD.[355] Similarly, several other studies have also shown that patients with AD are impaired on difficult problem solving tests that require mental manipulation, such as the Tower of London puzzle,[359] the modified Wisconsin Card Sorting Task,[360] tests of relational integration,[361] and other tests of executive functions such as the Porteus Maze Task, part B of the Trail Making Test, and the Raven Progressive Matrices.[354] It has been hypothesized that these deficits in executive functioning reflect features of AD, especially neurofibrillary tangle burden, in PFC. This regional PFC disorder is particularly noticeable in a subset of patients with AD who predominantly present executive dysfunction in an early stage.[361,362] This finding again highlights the influence of anatomically specific findings on the disruption of distinct neocortical networks. Among the cognitive domains, some might be less known to neurologists, such as mental flexibility and the inhibition response (**Box 14**).

MENTAL FLEXIBILITY

One of the best tests to evaluate attention and cognitive flexibility is the Trail Making Test,[363] which is widely administered. In the part A of this test, patients are asked to connect a series of numbered circles arbitrarily distributed on a page. In part B, the patient is asked to alternate between connecting numbers and letters in a series (see **Table 1**). The scores are derived from the time the patient takes to complete each part. This test is principally sensitive to the progressive cognitive decline in dementia.[364] Poor performance on part B by an elderly person is likely to be associated with problems performing complex activities in daily living.[365]

Box 14
Keynotes in cognitive assessment for clinicians[253]

- Symptoms in cognitive disorders correspond with location, and not findings on pathology. Thus, for example, in AD, instead of the more commonly appreciated autobiographical memory disturbance, patients may show a focal language syndrome, despite identical pathology findings.

- Overall, the cognitive examination is intended to single out those patients for whom a definitive clinical diagnosis can be made from those who require further and more thorough investigations.

- It is essential to have access to the perspective of a reliable informant, because memory disturbance and impaired insight are commonly seen.

- Time is always an issue in any crowded clinic. In general, an hour is needed for a full cognitive assessment, including performance of various cognitive rating scales. Regardless of the time available, a clear focus is needed early in the consultation. This focus directs attention to the relevant cognitive domains that are in need of specific and more detailed examination.

- Skillful examiners often integrate their assessment into a natural, comfortable conversation with a patient, rendering it more enjoyable for both. Many of the specific tests described in this article can be modified into this style of assessment.

- It is impractical to examine everything exhaustively in the cognitive assessment, and, similar to most other areas of neurology, the patient's history remains preeminent in guiding the subsequent examination.

- What distinguishes this means of neurologic assessment is the central role of an informant, and the ability to immediately test hypotheses that are generated during the history taking.

- In some patients, it is not possible to reach a definitive diagnosis after a single cognitive assessment, despite having access to a formal neuropsychological report. This situation chiefly arises in the mild stages of neurodegenerative diseases, and is reflective of the relative insensitivity of both clinical and imaging assessment to early disorder. In such cases, the time-honored method of longitudinal follow-up and repeated assessment is invaluable, and should not be forgotten.

Data from Kipps C, Hodges J. Cognitive assessment for clinicians. J Neurol Neurosurg Psychiatr 2005;76(Suppl 1):i22–30.

INHIBITION RESPONSE

Through inhibition the patient is required to suppress an overlearned response or a noticeable environmental stimulus. To assess inhibition, Stroop interference tests are widely used. In this paradigm, patients are shown a series of color names printed in different color ink (eg, the word "RED" printed in blue ink). The patient is supposed to inhibit the overlearned tendency to read the word and instead name the color of the ink in which the word is printed. In other tasks, such as opposite responding, patients are required to inhibit their response to a salient stimulus and provide a competing response. Executive functions can be informally assessed by observing for signs of disinhibition, such as frequently interrupting or making socially inappropriate comments. Moreover, patients with executive dysfunction also commonly have difficulty shifting from one task to another. This difficulty can be observed during interview: when the topic of conversation or task changes, the patient might show difficulty, be perseverative, or have poor mental flexibility. Elements of executive function can be formally assessed by asking the patient to alternate between reciting or drawing lines on a piece of paper between 2 sequences (eg, alternate between counting by 7s and recite the months of the year; alternate between stating the letters of the alphabet starting at A and ending at Z and counting numbers from 1 to 26; alternate between connecting numbers and letters on a page, as in the Trail Making Test part B).[366] With regard to executive and administrative functions, reasoning, judgment, insight, and decision making, patients with AD experience progressive difficulties that often manifest in daily challenges. Such challenges are faced in organization, planning, problem solving, social interactions, doing or completing familiar tasks at home and at work, and making suitable judgments and decisions, and include the patients' appreciation of the extent and nature of their cognitive, functional, and behavioral changes and limitations.[32] Some individuals experience changes in their ability to develop and follow a plan; work with numbers and money; follow a familiar recipe; or keep track of and manage monthly bills, finances, and tax records. Patients may become less efficient or effective while accomplishing tasks that they previously did, or may have great difficulty learning how to handle new tools or procedures. For example, relative to the past, the work they produce may consistently be of inferior quality, to accomplish a task might not be as effortless or as time-efficient as before, or they may be unable to satisfactorily learn a new system or procedure (eg, writing a report, managing a budget, learning a new computer program or work flow at work). They may also frequently have difficulty with concentration, be easily distractible, and often lose their train of thought. In addition, they may manifest deterioration in their ability to comprehend information, manipulate it, and make important connections and deductions necessary to make reasoned judgments and appropriate decisions. For example, they may have poor judgment when dealing with money; give large amounts to telemarketers, strangers, or associates; make poor purchases; display major changes in their spending; and not fully grasp that their ability to function and make decisions has changed (ie, have anosognosia). In addition, they may be less able to temper their affect, have poor impulse control and insight with regard to their behavior, and become less aware of proper grooming and hygiene. Differentiation of the age-related cognitive deficits from very mild AD is one of the great challenges that clinicians face. Normal cognitive aging does not preclude occasionally making an error while balancing the checkbook; being late with a check; having to look up a recipe; needing greater time or help to use a new device, tool, or program; having to be reminded of details of a conversation; or sometimes losing concentration and being distracted during a task. However, the frequency of these occurrences is significantly greater in AD. Making an occasional poor decision, being easily distracted (especially in the context of multitasking or not being present in the moment), or making an occasional careless mistake is normal.

SUMMARY

Neuropsychology has made a crucial contribution to the characterization of the dementia associated with the neurologic disorder of AD, its differentiation from cognitive changes associated with normal aging, and its distinction from dementias related to other types of neurologic disorder. The earliest neuropsychological symptoms of a dementia reflect their associated neuroanatomic systems; however, the relationship between the symptoms and the underlying disease is less obvious. Therefore, in early stages, neuropsychological profiles are most informative.[367] It is true that the accumulation of fluid and neuroimaging biomarkers will improve diagnosis and ultimately be used to measure the efficacy of the treatment. However, neuropsychological characterization continues to be of essential importance in understanding the individual patient's deficits and be valuable as a noninvasive, inexpensive and available method. The implementation of such an approach might be influential in the development of more sophisticated diagnostic procedures and aid in more appropriate selection of nonpharmacologic and/or pharmacologic interventions.

ACKNOWLEDGMENTS

The valuable editing of this work by Dr Shahrzad Irannejad is greatly appreciated.

REFERENCES

1. Kandel E. Principles of neural science. 5th edition. McGraw-Hill Education; 2013.
2. Ritchie K, Lovestone S. The dementias. Lancet 2002;360(9347):1759–66.
3. Katzman R. The prevalence and malignancy of Alzheimer disease: a major killer. Arch Neurol 1976;33(4):217–8.
4. Wortmann M. Dementia: a global health priority - highlights from an ADI and World Health Organization report. Alzheimers Res Ther 2012;4(5):40.
5. Ravaglia G, Forti P, De Ronchi D, et al. Prevalence and severity of dementia among northern Italian centenarians. Neurology 1999;53(2):416–8.
6. Thomassen R, van Schaick HW, Blansjaar BA. Prevalence of dementia over age 100. Neurology 1998;50(1):283–6.
7. Lobo A, Launer LJ, Fratiglioni L, et al. Prevalence of dementia and major subtypes in Europe: a collaborative study of population-based cohorts. Neurologic Diseases in the Elderly Research Group. Neurology 2000;54(11 Suppl 5):S4–9.
8. Tijms BM, Moller C, Vrenken H, et al. Single-subject grey matter graphs in Alzheimer's disease. PLoS One 2013;8(3):e58921.
9. Weintraub S, Wicklund AH, Salmon DP. The neuropsychological profile of Alzheimer disease. Cold Spring Harb Perspect Med 2012;2(4):a006171.
10. Flicker C, Bartus RT, Crook TH, et al. Effects of aging and dementia upon recent visuospatial memory. Neurobiol Aging 1985;5(4):275–83.
11. Storandt M. Neuropsychological assessment in Alzheimer's disease. Exp Aging Res 1991;17(2):100–1.
12. Locascio JJ, Growdon JH, Corkin S. Cognitive test performance in detecting, staging, and tracking Alzheimer's disease. Arch Neurol 1995;52(11):1087–99.
13. Salmon DP, Bondi MW. Neuropsychological assessment of dementia. Annu Rev Psychol 2009;60:257–82.
14. Daviglus ML, Bell CC, Berrettini W, et al. National Institutes of Health State-of-the-Science Conference statement: preventing Alzheimer disease and cognitive decline. Ann Intern Med 2010;153(3):176–81.
15. Kok E, Haikonen S, Luoto T, et al. Apolipoprotein E–dependent accumulation of Alzheimer disease–related lesions begins in middle age. Ann Neurol 2009; 65(6):650–7.
16. Ghebremedhin E, Schultz C, Braak E, et al. High frequency of apolipoprotein E epsilon4 allele in young individuals with very mild Alzheimer's disease-related neurofibrillary changes. Exp Neurol 1998;153(1):152–5.
17. Sugarman MA, Woodard JL, Nielson KA, et al. Functional magnetic resonance imaging of semantic memory as a presymptomatic biomarker of Alzheimer's disease risk. Biochim Biophys Acta 2012;1822(3):442–56.
18. Kraepelin E. Psychiatrie; ein Lehrbuch für Studierende und Ärzte, vol. 3. Barth (Germany); 1914.
19. Maurer K, Volk S, Gerbaldo H. Auguste D and Alzheimer's disease. Lancet 1997;349(9064):1546–9.

20. Braak H, Braak E. Neuropathological stageing of Alzheimer-related changes. Acta Neuropathol 1991;82(4):239–59.
21. Jack CR, Petersen RC, Xu YC, et al. Medial temporal atrophy on MRI in normal aging and very mild Alzheimer's disease. Neurology 1997;49(3): 786–94.
22. de Toledo-Morrell L, Goncharova I, Dickerson B, et al. From healthy aging to early Alzheimer's disease: in vivo detection of entorhinal cortex atrophy. Ann N Y Acad Sci 2000;911(1):240–53.
23. Braak H, Braak E. Development of Alzheimer-related neurofibrillary changes in the neocortex inversely recapitulates cortical myelogenesis. Acta Neuropathol 1996;92(2):197–201.
24. Braak H, Braak E. Evolution of the neuropathology of Alzheimer's disease. Acta Neurol Scand 1996;94(S165):3–12.
25. Braak E, Arai K, Braak H. Cerebellar involvement in Pick's disease: affliction of mossy fibers, monodendritic brush cells, and dentate projection neurons. Exp Neurol 1999;159(1):153–63.
26. Jack C, Petersen R, Xu Y, et al. Rates of hippocampal atrophy correlate with change in clinical status in aging and AD. Neurology 2000;55(4):484–90.
27. McKhann G, Drachman D, Folstein M, et al. Clinical diagnosis of Alzheimer's disease Report of the NINCDS-ADRDA Work Group* under the auspices of Department of Health and Human Services Task Force on Alzheimer's Disease. Neurology 1984;34(7):939.
28. McKhann GM, Knopman DS, Chertkow H, et al. The diagnosis of dementia due to Alzheimer's disease: recommendations from the National Institute on Aging-Alzheimer's Association workgroups on diagnostic guidelines for Alzheimer's disease. Alzheimers Dement 2011;7(3):263–9.
29. Albert MS, DeKosky ST, Dickson D, et al. The diagnosis of mild cognitive impairment due to Alzheimer's disease: recommendations from the National Institute on Aging-Alzheimer's Association workgroups on diagnostic guidelines for Alzheimer's disease. Alzheimers Dement 2011;7(3):270–9.
30. Sperling RA, Aisen PS, Beckett LA, et al. Toward defining the preclinical stages of Alzheimer's disease: recommendations from the national institute on aging-Alzheimer's Association workgroups on diagnostic guidelines for Alzheimer's disease. Alzheimers Dement 2011;7(3):280–92.
31. Rubin EH, Storandt M, Miller JP, et al. A prospective study of cognitive function and onset of dementia in cognitively healthy elders. Arch Neurol 1998;55(3): 395–401.
32. Dickerson B, Atri A. Dementia: comprehensive principles and practice. New York: Oxford University Press; 2014.
33. Park DC, Smith AD, Lautenschlager G, et al. Mediators of long-term memory performance across the life span. Psychol Aging 1996;11(4):621.
34. Moran JM, Jolly E, Mitchell JP. Social-cognitive deficits in normal aging. J Neurosci 2012;32(16):5553–61.
35. Strub RL, Black FW. The mental status examination in neurology. FA Davis Company; 2000.
36. Daroff RB. Bradley's neurology in clinical practice: principles of diagnosis and management. Philadelphia: Elsevier Saunders; 2012.
37. Baddeley A. Working memory. Curr Biol 2010;20(4):R136–40.
38. Goldman-Rakic PS, Cools A, Srivastava K. The prefrontal landscape: implications of functional architecture for understanding human mentation and the central executive [and discussion]. Philos Trans R Soc B Biol Sci 1996;351(1346):1445–53.

39. Squire LR, Zola SM. Structure and function of declarative and nondeclarative memory systems. Proc Natl Acad Sci U S A 1996;93(24):13515–22.
40. Dickerson BC, Eichenbaum H. The episodic memory system: neurocircuitry and disorders. Neuropsychopharmacology 2010;35(1):86–104.
41. Budson AE, Price BH. Memory dysfunction. N Engl J Med 2005;352(7):692–9.
42. Squire LR, Zola-Morgan S. The medial temporal lobe memory system. Science 1991;253(5026):1380–6.
43. Tulving E. Organization of memory: Quo vadis?. In: Gazzaniga MS, editor. The Cognitive Neurosciences. Chapter 54. Cambridge (MA): MIT Press; 1995. p. 839–47.
44. Tulving E. Episodic and semantic memory 1. Organ Mem Lond Acad 1972; 381(e402):4.
45. Ashcraft MH. Cognitive psychology and simple arithmetic: a review and summary of new directions. Math Cognit 1995;1(1):3–34.
46. Albert ML, Feldman RG, Willis AL. The 'subcortical dementia' of progressive supranuclear palsy. J Neurol Neurosurg Psychiatr 1974;37(2):121–30.
47. Massman PJ, Delis DC, Butters N, et al. Are all subcortical dementias alike?: Verbal learning and memory in Parkinson's and Huntington's disease patients. J Clin Exp Neuropsychol 1990;12(5):729–44.
48. Storandt M, Hill RD. Very mild senile dementia of the Alzheimer type: II. Psychometric test performance. Arch Neurol 1989;46(4):383–6.
49. Wilson RS, Bacon LD, Fox JH, et al. Primary memory and secondary memory in dementia of the Alzheimer type. J Clin Exp Neuropsychol 1983;5(4): 337–44.
50. Fox NC, Schott JM. Imaging cerebral atrophy: normal ageing to Alzheimer's disease. Lancet 2004;363(9406):392–4.
51. Herholz K. PET studies in dementia. Ann Nucl Med 2003;17(2):79–89.
52. Corkin S. Functional MRI for studying episodic memory in aging and Alzheimer's disease. Geriatrics 1998;53(Suppl 1):S13–5.
53. Rombouts SA, Barkhof F, Veltman DJ, et al. Functional MR imaging in Alzheimer's disease during memory encoding. AJNR Am J Neuroradiol 2000; 21(10):1869–75.
54. Buckner R, Snyder A, Sanders A, et al. Functional brain imaging of young, non-demented, and demented older adults. J Cogn Neurosci 2000;12(Supplement 2):24–34.
55. Saykin AJ, Johnson SC, Flashman LA, et al. Functional differentiation of medial temporal and frontal regions involved in processing novel and familiar words: an fMRI study. Brain 1999;122(10):1963–71.
56. Squire LR. Memory and the hippocampus: a synthesis from findings with rats, monkeys, and humans. Psychol Rev 1992;99(2):195–231.
57. Köhler S, Black S, Sinden M, et al. Memory impairments associated with hippocampal versus parahippocampal-gyrus atrophy: an MR volumetry study in Alzheimer's disease. Neuropsychologia 1998;36(9):901–14.
58. Delis DC, Kaplan E, Kramer JH. Delis-Kaplan executive function system (D-KEFS). Psychological Corporation; 2001.
59. Rey A. L'examen psychologique dans les cas d'encéphalopathie traumatique. (Les problems.). Arch Psychol 1941;28:215–85.
60. Lezak MD. Neuropsychological assessment. New York: Oxford University Press; 2004.
61. Cullum CM, Thompson LL, Smernoff EN. Three-word recall as a measure of memory. J Clin Exp Neuropsychol 1993;15(2):321–9.

62. Moss MB, Albert MS, Butters N, et al. Differential patterns of memory loss among patients with Alzheimer's disease, Huntington's disease, and alcoholic Korsakoff's syndrome. Arch Neurol 1986;43(3):239–46.
63. Milberg W, Albert M. Cognitive differences between patients with progressive supranuclear palsy and Alzheimer's disease. J Clin Exp Neuropsychol 1989; 11(5):605–14.
64. Albert MS, Moss MB, Tanzi R, et al. Preclinical prediction of AD using neuropsychological tests. J Int Neuropsychol Soc 2001;7(05):631–9.
65. Chen P, Ratcliff G, Belle S, et al. Cognitive tests that best discriminate between presymptomatic AD and those who remain nondemented. Neurology 2000; 55(12):1847–53.
66. Howieson D, Camicioli R, Quinn J, et al. Natural history of cognitive decline in the old old. Neurology 2003;60(9):1489–94.
67. Kluger A, Ferris SH, Golomb J, et al. Neuropsychological prediction of decline to dementia in nondemented elderly. J Geriatr Psychiatry Neurol 1999;12(4): 168–79.
68. Petersen R, Smith G, Ivnik R, et al. Memory function in very early Alzheimer's disease. Neurology 1994;44(5):867.
69. Cappa SF. Imaging studies of semantic memory. Curr Opin Neurol 2008;21(6): 669–75.
70. McCarthy RA, Warrington EK. Cognitive neuropsychology: a clinical introduction. San Diego (CA): Academic Press; 1990.
71. Weingartner HJ, Kawas C, Rawlings R, et al. Changes in semantic memory in early stage Alzheimer's disease patients. Gerontologist 1993;33(5): 637–43.
72. Randolph C, Braun AR, Goldberg TE, et al. Semantic fluency in Alzheimer's, Parkinson's, and Huntington's disease: dissociation of storage and retrieval failures. Neuropsychology 1993;7(1):82.
73. Monsch AU, Bondi MW, Butters N, et al. A comparison of category and letter fluency in Alzheimer's disease and Huntington's disease. Neuropsychology 1994;8(1):25.
74. Rosser A, Hodges JR. Initial letter and semantic category fluency in Alzheimer's disease, Huntington's disease, and progressive supranuclear palsy. J Neurol Neurosurg Psychiatr 1994;57(11):1389–94.
75. Fleischman DA, Gabrieli JD. Repetition priming in normal aging and Alzheimer's disease: a review of findings and theories. Psychol Aging 1998;13(1):88.
76. Salmon DP, Heindel WC, Butters N. Semantic memory, priming, and skill learning in Alzheimer's disease. In: Bäckman, Lars, editors. Memory functioning in dementia. Advances in psychology. Oxford (England): North Holland; 1992. p. 99–118.
77. Rascovsky K, Salmon DP, Hansen LA, et al. Disparate letter and semantic category fluency deficits in autopsy-confirmed frontotemporal dementia and Alzheimer's disease. Neuropsychology 2007;21(1):20.
78. Terry RD, Katzman RK. Senile dementia of the Alzheimer type. Ann Neurol 1983; 14(5):497–506.
79. Mickanin J, Grossman M, Onishi K, et al. Verbal and nonverbal fluency in patients with probable Alzheimer's disease. Neuropsychology 1994;8(3): 385.
80. Beatty WW, Testa JA, English S, et al. Influences of clustering and switching on the verbal fluency performance of patients with Alzheimer's disease. Aging Neuropsychol Cognit 1997;4(4):273–9.

81. Ober BA, Dronkers NF, Koss E, et al. Retrieval from semantic memory in Alzheimer-type dementia. J Clin Exp Neuropsychol 1986;8(1):75–92.
82. Tröster AI, Fields JA, Testa JA, et al. Cortical and subcortical influences on clustering and switching in the performance of verbal fluency tasks. Neuropsychologia 1998;36(4):295–304.
83. Sailor KM, Bramwell A, Griesing TA. Evidence for an impaired ability to determine semantic relations in Alzheimer's disease patients. Neuropsychology 1998;12(4):555.
84. Hodges JR, Patterson K. Is semantic memory consistently impaired early in the course of Alzheimer's disease? Neuroanatomical and diagnostic implications. Neuropsychologia 1995;33(4):441–59.
85. Hodges JR, Salmon DP, Butters N. Differential impairment of semantic and episodic memory in Alzheimer's and Huntington's diseases: a controlled prospective study. J Neurol Neurosurg Psychiatr 1990;53(12):1089–95.
86. Almkvist O, Bäckman L. Detection and staging of early clinical dementia. Acta Neurol Scand 1993;88(1):10–5.
87. Aggarwal N, Wilson R, Beck T, et al. Mild cognitive impairment in different functional domains and incident Alzheimer's disease. J Neurol Neurosurg Psychiatr 2005;76(11):1479–84.
88. Trachtenberg AJ, Filippini N, Mackay CE. The effects of APOE-ε4 on the BOLD response. Neurobiol Aging 2012;33(2):323–34.
89. Bondi MW, Kaszniak AW. Implicit and explicit memory in Alzheimer's disease and Parkinson's disease. J Clin Exp Neuropsychol 1991;13(2):339–58.
90. Irle E, Kaiser P, Naumann-Stoll G. Differential patterns of memory loss in patients with Alzheimer's disease and Korsakoff's disease. Int J Neurosci 1990;52(1–2):67–77.
91. Petersen RC, Smith GE, Waring SC, et al. Mild cognitive impairment: clinical characterization and outcome. Arch Neurol 1999;56(3):303–8.
92. Petersen R, Stevens J, Ganguli M, et al. Practice parameter: Early detection of dementia: mild cognitive impairment (an evidence-based review) report of the quality standards subcommittee of the American Academy of Neurology. Neurology 2001;56(9):1133–42.
93. Nilsson LG. Memory function in normal aging. Acta Neurol Scand 2003;107(s179):7–13.
94. Bookheimer SY, Strojwas MH, Cohen MS, et al. Patterns of brain activation in people at risk for Alzheimer's disease. N Engl J Med 2000;343(7):450–6.
95. Persson J, Nyberg L, Lind J, et al. Structure-function correlates of cognitive decline in aging. Cereb Cortex 2006;16(7):907–15.
96. O'Brien J, O'Keefe K, LaViolette P, et al. Longitudinal fMRI in elderly reveals loss of hippocampal activation with clinical decline. Neurology 2010;74(24):1969–76.
97. Baird A, Samson S. Memory for music in Alzheimer's disease: unforgettable? Neuropsychol Rev 2009;19(1):85–101.
98. Gabrieli JD, Corkin S, Mickel SF, et al. Intact acquisition and long-term retention of mirror-tracing skill in Alzheimer's disease and in global amnesia. Behav Neurosci 1993;107(6):899–910.
99. Knopman D. Unaware learning versus preserved learning in pharmacologic amnesia: similarities and differences. J Exp Psychol Learn Mem Cogn 1991;17(5):1017.
100. Miller G, Galanter E, Pribram KH. Plans and the structure of behavior. New York: Books on Demand; 1960.

101. Atkinson RC, Shiffrin RM. Human memory: a proposed system and its control processes. Psychol Learn Motiv 1968;2:89–195.
102. Baddeley AD, Hitch G. Working memory. Psychol Learn Motiv 1974;8:47–89.
103. Baddeley A. Working memory: theories, models, and controversies. Annu Rev Psychol 2012;63:1–29.
104. Baddeley A. The episodic buffer: a new component of working memory? Trends Cogn Sci 2000;4(11):417–23.
105. Baddeley A. Working memory: looking back and looking forward. Nature reviews. Neuroscience 2003;4(10):829–39.
106. Baddeley A, Bressi S, Della Sala S, et al. The decline of working memory in Alzheimer's disease. Brain 1991;114(6):2521–42.
107. Collette F, Van der Linden M, Salmon E. Executive dysfunction in Alzheimer's disease. Cortex 1999;35(1):57–72.
108. Kaschel R, Logie RH, Kazén M, et al. Alzheimer's disease, but not ageing or depression, affects dual-tasking. J Neurol 2009;256(11):1860–8.
109. Baddeley AD, Bressi S, Della Sala S, et al. The decline of working memory in Alzheimer's disease. A longitudinal study. Brain 1991;114(Pt 6):2521–42.
110. Parasuraman R, Haxby JV. Attention and brain function in Alzheimer's disease: a review. Neuropsychology 1993;7(3):242.
111. Perry RJ, Hodges JR. Attention and executive deficits in Alzheimer's disease. A critical review. Brain 1999;122(3):383–404.
112. Cherry BJ, Buckwalter JG, Henderson VW. Better preservation of memory span relative to supraspan immediate recall in Alzheimer's disease. Neuropsychologia 2002;40(7):846–52.
113. Kramer JH, Schuff N, Reed BR, et al. Hippocampal volume and retention in Alzheimer's disease. J Int Neuropsychol Soc 2004;10(04):639–43.
114. Perry R, Hodges J. Differentiating frontal and temporal variant frontotemporal dementia from Alzheimer's disease. Neurology 2000;54(12):2277–84.
115. Ala TA, Hughes LF, Kyrouac GA, et al. The mini-mental state exam may help in the differentiation of dementia with Lewy bodies and Alzheimer's disease. Int J Geriatr Psychiatry 2002;17(6):503–9.
116. Kramer JH, Jurik J, Sharon JS, et al. Distinctive neuropsychological patterns in frontotemporal dementia, semantic dementia, and Alzheimer disease. Cogn Behav Neurol 2003;16(4):211–8.
117. Diehl J, Monsch A, Aebi C, et al. Frontotemporal dementia, semantic dementia, and Alzheimer's disease: the contribution of standard neuropsychological tests to differential diagnosis. J Geriatr Psychiatry Neurol 2005;18(1):39–44.
118. Wicklund AH, Johnson N, Rademaker A, et al. Word list versus story memory in Alzheimer disease and frontotemporal dementia. Alzheimer Dis Assoc Disord 2006;20(2):86–92.
119. Welsh K, Butters N, Hughes J, et al. Detection of abnormal memory decline in mild cases of Alzheimer's disease using CERAD neuropsychological measures. Arch Neurol 1991;48(3):278–81.
120. Delis DC, Massman PJ, Butters N, et al. Profiles of demented and amnesic patients on the California Verbal Learning Test: implications for the assessment of memory disorders. Psychol Assess 1991;3(1):19.
121. Butters N, Salmon DP, Cullum CM, et al. Differentiation of amnesic and demented patients with the Wechsler Memory Scale-Revised. Clin Neuropsychol 1988;2(2):133–48.
122. Knopman DS, Ryberg S. A verbal memory test with high predictive accuracy for dementia of the Alzheimer type. Arch Neurol 1989;46(2):141–5.

123. Tröster AI, Butters N, Salmon DP, et al. The diagnostic utility of savings scores: differentiating Alzheimer's and Huntington's diseases with the logical memory and visual reproduction tests. J Clin Exp Neuropsychol 1993;15(5):773–88.
124. Fuld PA, Katzman R, Davies P, et al. Intrusions as a sign of Alzheimer dementia chemical and pathological verification. Ann Neurol 1982;11(2):155–9.
125. Jacobs D, Salmon DP, Tröster AI, et al. Intrusion errors in the figural memory of patients with Alzheimer's and Huntington's disease. Arch Clin Neuropsychol 1990;5(1):49–57.
126. Dalla Barba G, Wong C. Encoding specificity and intrusion in Alzheimers-disease and amnesia. Brain Cogn 1995;27(1):1–16.
127. Dalla Barba G, Goldblum M-C. The influence of semantic encoding on recognition memory in Alzheimer's disease. Neuropsychologia 1996;34(12):1181–6.
128. Bondi MW, Monsch AU, Galasko D, et al. Preclinical cognitive markers of dementia of the Alzheimer type. Neuropsychology 1994;8(3):374.
129. Jacobs DM, Sano M, Dooneief G, et al. Neuropsychological detection and characterization of preclinical Alzheimer's disease. Neurology 1995;45(5):957–62.
130. Howieson DB, Dame A, Camicioli R, et al. Cognitive markers preceding Alzheimer's dementia in the healthy oldest old. J Am Geriatr Soc 1997;45(5):584–9.
131. Small BJ, Fratiglioni L, Viitanen M, et al. The course of cognitive impairment in preclinical Alzheimer disease: three- and 6-year follow-up of a population-based sample. Arch Neurol 2000;57(6):839–44.
132. Kawas C, Corrada M, Brookmeyer R, et al. Visual memory predicts Alzheimer's disease more than a decade before diagnosis. Neurology 2003;60(7):1089–93.
133. Bäckman L, Small BJ, Fratiglioni L. Stability of the preclinical episodic memory deficit in Alzheimer's disease. Brain 2001;124(1):96–102.
134. Chen P, Ratcliff G, Belle SH, et al. Patterns of cognitive decline in presymptomatic Alzheimer disease: a prospective community study. Arch Gen Psychiatry 2001;58(9):853–8.
135. Lange KL, Bondi MW, Salmon DP, et al. Decline in verbal memory during preclinical Alzheimer's disease: examination of the effect of APOE genotype. J Int Neuropsychol Soc 2002;8(07):943–55.
136. Java RI, Gardiner JM. Priming and aging: further evidence of preserved memory function. Am J Psychol 1991;104:89–100.
137. Jelicic M. Effects of ageing on different explicit and implicit memory tasks. Eur J Cognit Psychol 1996;8(3):225–34.
138. BÄCkman L, Wahlin A. Influences of item organizability and semantic retrieval cues on word recall in very old age. Aging Neuropsychol Cognit 1995;2(4):312–25.
139. Hart RP, Colenda CC, Dougherty LM, et al. Recall of clustered and unclustered word lists in elderly adults. J Clin Psychol 1992;48(3):341–54.
140. Monti LA, Gabrieli JD, Reminger SL, et al. Differential effects of aging and Alzheimer's disease on conceptual implicit and explicit memory. Neuropsychology 1996;10(1):101.
141. La Voie D, Light LL. Adult age differences in repetition priming: a meta-analysis. Psychol Aging 1994;9(4):539.
142. Chertkow H, Bub D. Semantic memory loss in dementia of Alzheimer's type what do various measures measure? Brain 1990;113(2):397–417.
143. Russo R, Spinnler H. Implicit verbal memory in Alzheimer's disease. Cortex 1994;30(3):359–75.

144. Abbenhuis MA, Raaijmakers W, Raaijmakers J, et al. Episodic memory in dementia of the Alzheimer type and in normal ageing: similar impairment in automatic processing. Q J Exp Psychol 1990;42(3):569–83.

145. Deweer B, Pillon B, Michon A, et al. Mirror reading in Alzheimer's disease: normal skill learning and acquisition of item-specific information. J Clin Exp Neuropsychol 1993;15(5):789–804.

146. Eslinger PJ, Damasio AR. Preserved motor learning in Alzheimer's disease: implications for anatomy and behavior. J Neurosci 1986;6(10):3006–9.

147. Grosse DA, Wilson RS, Fox JH. Preserved word-stem-completion priming of semantically encoded information in Alzheimer's disease. Psychol Aging 1990;5(2):304.

148. Koivisto M, Portin R, Rinne JO. Perceptual priming in Alzheimer's and Parkinson's diseases. Neuropsychologia 1996;34(5):449–57.

149. Greene JD, Baddeley AD, Hodges JR. Analysis of the episodic memory deficit in early Alzheimer's disease: evidence from the doors and people test. Neuropsychologia 1996;34(6):537–51.

150. Keane MM, Gabrieli JD, Growdon JH, et al. Priming in perceptual identification of pseudowords is normal in Alzheimer's disease. Neuropsychologia 1994; 32(3):343–56.

151. Helkala E-L, Laulumaa V, Soininen H, et al. Different error pattern of episodic and semantic memory in Alzheimer's disease and Parkinson's disease with dementia. Neuropsychologia 1989;27(10):1241–8.

152. Brandt J, Corwin J, Krafft L. Is verbal recognition memory really different in Huntington's and Alzheimer's disease? J Clin Exp Neuropsychol 1992;14(5): 773–84.

153. Bayles KA, Kaszniak AW, Tomoeda CK. Communication and cognition in normal aging and dementia. Boston (MA): College-Hill Press/Little, Brown; 1987.

154. Elias MF, Beiser A, Wolf PA, et al. The preclinical phase of Alzheimer disease: a 22-year prospective study of the Framingham Cohort. Arch Neurol 2000;57(6): 808–13.

155. Linn RT, Wolf PA, Bachman DL, et al. The preclinical phase of probable Alzheimer's disease: a 13-year prospective study of the Framingham cohort. Arch Neurol 1995;52(5):485–90.

156. Almkvist O. Neuropsychological features of early Alzheimer's disease: preclinical and clinical stages. Acta Neurol Scand 1996;94(S165):63–71.

157. Masur DM, Sliwinski M, Lipton R, et al. Neuropsychological prediction of dementia and the absence of dementia in healthy elderly persons. Neurology 1994; 44(8):1427.

158. Newman S, Warrington E, Kennedy A, et al. The earliest cognitive change in a person with familial Alzheimer's disease: presymptomatic neuropsychological features in a pedigree with familial Alzheimer's disease confirmed at necropsy. J Neurol Neurosurg Psychiatr 1994;57(8):967–72.

159. Small BJ, Herlitz A, Fratiglioni L, et al. Cognitive predictors of incident Alzheimer's disease: a prospective longitudinal study. Neuropsychology 1997;11(3):413.

160. Fabrigoule C, Lafont S, Letenneur L, et al. WAIS similarities subtest performances as predictors of dementia in elderly community residents. Brain Cogn 1996;30(3):323–6.

161. Grober E, Kawas C. Learning and retention in preclinical and early Alzheimer's disease. Psychol Aging 1997;12(1):183.

162. Dartigues J, Commenges D, Letenneur L, et al. Cognitive predictors of dementia in elderly community residents. Neuroepidemiology 1997;16(1):29–39.

163. Almkvist O, Bråne G, Johanson A. Neuropsychological assessment of dementia: state of the art. Acta Neurol Scand 1996;94(s168):45–9.
164. Morris JC, McKeel D, Storandt M, et al. Very mild Alzheimer's disease: informant-based clinical, psychometric, and pathologic distinction from normal aging. Neurology 1991;41(4):469.
165. Collie A, Maruff P. The neuropsychology of preclinical Alzheimer's disease and mild cognitive impairment. Neurosci Biobehav Rev 2000;24(3):365–74.
166. Heaton RK, Grant I, Matthews CG. Comprehensive norms for an expanded Halstead-Reitan battery: demographic corrections, research findings, and clinical applications; with a supplement for the Wechsler Adult Intelligence Scale-Revised (WAIS-R). Odessa (FL): Psychological Assessment Resources; 1991.
167. Grober E, Lipton RB, Hall C, et al. Memory impairment on free and cued selective reminding predicts dementia. Neurology 2000;54(4):827–32.
168. Zonderman AB, Giambra LM, Arenberg D, et al. Changes in immediate visual memory predict cognitive impairment. Arch Clin Neuropsychol 1995;10(2):111–23.
169. Folstein MF, Folstein SE, McHugh PR. "Mini-mental state": a practical method for grading the cognitive state of patients for the clinician. J Psychiatr Res 1975; 12(3):189–98.
170. Crum RM, Anthony JC, Bassett SS, et al. Population-based norms for the Mini-Mental State Examination by age and educational level. JAMA 1993;269(18): 2386–91.
171. Wilson RS, Gilley DW, Bennett DA, et al. Person-specific paths of cognitive decline in Alzheimer's disease and their relation to age. Psychol Aging 2000; 15(1):18.
172. Jefferson AL, Cosentino SA, Ball SK, et al. Errors produced on the Mini-Mental State Examination and neuropsychological test performance in Alzheimer's disease, ischemic vascular dementia, and Parkinson's disease. J Neuropsychiatry Clin Neurosci 2002;14(3):311–20.
173. Mungas D, Reed BR, Kramer JH. Psychometrically matched measures of global cognition, memory, and executive function for assessment of cognitive decline in older persons. Neuropsychology 2003;17(3):380.
174. Jefferson AL, Paul RH, Ozonoff A, et al. Evaluating elements of executive functioning as predictors of instrumental activities of daily living (IADLs). Arch Clin Neuropsychol 2006;21(4):311–20.
175. Reisberg B, Finkel S, Overall J, et al. The Alzheimer's disease Activities of Daily Living International Scale (ADL-IS). Int Psychogeriatr 2001;13(02):163–81.
176. Cahn-Weiner DA, Malloy PF, Boyle PA, et al. Prediction of functional status from neuropsychological tests in community-dwelling elderly individuals. Clin Neuropsychol 2000;14(2):187–95.
177. Cahn-Weiner DA, Boyle PA, Malloy PF. Tests of executive function predict instrumental activities of daily living in community-dwelling older individuals. Appl Neuropsychol 2002;9(3):187–91.
178. Cahn-Weiner DA, Ready RE, Malloy PF. Neuropsychological predictors of everyday memory and everyday functioning in patients with mild Alzheimer's disease. J Geriatr Psychiatry Neurol 2003;16(2):84–9.
179. Boyle PA, Malloy PF, Salloway S, et al. Executive dysfunction and apathy predict functional impairment in Alzheimer disease. Am J Geriatr Psychiatry 2003;11(2): 214–21.
180. Noroozian M, Shakiba A, Iran-Nejad S. The impact of illiteracy on the assessment of cognition and dementia: a critical issue in the developing countries. Int Psychogeriatr 2014;26(12):2051–60.

181. Widmann CN, Beinhoff U, Riepe MW. Everyday memory deficits in very mild Alzheimer's disease. Neurobiol Aging 2012;33(2):297–303.
182. Hodges JR. Alzheimer's centennial legacy: origins, landmarks and the current status of knowledge concerning cognitive aspects. Brain 2006;129(11):2811–22.
183. Van Der Elst W, Van Boxtel MP, Van Breukelen GJ, et al. Rey's Verbal Learning Test: normative data for 1855 healthy participants aged 24–81 years and the influence of age, sex, education, and mode of presentation. J Int Neuropsychol Soc 2005;11(03):290–302.
184. Norman MA, Evans JD, Miller WS, et al. Demographically corrected norms for the California Verbal Learning Test. J Clin Exp Neuropsychol 2000;22(1):80–94.
185. Chaytor N, Schmitter-Edgecombe M. The ecological validity of neuropsychological tests: a review of the literature on everyday cognitive skills. Neuropsychol Rev 2003;13(4):181–97.
186. Simic G, Kostovic I, Winblad B, et al. Volume and number of neurons of the human hippocampal formation in normal aging and Alzheimer's disease. J Comp Neurol 1997;379(4):482–94.
187. Arnold SE, Hyman BT, Flory J, et al. The topographical and neuroanatomical distribution of neurofibrillary tangles and neuritic plaques in the cerebral cortex of patients with Alzheimer's disease. Cereb Cortex 1991;1(1):103–16.
188. Lewis DA, Campbell MJ, Terry RD, et al. Laminar and regional distributions of neurofibrillary tangles and neuritic plaques in Alzheimer's disease: a quantitative study of visual and auditory cortices. J Neurosci 1987;7(6):1799–808.
189. Golby A, Silverberg G, Race E, et al. Memory encoding in Alzheimer's disease: an fMRI study of explicit and implicit memory. Brain 2005;128(4):773–87.
190. Small SA, Perera GM, DeLaPaz R, et al. Differential regional dysfunction of the hippocampal formation among elderly with memory decline and Alzheimer's disease. Ann Neurol 1999;45(4):466–72.
191. Grön G, Bittner D, Schmitz B, et al. Subjective memory complaints: objective neural markers in patients with Alzheimer's disease and major depressive disorder. Ann Neurol 2002;51(4):491–8.
192. Sperling R, Bates J, Chua E, et al. fMRI studies of associative encoding in young and elderly controls and mild Alzheimer's disease. J Neurol Neurosurg Psychiatr 2003;74(1):44–50.
193. Ellis AW. Normality and pathology in cognitive functions. London: Academic Press; 1982.
194. Warrington EK, James M, Maciejewski C. The WAIS as a lateralizing and localizing diagnostic instrument: A study of 656 patients with unilateral cerebral lesions. Neuropsychologia 1986;24(2):223–39.
195. Nielson KA, Cummings BJ, Cotman CW. Constructional apraxia in Alzheimer's disease correlates with neuritic neuropathology in occipital cortex. Brain Res 1996;741(1):284–93.
196. Rapcsak SZ, Ochipa C, Anderson KC, et al. Progressive ideomotor apraxia - evidence for a selective impairment of the action production system. Brain Cogn 1995;27(2):213–36.
197. Fernandez-Duque D, Black SE. Selective attention in early dementia of Alzheimer type. Brain Cogn 2008;66(3):221–31.
198. Rizzo M, Anderson S, Dawson J, et al. Visual attention impairments in Alzheimer's disease. Neurology 2000;54(10):1954–9.
199. Ober BA, Jagust WJ, Koss E, et al. Visuoconstructive performance and regional cerebral glucose metabolism in Alzheimer's disease. J Clin Exp Neuropsychol 1991;13(5):752–72.

200. Parasuraman R, Greenwood PM, Haxby JV, et al. Visuospatial attention in dementia of the Alzheimer type. Brain 1992;115(3):711–33.
201. Della Sala S, Lucchelli F, Spinnler H. Ideomotor apraxia in patients with dementia of Alzheimer type. J Neurol 1987;234(2):91–3.
202. Nebes RD, Brady CB. Focused and divided attention in Alzheimer's disease. Cortex 1989;25(2):305–15.
203. Nestor PG, Parasuraman R, Haxby JV, et al. Divided attention and metabolic brain dysfunction in mild dementia of the Alzheimer's type. Neuropsychologia 1991;29(5):379–87.
204. Filoteo JV, Delis DC, Massman PJ, et al. Directed and divided attention in Alzheimer's disease: impairment in shifting of attention to global and local stimuli. J Clin Exp Neuropsychol 1992;14(6):871–83.
205. Zomeren AH, Brouwer WH. Clinical neuropsychology of attention. New York: Oxford University Press; 1994.
206. Rapoport S. Positron emission tomography in Alzheimer's disease in relation to disease pathogenesis: a critical review. Cerebrovasc Brain Metab Rev 1990;3(4):297–335.
207. Braak H, Braak E. Alzheimer's disease affects limbic nuclei of the thalamus. Acta Neuropathol 1991;81(3):261–8.
208. LaPointe LL. Aphasia and related neurogenic language disorders. New York: Thieme; 2011.
209. LaBarge E, Smith DS, Dick L, et al. Agraphia in dementia of the Alzheimer type. Arch Neurol Nov 1992;49(11):1151–6.
210. Horner J, Heyman A, Dawson D, et al. The relationship of agraphia to the severity of dementia in Alzheimer's disease. Arch Neurol Jul 1988;45(7):760–3.
211. Henderson VW, Buckwalter JG, Sobel E, et al. The agraphia of Alzheimer's disease. Neurology 1992;42(4):777–84.
212. Croisile B, Carmoi T, Adeleine P, et al. Spelling in Alzheimer's disease. Behav Neurol 1995;8(3–4):135–43.
213. Crossley M, Hiscock M, Foreman JB. Dual-task performance in early stage dementia: differential effects for automatized and effortful processing. J Clin Exp Neuropsychol 2004;26(3):332–46.
214. Roeltgen DP, Lacey EH. Alexias and agraphias. The roots of cognitive neuroscience: behavioral neurology and neuropsychology. New York: Oxford University Press; 2013. p. 89.
215. Fernandez-Duque D, Black SE. Attentional networks in normal aging and Alzheimer's disease. Neuropsychology 2006;20(2):133.
216. Levinoff EJ, Saumier D, Chertkow H. Focused attention deficits in patients with Alzheimer's disease and mild cognitive impairment. Brain Cogn 2005;57(2):127–30.
217. Festa EK, Heindel WC, Ott BR. Dual-task conditions modulate the efficiency of selective attention mechanisms in Alzheimer's disease. Neuropsychologia 2010;48(11):3252–61.
218. Giannakopoulos P, Duc M, Gold G, et al. Pathologic correlates of apraxia in Alzheimer disease. Arch Neurol 1998;55(5):689–95.
219. Johannsen P, Jakobsen J, Bruhn P, et al. Cortical responses to sustained and divided attention in Alzheimer's disease. Neuroimage 1999;10(3):269–81.
220. Waters GS, Caplan D, Rochon E. Processing capacity and sentence comprehension in patients with Alzheimer's disease. Cogn Neuropsychol 1995;12(1):1–30.
221. Albert MS. Cognitive and neurobiologic markers of early Alzheimer disease. Proc Natl Acad Sci U S A 1996;93(24):13547–51.

222. Perry RJ, Watson P, Hodges JR. The nature and staging of attention dysfunction in early (minimal and mild) Alzheimer's disease: relationship to episodic and semantic memory impairment. Neuropsychologia 2000;38(3):252–71.
223. Keefe JO, Nadel L. The hippocampus as a cognitive map. Oxford (United Kingdom): Clarendon Press; 1978.
224. Moscovitch M, Rosenbaum RS, Gilboa A, et al. Functional neuroanatomy of remote episodic, semantic and spatial memory: a unified account based on multiple trace theory. J Anat 2005;207(1):35–66.
225. Cabeza R, Nyberg L. Imaging cognition II: An empirical review of 275 PET and fMRI studies. J Cogn Neurosci 2000;12(1):1–47.
226. Grön G, Bittner D, Schmitz B, et al. Variability in memory performance in aged healthy individuals: an fMRI study. Neurobiol Aging 2003;24(3):453–62.
227. Cushman LA, Stein K, Duffy CJ. Detecting navigational deficits in cognitive aging and Alzheimer disease using virtual reality. Neurology 2008;71(12):888–95.
228. Treisman A. The binding problem. Curr Opin Neurobiol 1996;6(2):171–8.
229. Foster J, Behrmann M, Stuss D. Visual attention deficits in Alzheimer's disease: simple versus conjoined feature search. Neuropsychology 1999;13(2):223.
230. Parasuraman R, Greenwood PM, Alexander GE. Selective impairment of spatial attention during visual search in Alzheimer's disease. Neuroreport 1995;6(14): 1861–4.
231. Parasuraman R, Greenwood PM, Alexander GE. Alzheimer disease constricts the dynamic range of spatial attention in visual search. Neuropsychologia 2000;38(8):1126–35.
232. Burack JA. Attention, Development, and Psychopathology. In: Greenwood PM, Parasuraman R, editors. Attention in aging and Alzheimer's disease: Behavior and neural systems. Chapter 12. Guilford Press; 1997. p. 288–317.
233. Parasuraman R. The attentive brain. In: Greenwood PM, Parasuraman R, editors. Selective attention in aging and dementia. Chapter 21. Cambridge (MA): The MIT Press; 1998. p. xii, 577.
234. Mapstone M, Steffenella TM, Duffy CJ. A visuospatial variant of mild cognitive impairment: getting lost between aging and AD. Neurology 2003;60(5):802–8.
235. Fatehi F, Nafissi S, Noroozian M, et al. P53: Blink reflex: differentiating between Alzheimer disease and vascular dementia. Clin Neurophysiol 2014;125:S63–4.
236. Karrasch M, Sinervä E, Grönholm P, et al. CERAD test performances in amnestic mild cognitive impairment and Alzheimer's disease. Acta Neurol Scand 2005; 111(3):172–9.
237. Rouleau I, Salmon DP, Butters N, et al. Quantitative and qualitative analyses of clock drawings in Alzheimer's and Huntington's disease. Brain Cogn 1992;18(1): 70–87.
238. Kurylo DD, Corkin S, Growdon JH. Perceptual organization in Alzheimer's disease. Psychol Aging 1994;9(4):562.
239. Rouleau I, Salmon DP, Butters N. Longitudinal analysis of clock drawing in Alzheimer's disease patients. Brain Cogn 1996;31(1):17–34.
240. Heinik J, Solomesh I, Shein V, et al. Clock drawing test in mild and moderate dementia of the Alzheimer's type: a comparative and correlation study. Int J Geriatr Psychiatry 2002;17(5):480–5.
241. Powlishta K, Von Dras D, Stanford A, et al. The clock drawing test is a poor screen for very mild dementia. Neurology 2002;59(6):898–903.
242. Seigerschmidt E, Mösch E, Siemen M, et al. The clock drawing test and questionable dementia: reliability and validity. Int J Geriatr Psychiatry 2002;17(11): 1048–54.

243. Nasreddine ZS, Phillips NA, Bédirian V, et al. The Montreal Cognitive Assessment, MoCA: a brief screening tool for mild cognitive impairment. J Am Geriatr Soc 2005;53(4):695–9.
244. Noroozian M. The role of the cerebellum in cognition: beyond coordination in the central nervous system. Neurol Clin 2014;32(4):1081–104.
245. Miller BL, Boeve BF. The behavioral neurology of dementia. New York: Cambridge University Press; 2009.
246. Hof PR, Vogt BA, Bouras C, et al. Atypical form of Alzheimer's disease with prominent posterior cortical atrophy: a review of lesion distribution and circuit disconnection in cortical visual pathways. Vision Res 1997;37(24):3609–25.
247. Davie JE, Azuma T, Goldinger SD, et al. Sensitivity to expectancy violations in healthy aging and mild cognitive impairment. Neuropsychology 2004;18(2):269.
248. Zamarian L, Semenza C, Domahs F, et al. Alzheimer's disease and mild cognitive impairment: effects of shifting and interference in simple arithmetic. J Neurol Sci 2007;263(1–2):79–88.
249. Jackson GM, Jackson SR, Harrison J, et al. Serial reaction time learning and Parkinson's disease: evidence for a procedural learning deficit. Neuropsychologia 1995;33(5):577–93.
250. Campbell JI. Mechanisms of simple addition and multiplication: a modified network-interference theory and simulation. Math Cognit 1995;1(2):121–64.
251. Verguts T, Fias W. Interacting neighbors: a connectionist model of retrieval in single-digit multiplication. Mem Cognit 2005;33(1):1–16.
252. Ochipa C, Rothi LJG, Heilman KM. Conceptual apraxia in Alzheimer's disease. Brain 1992;115(4):1061–71.
253. Kipps C, Hodges J. Cognitive assessment for clinicians. J Neurol Neurosurg Psychiatr 2005;76(Suppl 1):i22–30.
254. Kleist K. Kortikale (innervatorische) apraxie. Jahrbuch für Psychiatrie und Neurologie 1907;28:46–112.
255. Zadikoff C, Lang AE. Apraxia in movement disorders. Brain 2005;128(7):1480–97.
256. Fukui T, Sugita K, Kawamura M, et al. Primary progressive apraxia in Pick's disease a clinicopathologic study. Neurology 1996;47(2):467–73.
257. Tsuchiya K, Ikeda K, Uchihara T, et al. Distribution of cerebral cortical lesions in corticobasal degeneration: a clinicopathological study of five autopsy cases in Japan. Acta Neuropathol 1997;94(5):416–24.
258. De Renzi E, Lucchelli F. Ideational apraxia. Brain 1988;111(5):1173–85.
259. Kertesz A, Ferro JM. Lesion size and location in ideomotor apraxia. Brain 1984;107(3):921–33.
260. Azouvi P, Bergego C, Robell L, et al. Slowly progressive apraxia: two case studies. J Neurol 1993;240(6):347–50.
261. Rapcsak SZ, Croswell SC, Rubens AB. Apraxia in Alzheimer's disease. Neurology 1989;39(5):664.
262. Liepmann H. Apraxie. Ergb Gesamte Med 1920;1:519–43.
263. Giannakopoulos P, Gold G, Duc M, et al. Neuroanatomic correlates of visual agnosia in Alzheimer's disease: a clinicopathologic study. Neurology 1999;52(1):71–7.
264. Ceccaldi M, Poncet M, Gambarelli D, et al. Progressive severity of left unilateral apraxia in 2 cases of Alzheimer disease. Rev Neurol (Paris) 1995;151(4):240–6 [in French].
265. Hier DB, Mondlock J, Caplan LR. Recovery of behavioral abnormalities after right hemisphere stroke. Neurology 1983;33(3):345.

266. Schnider A, Hanlon RE, Alexander DN, et al. Ideomotor apraxia: behavioral dimensions and neuroanatomical basis. Brain Lang 1997;58(1):125–36.
267. Johnen A, Tokaj A, Kirschner A, et al. Apraxia profile differentiates behavioural variant frontotemporal from Alzheimer's dementia in mild disease stages. J Neurol Neurosurg Psychiatr 2014;86(7):809–15.
268. Cotelli M, Manenti R, Brambilla M, et al. Limb apraxia and verb processing in Alzheimer's disease. J Clin Exp Neuropsychol 2014;36(8):843–53.
269. Förstl H, Burns A, Levy R, et al. Neuropathological basis for drawing disability (constructional apraxia) in Alzheimer's disease. Psychol Med 1993;23(03): 623–9.
270. Troyer AK. Normative data for clustering and switching on verbal fluency tasks. J Clin Exp Neuropsychol 2000;22(3):370–8.
271. Ruff RM, Light RH, Evans RW. The Ruff Figural Fluency Test: a normative study with adults. Dev Neuropsychol 1987;3(1):37–51.
272. Tariq S, Tumosa N, Chibnall J, et al. The Saint Louis University Mental Status (SLUMS) examination for detecting mild cognitive impairment and dementia is more sensitive than the Mini-Mental Status Examination (MMSE)–a pilot study. Am J Geriatr Psychiatry 2006;14(11):900–10.
273. Mathuranath P, Nestor P, Berrios G, et al. A brief cognitive test battery to differentiate Alzheimer's disease and frontotemporal dementia. Neurology 2000; 55(11):1613–20.
274. Mioshi E, Dawson K, Mitchell J, et al. The Addenbrooke's Cognitive Examination revised (ACE-R): a brief cognitive test battery for dementia screening. Int J Geriatr Psychiatry 2006;21(11):1078–85.
275. Dahlgren DJ. Impact of knowledge and age on tip-of-the-tongue rates. Exp Aging Res 1998;24(2):139–53.
276. Heine MK, Ober BA, Shenaut GK. Naturally occurring and experimentally induced tip-of-the-tongue experiences in three adult age groups. Psychol Aging 1999;14(3):445.
277. Schwartz BL, Metcalfe J. Tip-of-the-tongue (TOT) states: retrieval, behavior, and experience. Mem Cognit 2011;39(5):737–49.
278. Brown AS. The tip of the tongue state. New York: Taylor & Francis; 2012.
279. Schwartz BL, Brown AS. Tip-of-the-tongue states and related phenomena. New York: Cambridge University Press; 2014.
280. Carbone G, Barreca F, Mancini G, et al. A home assistance model for dementia: outcome in patients with mild-to-moderate Alzheimer's disease after three months. Ann Ist Super Sanita 2013;49(1):34–41.
281. Ricci S, Fuso A, Ippoliti F, et al. Stress-induced cytokines and neuronal dysfunction in Alzheimer's disease. J Alzheimers Dis 2012;28(1):11–24.
282. Onofri E, Mercuri M, Salesi M, et al. Cognitive performance deficits and dysgraphia in Alzheimer's disease patients. J Neurol Neurophysiol 2014;5:223.
283. Stelzmann RA, Norman Schnitzlein H, Reed Murtagh F. An English translation of Alzheimer's 1907 paper,"Über eine eigenartige Erkankung der Hirnrinde". Clin Anat 1995;8(6):429–31.
284. Croisile B. Writing, aging and Alzheimer's disease. Psychol Neuropsychiatr Vieil 2005;3(3):183–97 [in French].
285. Lambert J, Giffard B, Nore F, et al. Central and peripheral agraphia in Alzheimer's disease: from the case of Auguste D. to a cognitive neuropsychology approach. Cortex 2007;43(7):935–51.
286. Kumar V, Giacobini E. Use of agraphia in subtyping of Alzheimer's disease. Arch Gerontol Geriatr 1990;11(2):155–9.

287. Kemper S, LaBarge E, Ferraro FR, et al. On the preservation of syntax in Alzheimer's disease. Evidence from written sentences. Arch Neurol 1993;50(1):81–6.
288. Neils J, Boller F, Gerdeman B, et al. Descriptive writing abilities in Alzheimer's disease. J Clin Exp Neuropsychol 1989;11(5):692–8.
289. Heilman MDKM, Valenstein E. Clinical neuropsychology. New York: Oxford University Press; 2011.
290. Fukui T, Lee E. Progressive agraphia can be a harbinger of degenerative dementia. Brain Lang 2008;104(3):201–10.
291. Neils-Strunjas J, Groves-Wright K, Mashima P, et al. Dysgraphia in Alzheimer's disease: a review for clinical and research purposes. J Speech Lang Hear Res 2006;49(6):1313–30.
292. Hughes JC, Graham N, Patterson K, et al. Dysgraphia in mild dementia of Alzheimer's type. Neuropsychologia 1997;35(4):533–45.
293. Small JA, Sandhu N. Episodic and semantic memory influences on picture naming in Alzheimer's disease. Brain Lang 2008;104(1):1–9.
294. Yasuda K, Beckmann B, Nakamura T. Brain processing of proper names. Aphasiology 2000;14(11):1067–89.
295. Silveri MC, Corda F, Di Nardo M. Central and peripheral aspects of writing disorders in Alzheimer's disease. J Clin Exp Neuropsychol 2007;29(2):179–86.
296. Croisile B, Brabant M-J, Carmoi T, et al. Comparison between oral and written spelling in Alzheimer's disease. Brain Lang 1996;54(3):361–87.
297. Yoon JH, Kim H, Seo SW, et al. Dysgraphia in Korean patients with Alzheimer's disease as a manifestation of bilateral hemispheric dysfunction. J Neurol Sci 2012;320(1):72–8.
298. Hayashi A, Nomura H, Mochizuki R, et al. Neural substrates for writing impairments in Japanese patients with mild Alzheimer's disease: A SPECT study. Neuropsychologia 2011;49(7):1962–8.
299. Sakurai Y, Mimura I, Mannen T. Agraphia for kanji resulting from a left posterior middle temporal gyrus lesion. Behav Neurol 2008;19(3):93–106.
300. Sakurai Y, Onuma Y, Nakazawa G, et al. Parietal dysgraphia: characterization of abnormal writing stroke sequences, character formation and character recall. Behav Neurol 2007;18(2):99–114.
301. Yaguchi H, Yaguchi M, Bando M. A case of pure agraphia due to left parietal lobe infarction. No To Shinkei 2006;58(10):885–92 [in Japanese].
302. Archer T. Physical exercise alleviates debilities of normal aging and Alzheimer's disease. Acta Neurol Scand 2011;123(4):221–38.
303. Archer T, Kostrzewa RM. Staging neurological disorders: expressions of cognitive and motor disorder. Neurotox Res 2010;18(2):107–11.
304. Bonni S, Lupo F, Lo Gerfo E, et al. Altered parietal-motor connections in Alzheimer's disease patients. J Alzheimers Dis 2013;33(2):525–33.
305. Terranova C, SantAngelo A, Morgante F, et al. Impairment of sensory-motor plasticity in mild Alzheimer's disease. Brain Stimul 2013;6(1):62–6.
306. Archer T, Kostrzewa RM, Beninger RJ, et al. Staging neurodegenerative disorders: structural, regional, biomarker, and functional progressions. Neurotox Res 2011;19(2):211–34.
307. Baddeley A, Sala SD, Spinnler H. The two-component hypothesis of memory deficit in Alzheimer's disease. J Clin Exp Neuropsychol 1991;13(2):372–80.
308. Rochon E, Waters GS, Caplan D. Sentence comprehension in patients with Alzheimer' s disease. Brain Lang 1994;46(2):329–49.
309. Grober E, Bang S. Sentence comprehension in Alzheimer's disease. Dev Neuropsychol 1995;11(1):95–107.

310. MacDonald MC, Almor A, Henderson VW, et al. Assessing working memory and language comprehension in Alzheimer's disease. Brain Lang 2001;78(1):17–42.
311. Bowles NL, Obler LK, Albert ML. Naming errors in healthy aging and dementia of the Alzheimer type. Cortex 1987;23(3):519–24.
312. Hodges JR, Salmon DP, Butters N. The nature of the naming deficit in Alzheimer's and Huntington's disease. Brain 1991;114(4):1547–58.
313. Monsch AU, Bondi MW, Butters N, et al. Comparisons of verbal fluency tasks in the detection of dementia of the Alzheimer type. Arch Neurol 1992;49(12):1253–8.
314. Aronoff JM, Gonnerman LM, Almor A, et al. Information content versus relational knowledge: semantic deficits in patients with Alzheimer's disease. Neuropsychologia 2006;44(1):21–35.
315. Craik FI, Salthouse TA. The handbook of aging and cognition. 3rd Edition. New York: Psychology Press; 2011.
316. Hodges JR, Salmon DP, Butters N. Semantic memory impairment in Alzheimer's disease: failure of access or degraded knowledge? Neuropsychologia 1992; 30(4):301–14.
317. Chan AS, Butters N, Paulsen JS, et al. An assessment of the semantic network in patients with Alzheimer's disease. J Cogn Neurosci 1993;5(2):254–61.
318. Grossman M, Robinson K, Biassou N, et al. Semantic memory in Alzheimer's disease: representativeness, ontologic category, and material. Neuropsychology 1998;12(1):34.
319. Chan AS, Butters N, Salmon DP, et al. Comparison of the semantic networks in patients with dementia and amnesia. Neuropsychology 1995;9(2):177.
320. Chan AS, Butters N, Salmon DP. The deterioration of semantic networks in patients with Alzheimer's disease: a cross-sectional study. Neuropsychologia 1997;35(3):241–8.
321. Tippett LJ, Grossman M, Farah MJ. The semantic memory impairment of Alzheimer's disease: category-specific? Cortex 1996;32(1):143–53.
322. Henry JD, Crawford JR, Phillips LH. Verbal fluency performance in dementia of the Alzheimer's type: a meta-analysis. Neuropsychologia 2004;42(9):1212–22.
323. Henry JD, Crawford JR, Phillips LH. A meta-analytic review of verbal fluency deficits in Huntington's disease. Neuropsychology 2005;19(2):243.
324. Rohrer D, Salmon DP, Wixted JT, et al. The disparate effects of Alzheimer's disease and Huntington's disease on semantic memory. Neuropsychology 1999; 13(3):381.
325. Rohrer D, Wixted JT, Salmon DP, et al. Retrieval from semantic memory and its implications for Alzheimer's disease. J Exp Psychol Learn Mem Cogn 1995; 21(5):1127.
326. Silveri MC, Daniele A, Giustolisi L, et al. Dissociation between knowledge of living and nonliving things in dementia of the Alzheimer type. Neurology 1991; 41(4):545.
327. Rizzo M, Anderson SW, Dawson J, et al. Vision and cognition in Alzheimer's disease. Neuropsychologia 2000;38(8):1157–69.
328. Hof PR, Bouras C, Constantinidis J, et al. Selective disconnection of specific visual association pathways in cases of Alzheimer's disease presenting with Balint's syndrome. J Neuropathol Exp Neurol 1990;49(2):168–84.
329. Kéri S, Antal A, Kálmán J, et al. Early visual impairment is independent of the visuocognitive and memory disturbances in Alzheimer's disease. Vision Res 1999;39(13):2261–5.
330. Lakshminarayanan V, Lagrave J, Kean ML, et al. Vision in dementia: contrast effects. Neurol Res 1996;18(1):9–15.

331. Cronin-Golomb A, Corkin S, Rizzo JF, et al. Visual dysfunction in Alzheimer's disease: relation to normal aging. Ann Neurol 1991;29(1):41–52.
332. Cronin-Golomb A, Sugiura R, Corkin S, et al. Incomplete achromatopsia in Alzheimer's disease. Neurobiol Aging 1993;14(5):471–7.
333. Gilmore GC, Wenk HE, Naylor LA, et al. Motion perception and Alzheimer's disease. J Gerontol 1994;49(2):P52–7.
334. Trick GL, Silverman SE. Visual sensitivity to motion age-related changes and deficits in senile dementia of the Alzheimer type. Neurology 1991;41(9):1437.
335. Cronin-Golomb A, Rizzo JF, Corkin S, et al. Visual function in Alzheimer's disease and normal aging. Ann N Y Acad Sci 1991;640:28–35.
336. Kurylo DD, Corkin S, Rizzo JF III, et al. Greater relative impairment of object recognition than of visuospatial abilities in Alzheimer's disease. Neuropsychology 1996;10(1):74.
337. Mendola JD, Cronin-Golomb A, Corkin S, et al. Prevalence of visual deficits in Alzheimer's disease. Optom Vis Sci 1995;72(3):155–67.
338. Pantel J. Alzheimer's disease presenting as slowly progressive aphasia and slowly progressive visual agnosia: two early reports. Arch Neurol 1995;52(1):10.
339. Tetewsky SJ, Duffy CJ. Visual loss and getting lost in Alzheimer's disease. Neurology 1999;52(5):958.
340. Cronin-Golomb A, Corkin S, Growdon JH. Visual dysfunction predicts cognitive deficits in Alzheimer's disease. Optom Vis Sci 1995;72(3):168–76.
341. Barkley RA. Genetics of childhood disorders: XVII. ADHD, Part 1: The executive functions and ADHD. J Am Acad Child Adolesc Psychiatry 2000;39(8):1064–8.
342. Elliott R. Executive functions and their disorders imaging in clinical neuroscience. Br Med Bull 2003;65(1):49–59.
343. Stuss DT, Alexander MP. Executive functions and the frontal lobes: a conceptual view. Psychol Res 2000;63(3–4):289–98.
344. Funahashi S. Neuronal mechanisms of executive control by the prefrontal cortex. Neurosci Res 2001;39(2):147–65.
345. Anderson CV, Bigler ED, Blatter DD. Frontal lobe lesions, diffuse damage, and neuropsychological functioning in traumatic brain-injured patients. J Clin Exp Neuropsychol 1995;17(6):900–8.
346. Baker S, Rogers R, Owen A, et al. Neural systems engaged by planning: a PET study of the Tower of London task. Neuropsychologia 1996;34(6):515–26.
347. Walker R, Husain M, Hodgson T, et al. Saccadic eye movement and working memory deficits following damage to human prefrontal cortex. Neuropsychologia 1998;36(11):1141–59.
348. McMillan C, Gee J, Moore P, et al. Confrontation naming and morphometric analyses of structural MRI in frontotemporal dementia. Dement Geriatr Cogn Disord 2004;17(4):320–3.
349. Griffith H, Belue K, Sicola A, et al. Impaired financial abilities in mild cognitive impairment: a direct assessment approach. Neurology 2003;60(3):449–57.
350. Baddeley A, Logie R, Bressi S, et al. Dementia and working memory. Q J Exp Psychol 1986;38(4):603–18.
351. Bondi MW, Serody AB, Chan AS, et al. Cognitive and neuropathologic correlates of Stroop Color-Word Test performance in Alzheimer's disease. Neuropsychology 2002;16(3):335.
352. Lafleche G, Stuss D, Nelson R, et al. Memory scanning and structured learning in Alzheimer's disease and Parkinson' disease. Can J Aging 1990;9(02):120–34.

353. Morris RG, Baddeley AD. Primary and working memory functioning in Alzheimer-type dementia. J Clin Exp Neuropsychol 1988;10(2):279–96.
354. Grady CL, Haxby J, Horwitz B, et al. Longitudinal study of the early neuropsychological and cerebral metabolic changes in dementia of the Alzheimer type. J Clin Exp Neuropsychol 1988;10(5):576–96.
355. Lafleche G, Albert MS. Executive function deficits in mild Alzheimer's disease. Neuropsychology 1995;9(3):313.
356. Saxton J, Lopez O, Ratcliff G, et al. Preclinical Alzheimer disease Neuropsychological test performance 1.5 to 8 years prior to onset. Neurology 2004;63(12): 2341–7.
357. Milham MP, Erickson KI, Banich MT, et al. Attentional control in the aging brain: insights from an fMRI study of the Stroop task. Brain Cogn 2002;49(3):277–96.
358. Morrison JH, Hof PR. Selective vulnerability of corticocortical and hippocampal circuits in aging and Alzheimer's disease. Prog Brain Res 2002;136:467–86.
359. Lange K, Sahakian B, Quinn N, et al. Comparison of executive and visuospatial memory function in Huntington's disease and dementia of Alzheimer type matched for degree of dementia. J Neurol Neurosurg Psychiatry 1995;58(5): 598–606.
360. Bondi MW, Monsch AU, Butters N, et al. Utility of a modified version of the Wisconsin Card Sorting Test in the detection of dementia of the Alzheimer type. Clin Neuropsychol 1993;7(2):161–70.
361. Waltz JA, Knowlton BJ, Holyoak KJ, et al. Relational integration and executive function in Alzheimer's disease. Neuropsychology 2004;18(2):296.
362. Johnson JK, Head E, Kim R, et al. Clinical and pathological evidence for a frontal variant of Alzheimer disease. Arch Neurol 1999;56(10):1233–9.
363. Reitan RM. Trail Making Test: manual for administration and scoring. South Tucson (AZ): Reitan Neuropsychology Laboratory; 1992.
364. Greenlief CL, Margolis RB, Erker GJ. Application of the Trail Making Test in differentiating neuropsychological impairment of elderly persons. Percept Mot Skills 1985;61(3f):1283–9.
365. Bell-McGinty S, Podell K, Franzen M, et al. Standard measures of executive function in predicting instrumental activities of daily living in older adults. Int J Geriatr Psychiatry 2002;17(9):828–34.
366. Reitan RM, Wolfson D. The Halstead-Reitan neuropsychological test battery: theory and clinical interpretation, vol. 4. Tucson (AZ): Reitan Neuropsychology; 1985.
367. Weintraub S, Morhardt D. Treatment, education, and resources for non-Alzheimer dementia: one size does not fit all. Alzheimer's Care Today 2005; 6(3):201–14.
368. Meyers J. The Meyers Scoring System for the Rey Complex Figure and the recognition trial: professional manual. Odessa (FL): Psychological Assessment Resources; 1995.

Medicinal-Induced Behavior Disorders

Sai Krishna J. Munjampalli, MBBS, Debra E. Davis, MD*

KEYWORDS

- Behavioral • Encephalopathy • Medication • Nervous system • Psychiatric
- Side effects • Toxicity • Withdrawal

KEY POINTS

- The neurobehavioral effects of medications are relatively common and potentially life threatening.
- The nervous system can be affected whether the drug is targeted to treat a brain disorder or not.
- Sometimes the presentation follows a well-known pattern and the toxicity is relatively easy to diagnose.
- Other signs and symptoms may be subtle, not recognized by patients or caregivers, or ignored, leading to prolonged problems and risk of more serious complications.

MEDICATION-INDUCED BEHAVIORAL SIDE EFFECTS

In daily neurology practice, we see patients who present with behavioral changes that may not be explained by the primary diagnosis. Because some of our patients also have psychiatric diagnoses, the practitioner must have an open mind to find the cause of behavioral changes. When the secondary causes are being worked up, a complete list of the medications of each patient should be looked at closely, because medication side effects include behavioral changes. Some medications act as neurotoxins that can cause symptoms and signs along a spectrum that includes mild confusion, attention deficits, mood disturbances, fatigue, cognitive dysfunction, and encephalopathy.[1] Behavioral symptoms may resolve with removal from the exposure. However, depending on the toxin, the dose, and the individual, a single exposure of some toxins can result in permanent deficits. The patient may exhibit insidious symptoms and signs that go unrecognized as being attributed to the exposure and may not manifest until years after exposure begins. Significant recovery can take months or years after removal of the toxin, and recovery may never occur. Almost every group

The authors have nothing to disclose.
Department of Neurology, Louisiana State University Health Sciences Center – Shreveport, 1501 Kings Highway, Shreveport, LA 71103, USA
* Corresponding author.
E-mail address: delli1@lsuhsc.edu

Neurol Clin 34 (2016) 133–169
http://dx.doi.org/10.1016/j.ncl.2015.08.006
0733-8619/16/$ – see front matter © 2016 Elsevier Inc. All rights reserved.

of medications ranging from simple antihypertensive medications to the more complex antineoplastic/immunomodulatory medications, may cause some form of behavioral effects.[2,3] The central nervous system (CNS) is to some extent protected from toxic exposure by the blood–brain barrier (BBB), but remains vulnerable to many toxins nonetheless. Nonpolar lipid-soluble substances gain easiest access and, once that occurs, neurons are easy targets owing to their high lipid content and high metabolism. White matter can also be easily damaged by the lipophilic toxins.[2]

When a patient presents with behavioral changes, the differential diagnosis is initially very broad, and arriving at the correct diagnosis is often a diagnostic challenge. The importance of taking a good history and performing a comprehensive examination cannot be overemphasized. Medication side effects and drug–drug interactions are often overlooked, partly owing to physician oversight and partly owing to the lack of access to the complete medication list. Reviewing both the current and the past medication list is helpful.

CENTRAL NERVOUS SYSTEM TOXICITY

"That guy has delta MS." The meaning of this phrase is easily understood by medical personnel from the lowest levels of training to the most senior clinicians. Unfortunately, however, as a diagnosis it is about as helpful as saying that a patient is sick. Recognition of the syndrome of CNS toxicity is relatively simple; determining the cause and therefore the appropriate management can be a challenge.

A change in mental status can be thought of as too excited (agitation, mania, hallucinosis, psychosis, and seizure) or too sedated (depression, drowsiness, confusion, obtundation, and coma). These can occur in almost any combination, and may wax and wane. The clinician identifies the type as well as other concomitant neurologic and physical findings to steer the diagnostic exploration. These may include autonomic changes such as blood pressure, pulse rate, cardiac arrhythmia, diaphoresis, and pupillary size; or evidence of global neurologic dysfunction such as ataxia, dysarthria, or tremors. **Table 1** lists the major drug classes that affect consciousness.[4]

Depressed Level of Consciousness Owing to Pharmacologic Agents

Ruha and Levine[4] have published a very detailed discussion of the common toxidromes comprising CNS toxicity. In it, they explain that the sedated patient is reacting to an excess of inhibitory influences, most commonly at GABA, opioid, alpha2-adrenergic, and D2 dopaminergic receptors as well as sodium and potassium ion channels. The GABA-A agonists include benzodiazepines, nonbenzodiazepine sedative–hypnotics, barbiturates, meprobamate, ethanol, and anesthetics. Clues as to which agent has been ingested include the degree of sedation (barbiturates are more potent than sedative hypnotics), respiratory depression (barbiturates and opioids more likely), mild hypotension, bradycardia, or hypothermia (implicating a GABA-A agonist), or alternating agitation/sedation which can suggest the toxic effect of a benzodiazepine. GABA-B antagonists include baclofen and gamma hydroxybutirate (GHB). Baclofen causes a complex combination of excitation (seizures, hyperreflexia, clonus, heart arrhythmia) and sedation (bradycardia and hypothermia). GHB has a short half-life and causes a deep coma, which may last several hours, but from which the patient quickly recovers.[4]

The mu opioid agonists (morphine, codeine, heroin, oxycodone, buprenorphine, methadone, fentanyl, and meperidine) cause a classic opioid toxidrome of CNS and respiratory depression with miosis, with or without mild bradycardia, hypotension, or hypothermia. The effects are reversible with naloxone. Comorbid QT prolongation

Table 1 Drugs associated with CNS toxicity	
Class	**Examples**
Alpha-adrenergic antagonists	Reserpine, methyldopa
Antibiotics	Penicillin, aminoglycosides, cephalosporins, others
Anticonvulsants	Carbamazepine, topiramate, levetiracetam, others
Antidepressants	Tricyclics, venlafaxine, SSRIs
Antipsychotics	Chlorpromazine, haloperidol, risperidone, others
Antiretroviral drugs	Zidovudine, didanosine, lamivudine, others
Central alpha-2 agonists	Clonidine, tizanidine
Chemotherapeutic agents	Multiple
Dopamine agonists	Levodopa, ropinirole, pramipexole
GABA receptor agonists	Benzodiazepines
Interferon-alpha agents	Hepatits C treatments
Interferon-beta agents	Disease modulating agents for multiple sclerosis
Lipophilic beta-blockers	Metoprolol, propranolol
Muscarinic receptor antagonists	Atropine, scopolamine
Non-opioid analgesics (high doses)	Salicylates, NSAIDs
Opioid receptor agonists	Morphine, meperidine, tramadol
Serotonergic agents	SSRIs, SNRIs, ergotamine
Steroids	Prednisone, dexamethasone
Sympathomimetics	Cocaine, amphetamine, caffeine

Adapted from Ruha A, Levine M. Central nervous system toxicity. Emerg Med Clin North Am 2014;32:205–21.

suggests methadone (K^+ channel blockade) is the culprit; delirium is associated with meperidine (anticholinergic activity) ingestion, and seizures are associated with meperidine, tramadol, and propoxyphene. Central alpha-2 adrenergic agonists such as clonidine, tizanidine, guanfacine, and dexmedetomidine inhibit norepinephrine release. The clinical syndrome produced with alpha agonist toxicity is the same as that with opioids, with the addition of bradycardia and hypotension, or rarely, hypertension (as with a baclofen pump). Nonopioid analgesics also cause CNS depression. Salicylate toxicity causes confusion, lethargy, and coma along with metabolic disturbances, tachycardia, and tinnitus. Ibuprofen toxicity can lead to coma with metabolic acidosis. Acetaminophen causes coma with metabolic acidosis early, and hepatic encephalopathy later. Children may suffer from CNS depression owing to exposure to tetrahydrocannabinol or cannabis, which is increasingly prescribed as a therapeutic agent in those states in which it is legal.

Both the typical antipsychotics (D2 antagonists), such as haloperidol, droperidol, and the phenothiazines, and the atypical antipsychotics (less D2 antagonism and 5-hydroxytryptophan [5HT] 2A serotonin agonism) such as clozapine, quetiapine, and risperidone, may produce sedation in a dose-dependent fashion. Blockade of cardiac sodium channels with widened QRS intervals or ventricular dysrhythmia is possible with some phenothiazines. Other phenothiazines cause risk of torsades des pointes owing to a prolonged QT interval associated with potassium channel inhibition. Agitated delirium with coma can occur owing to muscarinic antagonism effects of chlorpromazine, clozapine, olanzapine, and quetiapine. Lithium is another antipsychotic medication that causes both excitation and sedation, with gastrointestinal symptoms, CNS depression, confusion, dysarthria, tremor, hyperreflexia, clonus, and seizures. All anticonvulsants are CNS depressants, and can also cause cerebellar dysfunction (ataxia, nystagmus), confusion, and seizures at very high doses. Concomitant cardiac dysrhythmia or heart block occurs with carbamazepine, lamotrigine, and phenytoin (PHT). Topamax can be associated with a non-anion gap acidosis and valproate (VPA) causes hyperammonemia.[4]

Agitation Owing to Pharmacologic Agents

Just as with CNS depression, agitation can present in a spectrum of mild anxiety or severe agitation or "excited delirium syndrome." It can also manifest as restlessness, hallucinations, paranoia, confusion, combativeness, and physical signs of diaphoresis, tachycardia or tachypnea, hypertension, and hyperthermia. There is an increased risk of sudden cardiovascular failure or arrest in the excited delirium syndrome. Medications that are muscarinic acetylcholine antagonists (tricyclic antidepressants [TCAs] and related compounds, atropine and scopolamine), 5HT-2A serotonin agonists (selective serotonin reuptake inhibitors [SSRIs], serotonin–norepinephrine reuptake inhibitors, atypical antidepressants such as trazodone and mirtazapine, monoamine oxidase inhibitors, meperidine, dextromethorphan, linezolid, tramadol, and amphetamines), and sympathomimetics (amphetamine, cocaine) can cause agitated delirium.

Central anticholinergic toxicity with no peripheral anticholinergic symptoms or signs occurs owing to TCAs, cyclobenzaprine, carbamazepine, older H1 antihistamines (diphenhydramine, doxylamine), phenothiazines, some atypical antipsychotics, and belladonna alkaloids (atropine, scopolamine). All other anticholinergics cause an agitated delirium associated with some or all of the following: tachycardia, flushing, mydriasis, constipation, hyperthermia, urinary retention, and dry skin. The TCAs are also dangerous owing to sodium channel inhibition, which causes widening of the QRS interval and ventricular arrhythmias, potassium channel inhibition causing QT prolongation, alpha1 antagonism causing hypotension, and inhibition of norepinephrine and serotonin reuptake causing dysrhythmias and seizures.[4]

Serotonin Syndrome

Serotonin syndrome is a result of overactivation of 5HT2 receptors, causing symptoms of nausea, vomiting, diarrhea, dizziness, anxiety, agitation, or lethargy early on. If it is allowed to continue and persist, it can cause altered levels of consciousness, tachycardia, hypertension, sweating, fever, shivering, tremor, myoclonus, and hyperreflexia with clonus. Life-threatening hyperthermia, muscle rigidity of the lower (more than the upper) extremities, and coma may occur. It is important to distinguish this syndrome from neuroleptic malignant syndrome owing to dopamine toxicity, in which all extremities are involved more equally.[4]

Seizures

There is a fine line between "behavioral" manifestations versus "neurologic" manifestations of drug toxicity. A discussion of seizures is included because there are occasions when the altered awareness from seizures is difficult to distinguish from another psychobiological process. Seizures owing to drug toxicity occur within a few hours of overdose. They are generalized in semiology, brief (minutes), and do not recur after the offending drug is removed. Nonconvulsive status epilepticus (NCSE) has been reported, and this would cause a depressed or altered mental state of unknown cause until an electroencephalogram (EEG) is performed. The list of medications associated with seizures includes benzonatate (a cough suppressant), camphor, buproprion, isoniazid, methylxanthines like caffeine and theophylline, and tramadol.[4]

Workup of the Patient with Central Nervous System Toxicity

There are some laboratory tests and imaging that may be helpful to the clinician in determining if drug toxicity is present in a patient with altered behavior or awareness (**Table 2**). This evaluation may lead the team to the specific offending agent, or may rule in or out other diagnoses. Sometimes such tests are ambiguous, however, such as a leukocytosis, which can be seen in both infection and after a seizure. Metabolic acidosis also accompanies convulsive seizures and can be associated with toxic alcohols. Rhabdomyolysis is seen in prolonged unconsciousness, agitation, or convulsions. If the patient's medication list is available, specific drug levels can be assayed. A urine drug screen is helpful to screen for opioids, barbiturates, cannabis, amphetamines, cocaine, and other substances.

Electrocardiograms help to confirm certain classes of drugs that cause prolonged QT or QRS intervals (sodium or potassium blockers), and rate or rhythm disturbances. A chest x-ray will suggest the presence of aspiration, pneumonia, heart failure, or a tumor, suggesting a paraneoplastic syndrome. A computed tomographic scan of the brain should be performed if there are focal neurologic findings or evidence of trauma. An EEG is helpful if there is suspicion of a seizure. A patient may benefit from a lumbar puncture to rule out subarachnoid hemorrhage or meningoencephalitis.[4]

Patient Management

As with all medical emergencies, the "ABC's" take precedence in patient management. An airway should be secured for patients with depressed consciousness. They should be hooked up to a cardiac monitor and an intravenous (IV) line started for hemodynamic management and medication administration. A urethral catheter is placed, and blood and urine sent to the laboratory. If the patient remains hypotensive after a fluid bolus of 1 to 2 L, norepinephrine is used as a vasopressor to counteract alpha1-adrenergic receptor antagonists. Dopamine is used if the toxin is a known alpha2 agonist. IV thiamine followed by dextrose is given for hypoglycemia. Sodium bicarbonate is given if the electrocardiogram shows QRS prolongation. Activated charcoal can be administered orally or via endogastric tube if the toxin was ingested a short time before admission. Care must be taken to avoid aspiration. All patients should be supported for any sequelae on a telemetry unit or intensive care unit.

Patients who may have been exposed to an opioid should be given naloxone to restore wakefulness and respiration in small enough doses to avoid drug withdrawal symptoms. The half-life of this drug is shorter than most opioids, so it needs to be repeated until the toxicity naturally subsides. Patients with overdose of monoamine oxidase inhibitors, methadone, VPA, or bupropion may have delayed onset of symptoms, and should be watched for a longer period.

Agitated patients may only need reassurance and gentle redirection, but pharmacologic sedation is often needed if that is inadequate to keep the patient quiet. Benzodiazepines are given to start with. If a dopaminergic drug is the intoxicant, then an antipsychotic is used, such as haloperidol or ziprasidone, although they may lower the seizure threshold. Phenobarbital is an option for withdrawal syndromes, taking care to maintain respirations. Dexmedetomidine and ketamine have been used for excited delirium syndrome. Patients with hyperthermia and rigidity are intubated, sedated, and paralyzed, with IV fluids and mechanical cooling.

Table 2
Useful diagnostic tests for altered mental state due to pharmacologic agents

Blood	Urine	Imaging	ECG	EEG	LP
CBC with differential	Drug screen	Chest X-ray	QT prolongation	Focal spikes or sharp waves	Cells
Electrolytes	Immunoassays	CT brain	Arrhythmia	Beta activity	Glucose
Renal/Liver Function	Heavy metals			Triphasic waves	Protein
Creatine phosphokinase	Strychnine			Slowing	Cultures
Thyroid stimulating hormone					PCRs
Prothrombin time					
Serum acetaminophen level					
Serum salicylate level					
Specific drug concentrations (antiepileptic agents, lithium, theophylline)					
Alcohol level					
Ammonia level					
Lead level					

Anticholinergic toxicity can be reversed with physostigmine given slowly over 2 to 3 minutes if there is no history of asthma or seizure disorder or concern for cardiac conduction delay. Care is taken to avoid cholinergic symptoms of vomiting or bronchospasm. Serotonin syndrome responds to supportive care and benzodiazepines most of the time. If there is severe sedation, paralysis and intubation are necessary. An isolated short-duration seizure does not require antiepileptic treatment. Recurrent seizures are treated with IV benzodiazepines first, and then the usual seizure protocol with PHT, or if not agitated then levetiracetam (LVT). Patients toxic with isoniazid or Gyromitra mushrooms will need reversal with pyridoxine.[4]

The different groups of medications that are used regularly and are known to cause significant behavioral changes are discussed in the subsequent sections.

ANTIHYPERTENSIVE AGENT–INDUCED BEHAVIORAL SIDE EFFECTS

Antihypertensive agents are among the most commonly prescribed medications to the general population. Among them, the commonly used β-adrenoreceptor antagonists (ß-blockers) have been reported to cause behavioral side effects such as drowsiness, fatigue, lethargy, sleep disorders, nightmares, depressive moods, and hallucinations. These undesirable actions indicate that ß-blockers affect not only peripheral autonomic activity, but also some CNS function. The various hypothesized centrally mediated actions include local actions on centrally located β-adrenergic receptors, actions on the terminals of "vigilance-enhancing" central noradrenergic pathways, actions of some ß-blockers on 5HT receptors, and other actions including membrane-stabilizing effects. It has been proven that the actions of the ß-blockers depend on various characteristics such as lipophilicity and hydrophilicity, the ratio of antagonist versus (partial) agonist properties, strength of membrane-stabilizing activity, stereospecific affinity, and potency.[3]

Hydrophilic ß-blockers, which appear at low concentrations in brain tissue, are less likely to produce CNS-related side effects than their lipophilic counterparts, which occur at greater concentrations in the brain. The lipophilic ß-blockers include metoprolol, oxprenolol, and propranolol. Examples of hydrophilic ß-blockers are atenolol, nadolol, and carvedilol. A double-blind, crossover study was done to study the behavioral side effects of the commonly used ß-blockers. The hydrophilic ß-blocker atenolol was compared with the lipophilic agents metoprolol and propranolol in 14 patients with a previous history of nightmares or hallucinations. When treated with lipophilic ß-blockers, nightmares or hallucinations were reported by all patients, but by only 3 patients receiving atenolol. The total number of episodes was significantly lower patients receiving atenolol[5] than for those receiving lipophilic ß-blockers.[6] It was concluded that atenolol is significantly less likely to provoke nightmares and hallucinations than are the lipophilic ß-blockers. It seems likely that this finding is owing to the differences in hydrophilicity among these drugs.[7]

Another study was performed to compare the incidence of CNS side effects with atenolol and metoprolol in hypertensive patients who had reported CNS side effects with lipophilic ß-blockers. Eleven women and 6 men completed the study, in which a psychiatric questionnaire was used to detect changes in psychological status and possible CNS side effects. Discontinuation of the original lipophilic ß-blocker produced improvement in quality of sleep, dreams, concentration, memory, energy, and anxiety. No significant CNS side effects were reported with atenolol, but metoprolol caused a significant increase in the incidence of sleep disturbances and restless nights (as well as failure to achieve satisfactory sexual intercourse).[8]

Other Antihypertensive Medications

Other antihypertensive agents commonly reported to cause depression include thiazide diuretics, antiadrenergic agents like clonidine, methyldopa, reserpine, and guanethidine; angiotensin-converting enzyme inhibitors; and calcium-channel blockers. Depression is among the reasons why reserpine, guanethidine, and methyldopa are no longer used.[5,9] There are multiple case reports describing clonidine's role in depression, but this was later refuted by the observation that its incidence was same as in the general population.[10]

OPIOID-INDUCED BEHAVIORAL SIDE EFFECTS

Chronic painful conditions are being increasingly treated with opioid medications in addition to their traditional role in the management of acute pain and cancer-related terminal pain. Psychological addiction, abuse, and diversion of these medications is a growing threat, because these agents are increasingly available to the general public. The commonly reported side effects of opioids include nausea, vomiting, constipation, dizziness, sedation, respiratory depression, tolerance, and physical dependence. Reducing the dose, switching to a different medication, or changing the route of administration may provide benefit when these side effects are seen. Adequate patient screening, proper patient education, and pre-emptive treatment of the side effects will help to maximize the efficacy of these medications.[11]

Opioid Tolerance and Physical Dependence

Tolerance is the loss of analgesic potency, which leads to an increase in the opioid dose requirement over time, with a corresponding decrease in the efficacy of the medication. Physical dependence is an altered physiologic state associated with autonomic and somatic hyperactivity upon opioid withdrawal. Two types of tolerance are reported: innate tolerance, which is determined genetically and present from the initial dosing of the opioid, and acquired tolerance to the pharmacokinetic properties, pharmacodynamics, or learned behavior.[12] Pharmacokinetic tolerance is caused by changes in drug metabolism, such as enzyme induction, after repeated opioid usage. Pharmacodynamic tolerance is caused by decreased effectiveness upon repeated usage of an opioid, possibly related to upregulation of receptors. Learned tolerance results in decreased efficacy of the medication as compensatory mechanisms are learned or incorporated.[13,14] There is a lack of complete cross-tolerance with opioids, which means that tolerance to one opioid does not confer tolerance to other opioids. This needs to be kept in mind when switching to other opioids, because overdosing may be seen even at equianalgesic doses.[15]

Opioid-Induced Hyperalgesia

Hyperalgesia is owing to an increase in pain sensitivity, which leads to increasing requirements of opioids.[16] It may be related to cell apoptosis and formation of metabolites such as morphine 3-gluceronide. Loss of GABA neurons from apoptosis, N-methyl-D-aspartate (NMDA) receptor agonism and glycine-induced postsynaptic inhibition of spinal neurons are postulated to be associated with hyperalgesia.[17,18] Studies done in opioid addicts confirmed that abnormal pain perception from chronic opioid use is a result of hyperalgesia.[19]

Opioid-Induced Sedation

Opioid-induced sedation and drowsiness is caused by anticholinergic activity. This can severely affect quality of life and activity level (and thus undermine the treatment goal). Treatment of opioid-induced sedation includes reduction of dosage, use of psychostimulants, and opioid rotation. Methylphenidate, a psychostimulant, is shown to improve subjective drowsiness and psychomotor performance scores.[20] Even though other treatments like caffeine, donepezil, modafinil, and dextroamphetamine are available, methylphenidate is considered first-line therapy.[21]

Opioid-Induced Sleep Disturbances

Opioids can cause a decrease in sleep efficiency, delta sleep, rapid eye movement (REM) sleep, and total sleep time.[22,23] Unfortunately, these side effects cannot always be differentiated from those caused by underlying diseases like cancer, addiction, dependence, or the pain itself. Cortical arousal and sleep–wake cycles are regulated via input of the brainstem and pontine–cholinergic pathway.[24] The neurotransmitters GABA, dopamine, serotonin, acetylcholine, melatonin, and histamine play a role in the sleep–wake cycle. Altering the balance of these neurotransmitters by any drugs, like opioids, can cause an alteration in the sleep–wake cycle. Morphine inhibits the release of acetylcholine in the medial pontine reticular formation by altering the GABAergic signaling. This alteration reduces the REM sleep duration and the resultant disruption of sleep architecture affects the arousal state during wakefulness.[25]

Psychomotor Performance in Opioid Therapy

The negative effects of opioids on psychomotor and driving performance are reported widely. The patient's ability to operate heavy equipment and drive an automobile may be impaired. Periodic assessment should be done to allow patients to drive, as with any CNS depressant medication.[26] Fishbain and colleagues[27] suggested that opioid-dependent or -tolerant patients on stable dose of opioids showed no impairment of psychomotor ability immediately after a dose of opioid.

ANTIBIOTIC-INDUCED BEHAVIORAL SIDE EFFECTS

Antibiotics are among the most commonly used medications in inpatient and outpatient settings. Various neuropsychiatric side effects are reported that may be dose dependent or idiosyncratic in nature.

Penicillins

Penicillin is known to cause a variety of neuropsychiatric side effects ranging from behavioral changes, seizures, NCSE, encephalopathy, and tardive seizures. Penicillins have a β-lactam ring structure, sharing a similar structure with GABA. This is believed to exert inhibitory effects on GABA transmission, resulting in a lowered seizure threshold.[28] Studies have shown that epileptic potential is lost after this β-lactam ring is cleaved enzymatically.[29] It is hypothesized that penicillins cause CNS disinhibition and lower the seizure threshold by inhibiting both the benzodiazepine receptors and the GABA-A receptor–chloride ionophore complex.[30] CNS kindling is proved to be primarily from GABA antagonism.[31] The risks of penicillin neurotoxicity are high when using higher doses, in patients with preexisting CNS disease, advanced age, IV or intrathecal usage, and renal insufficiency.[32]

Piperacillin-induced encephalopathy is characterized by behavioral changes, progressive confusion, dysarthria, generalized tonic–clonic seizures, and tremor, commonly seen in patients with end-stage renal disease.[33,34]

Hoigné syndrome, reported in 1950, is an acute psychotic reaction after the administration of intramuscular procaine penicillin.[30] After the injection, these patients develop psychiatric symptoms such as anxiety, hallucinations, and autonomic hyperactivity. This "pseudoanaphylactic" reaction lasts for 5 to 30 minutes and has a similar presentation to limbic and temporal lobe seizures. The pathophysiology was initially considered to be owing microembolization of procaine crystals or procaine neurotoxicity. Based on recent research, the current hypothesis is that these behavioral effects may be caused by temporolimbic kindling, owing to the behavioral and physiologic responses seen after repeated stimulation.[31]

Aminoglycosides

The common side effects of aminoglycosides involve ototoxicity and nephrotoxicity. Lesser known side effects include peripheral neuropathy, encephalopathy, and neuromuscular blockade. A case series of patients using gentamicin, who developed peripheral neuropathy and encephalopathy, showed lysosomal abnormalities on nerve biopsies similar to that seen in gentamicin-induced nephrotoxicity.[35] Another case series of patients receiving intrathecal gentamicin showed brain lesions in the pons and mesencephalon. These lesions were characterized by inflammatory reaction, as well as oligodendroglial, astrocytic, and axonal loss.[36]

Cephalosporins

The commonly used cephalosporins are cefuroxime, cefixime, and cefazolin. Their neuropsychiatric side effects include coma, tardive seizures, NCSE, myoclonus, truncal asterixis, and encephalopathy.[37] These effects may occur within 1 to 10 days of starting the medication, and are more frequent in cases of renal insufficiency and preexisting CNS disease. A case series involving 8 patients with renal failure, who developed neurotoxicity after using cephalosporins was reviewed. Patients developed the described myriad of symptoms and EEGs showed diffuse slowing with features of toxic–metabolic encephalopathy, including triphasic waves.[38]

The mechanism of neurotoxicity owing to cephalosporins includes increased excitatory amino acid and cytokine release, and decreased GABA release.[39,40] Neurotoxicity in patients with renal impairment is associated with elevated serum levels. Increased permeability of the BBB causes a buildup of toxic organic acids in the cerebrospinal fluid.[41]

Carbapenems

Carbapenems cause encephalopathy and seizures in patients with renal dysfunction. As with other β-lactam antibiotics, the seizures seen after carbapenem use are considered to be related to binding of glutamate and inhibition of GABA-A receptors.[42] A clinical trial of young children with bacterial meningitis treated with imipenem–cilastin described; acute seizures in 7 of 25 patients and the trial was stopped prematurely. High levels of the drug in the cerebrospinal fluid were associated with a lowered seizure threshold.[43]

Trimethoprim–Sulfonamindes

An association of encephalopathy and psychosis has been reported after the use of cotrimoxazole. A report of a patient who developed transient psychosis, delirium, and visual/auditory hallucinations after using trimethoprim–sulfamethoxazole reported that the symptoms resolved once the medication was stopped.[44] Another report described aseptic meningitis and encephalopathy in elderly and immunocompromised patients using cotrimoxazole.[45,46] Although these neurotoxic effects were partly considered to be related to the high CNS penetration of the drug, the exact mechanism is unknown.

Quinolones

Quinolones are a class of newer antibiotics currently on the market. Neuropsychiatric effects such as toxic psychosis, encephalopathy, seizures, and myoclonus have been reported. Patients with ciprofloxacin-induced neurotoxicity present with confusion and altered mental status. EEGs reveal NCSE or complex partial status in these cases.[47] In addition, a case of delirium with generalized myoclonus was reported in a patient on ciprofloxacin.[48] EEGs done in such patients did not always correlate with the CNS penetration and epileptogenic potential, and usually were normal or showed diffuse slowing.[49]

Ciprofloxacin and ofloxacin are reported to cause orofacial dyskinesias in older individuals.[50,51] Disruption of the GABAergic system is postulated to be the cause of these effects.[52] A Tourette-like syndrome in a 71-year-old man was described who presented with hypersalivation, spitting, insomnia, orofacial and limb automatisms, echolalia, and echopraxia. Extrapyramidal symptoms like choreiform movements, gait problems, and dysarthria are reported in quinolone treated patients. These symptoms suggest that the dopaminergic system is involved in patients on quinolones.[6,53]

Quinolone-mediated neuropsychiatric effects are also postulated to be mediated by GABA-A receptor inhibition and NMDA receptor activation.[54] Increased drug concentrations causing severe side effects are reported in patients with a breached BBB.[54] Such CNS effects can also be seen with an intact BBB as proved in a quantitative EEG study in rats treated with norfloxacin. These neurotoxic effects are dose dependent; abnormal behavior and increased epileptic discharges were seen more commonly in groups exposed to higher dosages of the antibiotics.[55]

ANTIEPILEPTIC MEDICATION–INDUCED BEHAVIORAL SIDE EFFECTS

The major categories of behavioral changes caused by antiepileptic drugs (AEDs) include mood alterations, withdrawal syndromes, intoxication and forced normalization (FN).[56] Psychotropic effects can be either positive or negative depending on the drug used, the dosage, duration, efficacy, and the patient's psychological predisposition. Owing to the variability of associated circumstances, the exact frequency of side effects is difficult to estimate. A case series of patients on AEDs who developed major depression or schizophreniform psychosis showed that 15% of the total psychotic episodes and 28% of depressive episodes were attributed to AED treatment.[56] A case series of patients who developed psychotic episodes in Japan showed that one-half of the episodes related to any medication use were caused by an AED. Many of the AEDs have a black-box warning by the FDA concerning an increased risk of suicide.

Forced Normalization

FN is an iatrogenic psychosis triggered by the "successful" suppression of epilepsy by AEDs. It was first described by Landolt[57] in 1953, who noted that the patients' EEG recordings had an "antagonistic relationship" to psychiatric episodes. Tellenbach[58] in 1965 further described it as "alternative psychosis," and it was also reported as "transformed epilepsy" and "epileptic equivalents" by Schmitz[59] in 1998.

The symptoms that patients with FN may present with include paranoia, hallucinations, catatonia, delusions, mania/hypomania or depression, anxiety including depersonalization and derealization phenomena, and conversion disorder including motor, sensory or gait disturbances (astasia–abasia).[60,61] What may be pseudobulbar affect ("weeping without reason") has also been seen. In all patients, if the offending AEDs are discontinued and the epileptic seizures return, the psychiatric symptoms resolve or improve greatly. Treatments with many different AEDs have been associated with FN, and the list of the ones found in the literature by one of the authors (D.D.) include carbamazepine, clobizam, ethosuximide, lacosamide, lamotrigine, LVT, phenobarbital, PHT, topiramate (TPM), VPA, and vigabatrin (VGB). The phenomenon is not limited to pharmacologic treatment, because it has also been seen after seizure improvement after vagal nerve stimulation and epilepsy surgery. In most instances, the quality of life of the patient seems so much more deficient during FN that the decision is made to lighten the treatment so that some seizure breakthrough occurs but the patient is psychiatrically back to their baseline.

CLASSIC ANTIEPILEPTIC DRUGS

It is not unusual for epileptic patients (both children and adults) to develop depression after starting AED treatment.[62–64] Children commonly develop a conduct disorder with features similar to attention deficit hyperactivity disorder. Hyperactivity is seen most commonly with phenobarbital. Developmentally delayed patients seem to be particularly susceptible to aggressive behavior and irritability when treated with barbiturates.

Phenytoin

PHT is among the most commonly used AEDs. High serum levels of this drug can cause a schizophrenia-like psychosis.[65] This toxicity syndrome is dose related, in contrast with cerebellar symptoms, which can be seen after long-term PHT use. A study of 45 patients who developed drug-related psychosis showed that 25 patients (56%) were undergoing treatment with PHT as opposed to another AED.[66] "Dilantin dementia" is a chronic encephalopathy characterized by a functional decline and altered mental status. It is seen in patients on chronic PHT therapy.[67]

Valproic Acid

Treating epilepsy patients with VPA has been shown to precipitate VPA-induced hyperammonemic hepatic encephalopathy (VHE). It was originally reported in 7 cases by Vossler and colleagues[68] and later substantiated by other authors. Signs of VHE include increased seizures, focal or diffuse neurologic signs and symptoms, confusion, lethargy, impaired consciousness, behavioral changes, NCSE, convulsive status epilepticus, stupor, ataxia, and coma.[69,70] Serum ammonia levels and serum and cerebrospinal fluid glutamine levels are elevated and EEG findings are consistent with metabolic encephalopathy in patients with VHE. A few cases of VHE in the absence of hyperammonemia have also been reported. The diagnosis was confirmed when complete recovery occurred after VPA therapy was discontinued.

The exact mechanism of VHE is not elucidated fully in the literature. Possible mechanisms include hyperammonemia causing inhibition of glutamate uptake by astrocytes leading to neuronal injury and cerebral edema. The glutamate, which is increased in the extracellular spaces, downregulates astrocytic glutamate receptors, leading to further impairment of astrocyte function.[71] VPA is postulated to cause elevations in ammonia levels through both hepatic and renal pathways. Ammonia levels are increased by VPA in the liver via the urea cycle. VPA and its metabolite, propionate inhibit ureagenesis at the mitochondrial level by inhibiting carbonyl phosphate synthetase 1. It is a mitochondrial enzyme necessary for removal of ammonia through the urea cycle, and its inhibition leads to hyperammonemia. At the renal level, ammonia is produced by the conversion of glutamine to glutamate by the enzyme glutaminase. VPA increases transport of glutamine across the mitochondrial membrane, making more available for producing more ammonia.[70,72] VPA is a short chain fatty acid metabolized by β-oxidation by involving carnitine leading to a secondary deficiency of carnitine in VPA toxicity.[71]

VHE was shown to resolve quickly on reducing or discontinuing VPA therapy. Carnitine supplementation has shown to provide some improvement in VHE owing to its role as an essential cofactor in the metabolism of VPA.[71,73,74]

Other Older Antiepileptic Drugs

Ethosuximide, used in the treatment of absence seizures in children, causes psychoses in 2% after seizures are controlled and there is normalization of the EEG (FN). The risk is much greater in adults and adolescents at about 8%.[75] Behavioral problems are comparatively rarer with carbamazepine treatment.[76] It is related chemically to the TCAs. Symptoms of mania and depression have been reported, and are considered to be a paradoxic effect of its antidepressant properties.[77]

Newer Antiepileptic Drugs

Vigabatrin

VGB is among the more recently introduced drugs. Seven percent of patients on VGB treatment were reported to have developed psychiatric complications.[78] Psychosis was described in 3 different patterns.[79] One group achieved seizure freedom (FN). The second group had a cluster of seizures after the initial seizure-control period, and then developed postictal psychosis. The third group developed psychosis after complete withdrawal of VGB. When it was used in children with learning disabilities, it caused a behavioral syndrome similar to barbiturates, with symptoms of aggression, excitation, hyperkinesia, and agitation. A French study showed that the incidence of this behavioral syndrome was about 26% in children.[80]

Lamotrigine

LTG usage causes positive psychotropic effects, improving cognitive function and mood. Behavioral side effects are reported rarely, including depression and psychosis.[81] Other side effects include insomnia, hypomania, irritability, and anxiety in 6% of patients on LTG monotherapy.[82] A "release phenomenon" was reported by Besag, where caregivers complained that developmentally delayed patients on LTG became more demanding and more alert through the day.[83,84] This was initially thought to be owing to the inadequacy of the rehabilitation facilities rather than a side effect of the medication, but was proved otherwise later. A reversible Tourette syndrome, characterized by obsessive–compulsive behavior, was reported with chronic LTG use.[85]

Gabapentin

Gabapentin (GBP) is a well-tolerated drug (despite the black-box warning) and, other than somnolence, positive or negative psychotropic side effects have not been reported in controlled studies of cognitively normal patients. Some studies reported that GBP may induce aggression in mentally handicapped adults and in children with learning disabilities.[86,87]

Tiagabine

The therapeutic window of tiagabine is very narrow and it has been shown to cause de novo NCSE by paradoxic provocation.[88] This complication was reported during early clinical trials and it was unclear whether this it was a side effect of the medication or owing to the underlying epileptic disease. An EEG should always be performed whenever new behavioral side effects are noted. In a few placebo-controlled studies, tiagabine-treated groups showed an increase in depressed mood (5% vs 1%) and nervousness (12% vs 3%).[89]

Topiramate

Behavioral side effects occur at a high rate in patients treated with TPM. A study comparing the side effects in patients treated with TPM, LTG, or GBP showed that psychotic episodes occurred in 12% of the TPM group compared with 0.7% and 0.5% in the LTG and GBP groups, respectively.[90] FN is believed to be the main cause of the TPM-associated psychosis.[91] Amnestic and motor aphasia are considered idiosyncratic side effects of TPM. A controlled study showed that symptoms of abnormal thinking occurred at a rate of 17% to 28%. These behavioral symptoms are dose dependent, with daily doses of 200 and 1000 mg showing an incidence of 9% and 19%, respectively.[92] Some highly functioning individuals notice word-finding difficulties at relatively low doses (50 mg/d; personal experience, D.D.).

Levetiracetam

Preclinical trials with LVT showed affective behavioral episodes in 2% of patients and psychotic episodes in 0.7%. These effects were considered to be a manifestation of FN. A common clinical side effect in both adults and children is irritability and aggressive behavior. An English case series of 517 patients on LVT showed that 10% developed a behavioral side effect, with aggression being the most common presentation.[93] This is more often seen in patients with preexisting dysphoria and irritability. Children seem to have a greater risk of developing aggressive behavior, including suicidal tendencies, than adults.

Zonisamide

Significant behavioral side effects, including psychotic episodes and affective problems, are reported with the use of zonisamide.[94]

Mechanisms of Side Effects of Antiepileptic Drugs

The important behavioral side effects related to the use of AEDs are idiosyncratic reactions and FN. Side effects owing to withdrawal syndromes and dose-related toxicity are less frequently seen, and cause less morbidity. Behavioral side effects, particularly depressive disorders, are more frequently seen in AEDs with GABA-ergic properties (barbiturates, benzodiazepines, VPA, GBP, TPM, tiagabine, and VGB).[95] Trimble first hypothesized the link between GABA-ergic AEDs and behavioral side effects. This was supported by Ketter and colleagues[96] who divided AEDs into 2 distinct categories. The first category includes GABA-ergic AEDs, which are known to have properties of anxiolysis, antimania, and sedation. Drugs in this group include those listed, excluding TPM. The second category includes antiglutamatinergic AEDs like LTG and felbamate, which have antidepressant and anxiogenic effects. TPM is unique; it has multiple mechanisms of action and holds an "intermediate" position. LVT has an atypical mechanism of action and cannot be included in these groups.

AEDs may have different behavioral effects in patients with different preexisting mental states. "Sedating category" drugs help in patients who are activated primarily, and these patients worsen when given "activating drugs" and vice versa. This effect may explain the development of paradoxic effects in patients treated with AEDs when due consideration is not given to the individual's primary psychopathologic status.[96]

Overall, the risk of behavioral side effects of AEDs is multifactorial, with drug dosing, rapid titration, and severity of disease each playing a significant role. Familial predisposition and previous behavioral and psychiatric issues also increase the incidence of these side effects. It is important to identify at-risk patients so that appropriate education can be provided to the patient, caregiver, and family. When appropriate, patients can be followed more frequently and titration schemes can be personalized to the individual needs of the patient if problems arise.

STEROID-INDUCED BEHAVIORAL SIDE EFFECTS

Corticosteroid (CS) treatment is important in both acute (eg, asthma exacerbation) and chronic medical conditions (eg, systemic lupus erythematosus). Somatic side effects have been researched extensively and described widely, but less attention has been paid to neuropsychiatric adverse effects.

Adverse psychological side effects (APSE) from CS range from mild mood or cognitive deficits and emotional lability to severe psychotic symptoms, such as persecutory delusions or auditory hallucinations.[97] They may depend on the patient's premorbid personality and may reflect an extreme version of the patient's usual stress reaction.[98] The side effects show a linear correlation with increased levels of endogenous CS.

Adults with Cushing disease on steroids show a very high rate of psychiatric symptoms (commonly anxiety and depression) at rates between 57% and 78%.[99,100] Side effects in children are less common (44%). Compulsive behavior is the predominant presentation.[101] "Steroid psychosis" is the most severe form of APSE. It occurs in an estimated 5% to 6% of adult patients on CS.[102] These behavioral changes often occur within a few days of treatment and are usually episodic with periods of altered mental status and disorientation. They vary in duration and remit when the steroid dose is decreased or stopped.[103,104]

CS are often prescribed when an underlying medical condition deteriorates, suggesting the possibility that behavioral symptoms (most commonly acute confusional state) may be secondary to the deterioration rather than the treatment itself. Many studies have quoted that adult patients with systemic lupus erythematosus have a low threshold to develop severe APSE. Halper made an important observation that these patients with systemic lupus erythematosus are often acutely sick with CNS symptoms, which have a similar presentation of CS-induced APSE.[105] Some authors observing adult cancer patients with severe APSE concluded that narcotics and medical complications may play an important role contributing to the APSE as well.[11,106]

The incidence of severe APSE is more common as the CS dose is increased.[105] The Boston Collaborative Drug Surveillance Program is a prospective case series conducted in multiple centers across the United States. Acute psychiatric reactions were recorded in 1.3% of patients on 40 mg prednisone, 4.6% of patients on 41 to 80 mg, and 18.4% of patients receiving greater than 80 mg.[107] Steroid-induced "psychological dependency" is well-recognized and is thought to be owing to euphoric effects.[105,106]

Steroid taper or cessation can also cause florid to mild APSE.[105,108] In adults, changes in mood and affect are common, followed less often by delirium or a psychotic state.[109] Suicidal behavior is also reported in patients on steroids, with a significant proportion occurring during withdrawal.[105] In children and adolescents reports of suicidal ideation exist, but because the data are limited, it is difficult to confirm a definite association.[97]

Potential Mechanisms Underlying Adverse Psychological Side Effects

Steroids are known to exert a wide range of effects on the CNS, primarily based on their effects on the adrenal steroid receptors and the neurotransmitters serotonin and dopamine.[105] At a molecular level, steroids cause direct nongenomic effects like altering the membrane permeability or receptor binding, as well as indirect genomic effects like repressive actions on gene transcription.[110,111]

Some studies suggest that hippocampal damage may be a source of underlying APSE. As an integral part of the limbic system, the hippocampus has a role in regulating emotions; emotional lability is the most common feature of APSE. It also has an important role in forming episodic and declarative memory, which are gravely affected in Cushing's disease patients, patients being treated with CS, and CS-treated normal healthy volunteers.[105,110,112]

The hippocampus has high levels of adrenal steroid receptors.[113,114] There is a linear correlation between high steroid levels, hippocampal atrophy/damage, and cognitive dysfunction.[105,115] Hippocampal damage has a "cascade effect," because it impairs the ability to give negative feedback (when endogenous steroid levels are elevated) to the hypothalamic–pituitary–adrenal (HPA) axis, leading to increased levels of CS and further damage to the hippocampus.[105,116] It is hypothesized that APSE may be caused by an increase in serotonin or amino acids, or by causing the hippocampal neurons to be more vulnerable to ischemic insults leading to impaired glucose uptake.[110,112,117] The reversibility of this damage or how it occurs is unclear.

On the other hand, steroids are also known to improve cognitive functioning that has been impaired by underlying illnesses.[105,118] Halper[105] proposed the presence of different CS dose–response curves for these beneficial effects in CS-responsive illnesses associated with cognitive dysfunction versus hippocampal damage. Other studies testing cognitive functioning in normal healthy adults, whose cortisol levels were altered pharmacologically, clearly showed that optimum physiologic levels of CS are necessary for memory and learning.[119]

Management

Management of CS-induced APSE should start with cessation or reduction of dosage. Complete cessation is usually not an option in patients on chronic CS treatment, so the dose is tapered initially to 40-mg prednisone equivalents per day, and titrated to 7.5-mg prednisone equivalents per day as quickly as is safe to do so.[120] Tapering needs to follow strict guidelines to avoid HPA axis suppression with resulting secondary adrenal insufficiency, recurrence of the underlying disease, and CS withdrawal syndrome (symptoms of adrenal insufficiency but normal HPA functionality). The CS tapering is usually based on total dosage, type of CS used, and duration of therapy. Some of the side effects of tapering or cessation (altered affective state, depression, or mania) may take 6 weeks for complete resolution after cessation of the offending agent.[120] After discontinuation, CS withdrawal syndrome and HPA suppression can be distinguished by the corticotropin stimulation test, which evaluates the integrity of the HPA axis.[121] If patients develop severe withdrawal symptoms during dose reduction, they may be alleviated with a temporary dose increase and slowing the taper as tolerated.[122]

BEHAVIORAL SIDE EFFECTS OF MEDICATIONS TO TREAT PARKINSON'S DISEASE

The main classes of drugs used to treat Parkinson's disease (PD) are levodopa, including carbidopa/levodopa combination pills, dopamine agonists (DAs), catechol-O-methyltransferase enzyme inhibitors, monoamine oxidase inhibitors, amantadine, and anticholinergics. The primary cause of behavioral disturbances in

PD is dopamine replacement treatment with excessive or aberrant dopamine receptor stimulation. Dopamine has many important functions, including motor function, a role in the brain's reward system, and behavior modulation. The main behavioral side effects of dopamine replacement treatment include dopamine dysregulation syndrome (DDS), which is also referred to as hedonistic homeostatic dysregulation; punding, and impulse control disorders (ICDs). Patients may not be able to stop compulsive reward-seeking behavior or assess the negative consequences, so the clinician must assume a primary role in identifying and managing these disorders.[123]

Per the Diagnostic and Statistical Manual of Mental Disorders, 4th edition, text revision (DSM-IV-TR), ICDs are a group of psychiatric disorders in which there is a failure to resist an impulse, drive, or temptation and may lead to performing an act that may be harmful to self or others.[124] The most common among these are compulsive buying, pathologic gambling (PG), binge eating, hypersexuality, and compulsive reckless driving/walking about.[125] These acts may give pleasure and so are performed repetitively or compulsively.

PG is the failure to resist the urge to gamble, leading to a maladaptive gambling behavior with dire consequences to interpersonal and occupational functioning. Punding is a syndrome of repetitive, stereotyped motor patterns that include ritualistic, disabling behavior or excessive "hobbyism," such as cleaning, collecting, gardening, writing, or excessive Internet use.[126] DDS or hedonistic homeostatic dysregulation caused by is the excessive use of dopaminergic medications, beyond the usual prescribed doses despite severe side effects on physical, psychiatric, and social function.[127]

Neurobiology

The pathophysiology of these effects is not clearly understood, but studies using PET and functional MRI have provided some information. It was hypothesized that ICDs occur in individuals having personality traits of impulsivity and high novelty-seeking behavior. They may have genetically determined neurobiological features (high ventral striatum activity) caused by dopaminergic medication-induced overstimulation of the mesocorticolimbic system.[128] Modulation of memory, positive and negative reinforcement, reward, inhibitory control and decision making, and motivation are under the control of the mesocorticolimbic dopamine system involved in reward-seeking behavior and impulse control.

An (11C)raclopride-PET study in healthy men showed that dopamine release was higher in high novelty-seeking subjects.[129] This study showed a clear correlation with long-term dopaminergic medication overuse, and supported the hypothesis of a neurobiological basis of increased novelty seeking, impulsivity, and high risk of addictive behaviors. This may be caused by hyperreactivity of the ventral striatum and its connected structures.[130,131]

D2 receptor availability was compared in a study of 2 groups of PD patients, with and without PG.[132] These patients were on treatment with DAs. They were tested during a gambling task and during a control task. It was shown that PD patients with PG had an increased release of dopamine in the ventral striatum during the gambling task, and lower binding in (11C)raclopride-PET during the control task, indicating lower D2 receptor availability. This mimics what is also seen in chemical addicts. It was concluded that DAs may produce a neuronal pattern that is abnormal, but only in PD patients who are vulnerable. This may be similar to the neuronal pattern seen in patients with drug addiction and nonparkinsonian PG. The loss of impulse control in these patients is shown to be caused by deactivation of inhibitory networks, induced by DA, which finally leads to PG.[130,131]

Diagnosis

The diagnosis of ICD is difficult in patients with cognitive impairment and no prior psychiatric history. It is underreported and many patients actually deny it. Education of the patient, caregiver, and family is very important for the prevention and early recognition of these behavioral side effects. The Questionnaire for Impulsive–Compulsive Disorders in Parkinson's disease (QUIP)[133] is a commonly used screening tool for ICD, DDS, and punding in PD patients.

Management

The main step in management is reducing or replacing DAs.[134,135] Amantadine, an NMDA-glutamate antagonist showed promising results in eliminating gambling behavior within days of usage.[136] Other approaches include the use of atypical antipsychotics, SSRIs (very helpful in patients with comorbid depression), and methylphenidate (an inhibitor of the dopamine transporter and enhancer of dopamine release in dorsal and/or ventral striatal regions). However, consistent evidence is unavailable for this to become standard of practice. The usefulness of deep brain stimulation surgery is also not substantiated as seen in a study of 21 patients where the ICD, punding, and DDS persisted and sometimes worsened.[137] Counseling, behavioral therapy, and supportive psychotherapy may help as adjuncts in the treatment of ICDs, but data are lacking to support their benefits.

BEHAVIORAL SIDE EFFECTS OF PSYCHIATRIC MEDICATIONS

Individuals vary in their response to psychotropic and antidepressant medications, a critical problem when trying to manage psychotic disorders. This variability is multifactorial and may be owing to age, gender, comorbid medical conditions, other concurrent medications, and environmental factors. Genetic polymorphism, variations in pharmacokinetics, and pharmacodynamics also influence the treatment response. Cytochrome (CYP) enzymes, serotonin, and dopamine gene variants are known to contribute to the various behavioral side effects of the psychotropic drugs.[138,139] Nearly 80% of the drugs used today are metabolized by these pathways. These differences account for the phase I metabolism variation of different drugs.[140]

Antidepressants

Because depression is an extremely common and disabling disease, treatment with antidepressants is almost ubiquitous. Epidemiologic studies have shown that depression is the second most common cause of disability among adult patients.[141] At any given time, up to 10% of the population may be depressed, and up to 45% of the population may suffer from an episode of depression in their lifetime. Most of these patients may undergo remission with antidepressant treatment, but some develop drug-induced side effects. These range from mild mood changes to severe life threatening neuropsychiatric complications.[142] Adverse drug reactions such as psychotic episodes, suicide, or homicide may develop. It is almost impossible to predict this owing to variations in pharmacogenetics and the varied metabolism of the drugs.

TCAs produce significant neuropsychiatric effects at therapeutic doses. They have a moderate therapeutic index and dangerous side effects are seen with overdosing. The prevalence of side effects is estimated to be around 5%, and acute poisoning is notably life threatening.[143] Common neuropsychiatric effects include seizures, agitation, mania, stupor, and coma. These correlate with the plasma levels of the drug. Significant CNS and cardiac toxicity is seen in patients overdosing on

TCAs like amitriptyline, imipramine, or doxepin, when the blood levels are greater than 1000 ng/mL.[144,145] TCA metabolites commonly exist as secondary or tertiary amines, which are active by themselves or may be activated to their hydroxylated metabolites. Secondary amines are metabolized by CYP2D6, and tertiary amines by the CYPP450s.

E-10-hydroxynortriptyline is an example of a major active metabolite produced by CYP2D6, which is known to produce some antidepressant effects similar to the parent drug, nortriptyline.[146]

Different CYP2D6 genotypes are present in different ethnic population groups and produce variations in nortriptyline clearance. CYP450 genes play a crucial role in the phase I oxidative metabolism of both exogenous and endogenous compounds. If these enzymes are dysfunctional, then the risk of the side effects is greater.[147,148] Based on pharmacogenetic research of various antidepressants, dose adjustment should be based on the CYP450 genotype variations, especially in treatment-resistant patients.[149–151]

Venlafaxine is biotransformed into its active metabolite, O-desmethylvenlafaxine by CYP450 enzymes. It can induce serotonin syndrome even at low doses.[152] Confusion and mydriasis are more commonly reported with venlafaxine than with SSRIs.[153] Patients who ingest high doses of venlafaxine deliberately tend to show greater suicide intent than those who overdose on SSRIs.[153]

Patients younger than 25 years have shown an association of increased suicidality when treated with antidepressants.[154] An analysis of 24 placebo-controlled antidepressant trials involving more than 4400 children and adolescents with obsessive–compulsive disorder, major depressive disorder (MDD), or other psychiatric disorder was undertaken. It showed that there is an increased risk of suicide in those treated with antidepressants. All antidepressant medications approved by the US Food and Drug Administration (FDA) for MDD come with a serious warning of suicide risk, and this risk should be considered while choosing a treatment for MDD and the patient should be monitored closely.

Antipsychotics

The first-generation antipsychotics (eg, chlorpromazine, haloperidol) cause irreversible brain damage by chronic dopamine blockade. This side effect has limited the prescription of dopamine blockers for schizophrenia spectrum illnesses. Second-generation antipsychotics (SGAs) like risperidone, aripiprazole, quetiapine, and lurasidone are commonly used for schizophrenia, bipolar disorder 1, MDD, and acute mania. SGAs are considered atypical because of more selective blockade of serotonin and dopamine receptors (compared with older antipsychotics). This dual action is purported to enhance utility and decrease neurotoxicity.[155]

Chronic dopamine blockade treatment causes an irreversible hypersensitivity of dopamine receptors in the brain, leading to abnormal involuntary motor movements and significant cognitive dysfunction. Side effects caused by chronic dopamine blockade are called extrapyramidal side effects (EPS), and include akathisia, acute dystonia, tardive dyskinesia (TD), and parkinsonism. These symptoms are often debilitating and require treatment. They occur in 2 phases. The early phase occurs upon beginning the treatment with antipsychotics or when the dose is increased. The later onset phase is caused by chronic treatment, which usually presents as TD.

Akathisia is a common motor manifestation of EPS, characterized by restlessness and pacing. It is seen within the first 3 months of treatment with antipsychotics. It is a poorly understood symptom and very difficult to treat. Akathisia does not respond to anticholinergics but benzodiazepines, lipid-soluble ß-blockers, and a reduction in the treatment dosage can ameliorate the symptoms.[156,157]

Acute dystonia is characterized by abnormal postures and muscle spasms of the head and neck and occur within the first few days of treatment with antipsychotics. Anticholinergic drugs like benztropine can reverse or prevent these symptoms.[156–158] Being a young male, having dystonia in the family, and substance abuse are considered the risk factors for developing dystonia.[159,160] It is more commonly seen in patients treated with first-generation antipsychotics like haloperidol and less common with SGAs.[161] Seven percent of patients treated with parenteral long-acting risperidone develop acute dystonic reactions.[162] There are also case reports of acute dystonia in patients treated with aripiprazole and ziprasidone.[163,164]

Parkinsonism induced by antipsychotics presents with bradykinesia, tremor, and skeletal muscle rigidity. It occurs within a few days to a few months after treatment initiation, and is commonly seen in older females and in patients with cognitive deficits.[165] It is reversible, but with variable duration. Dose reduction and anticholinergics are shown to be useful. However, anticholinergics are avoided in the elderly owing to glaucoma risk, dry mouth, urinary retention, and deterioration of cognitive function. Switching to an SGA is recommended, because parkinsonism rates with SGAs are comparatively lower (26% with olanzapine vs 55% with haloperidol).[166]

Tardive Dyskinesia

TD is characterized by repetitive, involuntary facial movements like puckering of lips, protruding of the tongue, grimacing, and oculogyric crisis, as well as torso and limb movements. It usually occurs months to years after antipsychotic treatment initiation. Risk factors include advanced age, female gender, non-Caucasian race, brain pathology, diabetes history, and persistent negative symptoms of schizophrenia.[167] TD occurs in schizophrenia patients at a rate of 0.5% per year.[168] The prevalence of TD in patients being treated with first-generation antipsychotics is between 0.5% and 70%, average (average 24% to 30%).[169,170] Management of TD is different from other EPS treatment, because anticholinergics are shown to increase the incidence of TD. Current guidelines include switching to an SGA agent, followed by medical management. An empirical treatment regimen that includes tapering of anticholinergic drugs, switching to another SGA, and adding tetrabenazine as needed has been suggested. If that does not provide relief, then adding an experimental regimen that includes vitamin B_6, vitamin E, donepezil, branched chain amino acids, and melatonin has shown some benefit.[171] Clozapine, an SGA, improves involuntary symptoms and is considered the safest and most beneficial drug in the treatment of TD.[172]

BEHAVIORAL SIDE EFFECTS OF HUMAN IMMUNODEFICIENCY VIRUS AND HIGHLY ACTIVE ANTIRETROVIRAL THERAPY

Patients with human immunodeficiency virus (HIV) infection can suffer from various neuropsychiatric symptoms. They may be caused by the direct toxic effects of the virus on the CNS, comorbid psychiatric conditions, substance abuse, immunodeficiency leading to CNS opportunistic infections, activity of immune mediators, metabolic decompensation, and/or the side effects of the antiretroviral therapy. The discovery of antiretroviral drugs has changed the outlook of HIV in developed countries. It is now considered a chronic disease that may be managed with lifelong therapy, although not necessarily without a cost.[173] Neuropsychiatric disorders like mood changes and depression have a prevalence rate of 20% to 30% in these patients.[174]

HIV-induced neuronal damage is mediated by immune activation and infection of the macrophages and microglia in the brain.[175] Conflicting evidence is available as to whether these neuropsychiatric disorders have decreased or increased since the initiation of highly active antiretroviral therapy (HAART).[176]

Antiretroviral Agents

The 5 groups of antiretroviral agents are protease inhibitors, nucleoside reverse transcriptase inhibitor (NRTI), nucleotide reverse transcriptase inhibitor, non-NRTI (NNRTI), and fusion or entry inhibitors. They are the mainstay of HIV treatment and are usually grouped based on their mechanisms of action. HAART is a combination of at least 3 antiretroviral drugs. Because the drugs are potent and the patient has to take more than 1 or 2, the potential for side effects and drug–drug interactions is huge.[173] The degree of penetration of these drugs across the BBB is very important. If they did not cross, then the brain would act as a viral reservoir, leading to severe CNS affects and the inability to clear the virus. The ability to invade the BBB relates to the antiretroviral medications' effect on neuropsychiatric symptoms related to HIV.[177] The underlying mechanisms of neuropsychiatric symptoms that develop in HIV are complex and multifactorial, and are poorly understood.

The degree of CNS penetration of protease inhibitors is limited and so the neuropsychiatric side effects are minimal.[173,178] Among this group, ritonavir and saquinavir may rarely produce neurologic effects like anxiety, depression, and sleep disturbances. The other drugs like indinavir, lopinavir, and amprenavir cause mood changes in only a minority of patients.[173] There are no neuropsychiatric effects reported with tenofovir, a nucleotide reverse transcriptase inhibitor. Enfuvirtide, a fusion/entry inhibitor, may cause anxiety and depression.[179]

Zidovudine was the first drug used for the treatment of HIV, belonging to the NRTI group. The neuropsychiatric effects of this drug are usually dose related.[173] Psychiatric effects are also seen with didanosine and lamivudine. Abacavir has fewer neuropsychiatric effects when used alone, but causes catatonia and psychosis when used in combination with other drugs.[180]

Efavirenz, which belongs to the NNRTI group, causes sudden and severe neuropsychiatric effects in up to 50% of patients treated.[181,182] Cognitive deficits, hostile behavior with personality changes, and twilight states are often described.[173,181] Suicidal ideation and major depression are also associated with this drug.[183] The majority of these side effects are seen during the first 4 weeks of treatment and may remit spontaneously despite persistent use.[184] High plasma levels of efavirenz seem to be a possible association. A comorbid psychiatric history also increases vulnerability to neuropsychiatric symptoms.[182] These behaviors may be ameliorated with nighttime dosing, but vivid dreams are often experienced. Delavirdine and nevirapine, belonging to the same group, have no neuropsychiatric effects.[173] Significant interactions have been reported with recreational drugs and antiretroviral agents. Metabolism of "rave" drugs like methylene dioxymethamphetamine (MDMA), ketamine, and amphetamines is inhibited by protease inhibitors, leading to severe toxic effects. Methadone withdrawal syndrome is seen in patients treated with protease inhibitors and NNRTIs, because they induce the metabolism leading to withdrawal symptoms. It is unclear if there is a bidirectional interaction.

Treatment of Psychiatric Complications Associated with Highly Active Antiretroviral Therapy

The neuropsychiatric effects of antiretroviral agents are usually a diagnosis of exclusion. Comorbid psychiatric conditions and the effects of other medications need to be excluded first. Monitoring the drug levels of antiretroviral medications may help in the diagnosis as well.

Treatment depends on the severity of the neuropsychiatric effects. Mild cases need monitoring or the addition of low-dose psychotropics as needed. Severe side effects may require the discontinuation of the medication completely or altering the HAART regimen. According to the current guidelines, HAART-induced depression should be treated aggressively by switching the HAART medications, especially in patients with a psychiatric history.[173] Efavirenz, which causes severe side effects as described previously, needs to be discontinued, because rapid improvement in symptomatology is usually noted after the cessation of treatment.[182,185]

Patients with depression may benefit from active treatment of the depression before the initiation of HAART therapy. This strategy tends to improve the compliance with HAART.[173] Various psychotropic medications may be used to treat the neuropsychiatric effects caused by HIV or treatment with HAART.[185] HIV patients have a greater sensitivity to psychotropics, and so the treatment should be individualized accordingly.[179]

Antiretroviral drugs and the psychotropics have interactions with the CYP450 family of hepatic enzymes. These interactions are very complex and sometimes bidirectional, leading to altered levels of either class of drugs.[186] Ritonavir, a protease inhibitor, is an inhibitor of the CYP2D6 isoenzyme. The same enzyme causes metabolism of risperidone, TCAs, and other antidepressants like fluvoxamine, venlafaxine, and paroxetine. Concomitant use of these psychotropics in patients on ritonavir may cause toxic blood levels of any of these drugs. Protease inhibitors and NNRTIs also interact with the CYP3A4 isoenzyme group, causing altered metabolism of various psychotropics and so medications need to be prescribed with utmost caution. Starting at a low dose of psychotropics (one-quarter to one-half of the optimum dose) and increasing gradually will decrease the incidence of these drug–drug interactions and the resulting side effects.[179]

SSRIs are used commonly for treating the neuropsychiatric effects of antiretroviral treatment, but may cause gastrointestinal side effects.[179] St John's wort, an herbal medication used to treat anxiety and depression, decreases the levels of NNRTIs and protease inhibitors, leading to failure of the treatment.[187] Benzodiazepines like alprazolam, zolpidem, midazolam, and diazepam have major interactions with protease inhibitors and NNRTIs, leading to marked increases in the benzodiazepine effects. As stated, HIV patients are highly sensitive to neuroleptics, and EPS are commonly reported on using these drugs.[188] Although the atypical antipsychotics also cause extrapyramidal reactions, they are much easier to use and the side effects are better tolerated.[173,188] Psychosis in HIV patients responds well to clozapine, but this is seldom used owing to the risk of bone marrow toxicity.[189] Clozapine is contraindicated in patients receiving protease inhibitors.[173,179,190]

CHEMOTHERAPY-INDUCED BEHAVIORAL SIDE EFFECTS

Although chemotherapeutic agents can achieve great success in the treatment of various cancers, some of these agents cause severe debilitating side effects that may warrant dose reduction or cessation of therapy. The commonly reported neuropsychiatric side effects of chemotherapy include fatigue, cognitive deficits, memory impairment, decreased attention span, deficiencies in executive functioning, and motivational deficits; they also cause neuropathy. These symptoms, which develop during therapy, can impact severely the quality of life and remain for a prolonged duration of time even after treatment cessation. Currently there are no FDA-approved treatments available for the prevention or treatment of these symptoms.[191]

The mechanisms underlying behavioral problems owing to chemotherapeutic toxicity are not clearly known. Many believe that neuroinflammation may be the cause of these symptoms.[192–194] The neuroinflammation seen after chemotherapy may be owing to the generation of peripheral inflammatory signals that cause an effect on peripheral tissues or the tumor directly. It has been shown in various clinical studies in noncancer patients that acute behavioral symptoms are propagated by peripheral inflammatory signals. These symptoms may be acute or chronic. During the acute phase, altered mood, increased fatigue, and pain are adaptive responses to disease or the inflammatory process. Persistence of these symptoms even after the disease has cleared show that they have transitioned into a chronic pathologic process.[195]

Fatigue

Fatigue is the most common symptom experienced during chemotherapy affecting up to 60% of patients.[192] Although fatigue often decreases after cessation of treatment, it may persist in some. An estimated 19% to 38% of cancer survivors suffer from fatigue long after the therapy has been discontinued.[196–198] Fatigue impairs quality of life at the physical, social, and psychological levels.[199] It can be divided into peripheral fatigue and central fatigue.[200,201] Peripheral fatigue is the lack of physical energy caused by physical exhaustion and muscle fatigue. Central fatigue refers to the cognitive processes associated with fatigue, including a lack of motivation to engage in or complete a given task. When the motivational components are included, studies have shown that there is an increase in the incidence of fatigue by 50% in cancer patients and survivors.[199,202,203]

Fatigue is also an integral part of the diagnostic criteria for depression. About 73% of depression patients report significant fatigue and lack of energy.[204] These rates are shown to be much higher in cancer patients with depression, with somatic depression-related symptoms being more common than affective symptoms.[205]

Neuroinflammation is proposed as the mechanism accounting for cancer-related fatigue.[193] This idea has been driven partly by the role of neuroinflammation and fatigue in noncancer diseases like multiple sclerosis and rheumatoid arthritis. Clinical studies have, however, failed to differentiate between fatigue induced by the disease or other treatment and chemotherapy-induced fatigue. A preclinical murine study compared fatigue-related behaviors in mice receiving etoposide afflicted with noninflammatory Lewis lung carcinoma cell tumor.[206] The mice treated with etoposide had significantly decreased voluntary wheel running activity (an index of fatigue), suggesting that the fatigue was related to the drug.[207]

Cognitive Dysfunction

Chemotherapy-induced cognitive impairment (CTCI) is seen in 15% to 80% of cancer patients and survivors. It is also referred to as "chemobrain" or "chemofog."[192] The variation in the incidence rates of CTCI is attributed to different treatment regimens used, different objective and subjective tests used across various studies, and different times of patient evaluation.[208,209] The most common effects are frontal lobe dysfunction (memory deficits, increased time to process, and decreased executive functioning).[192,210,211] Imaging studies done in breast cancer survivors after completion of chemotherapy showed subtle decreases in white and gray matter volume and density. They also had frontal hypoactivity as well as hyperactivity during memory-related cognitive tasks.[208,209,212] Although improvement in brain volume and activity is noted after cessation of chemotherapy, some subtle changes may be permanent.[213]

The proposed underlying mechanisms for cognitive impairment in chemotherapy patients include neuroinflammation, decreased neurogenesis, direct neurotoxic injury, and hormonal changes.[214] Both human and animal studies have shown that neuroinflammation can be a possible explanation for the cognitive dysfunction. An association between memory deficits and soluble tumor necrosis factor (TNF) receptor type II (sTNF-RII), a marker for TNF-α activity, was identified. It has a role in development of inflammation in CTCI in breast cancer survivors.[211,215] Greater memory deficits were associated with higher levels of sTNF-RII at 3 months after treatment. The improvement in memory function seen at 12 months after treatment correlated with a decrease in sTNF-RII. To summarize this, the cognitive deficits seen after chemotherapy may be owing to peripheral inflammation suggesting a role for neuroinflammation in CTCI.

Treatments for CTCI include the use of antioxidants, erythropoietin, stimulants like methylphenidate, and cognitive–behavioral therapy. These treatments are still theoretic, because the mechanisms underlying CTCI are still not clear.[216] Modafinil has been used as an off-label drug in trials of breast cancer survivors presenting with symptoms of CTCI. Modafinil is a wakefulness-promoting drug that improved concentration and alertness.[217,218] Estrogen hormone supplementation has shown to reverse the symptoms of CTCI in breast cancer survivors, but associated health risks have limited its use.[219]

IMMUNOTHERAPY-INDUCED BEHAVIORAL SIDE EFFECTS

Commonly used immunotherapy medications like mycophenolate, interferon (INF)-α, INF-β, and interleukin (IL)-2 have all been shown to have neuropsychiatric side effects, especially depression.[220]

Interferon-α

Currently multiple INF-α type formulations are available including recombinant INF-α2a, recombinant INF-α2b, INF-αn3, pegylated IFN-α2a, pegnterferon α2b, and INF alfacon-1, a recombinant synthetic product. These are commonly used in the treatment of hepatitis C, malignant melanoma, and other medical conditions. The commonly reported neuropsychiatric side effects include affective, behavioral, and cognitive deficits, depression, memory impairment, sexual dysfunction, sleep disturbances, anhedonia, fatigue, apathy, irritability, and weight loss.[221,222] Suicidal ideation and suicides have been reported during or after IFN-α therapy.[223] Depression and suicidal ideation are the main reasons for discontinuing or reducing the dose of medication.[223]

Several trials involving different INF-αs and their association with depression showed that the prevalence ranged from 16% to 96% in these patients.[224–226] Most of these studies did not exclude patients with a psychiatric history. An exception is a prospective study of 53 patients with hepatitis C that was specifically conducted to assess the incidence of IFN-α–induced MDD.[227] Patients in this study with a psychiatric history were excluded at screening. Depression was screened for using the Beck Depression Inventory before starting the IFN-α therapy and weekly thereafter.[228] The patients were treated with IFN-α2b and ribavarin combination therapy for 6 to 12 months. About one-third of the patients developed IFN-α–induced MDD.[227] Prior MDD diagnosis or substance abuse and advanced age were not more frequently associated in depressed patients. Caucasians and patients who had higher baseline depression ratings did have a higher incidence of pharmacologically induced MDD. The mean time of developing MDD symptoms from the time of initiation of IFN-α therapy was 12.1 weeks. The majority of patients showed escalation of depressive symptoms in 2 weeks or less thereafter. This study emphasized that patients being initiated on IFN-α therapy should be regularly screened for depression.

Etiology of Interferon-α–Induced Depression

The mechanisms of IFN-α–induced depression are not clearly understood. Various studies suggest it may be caused by cytokine, neuroendocrine, or neurotransmitter pathways.[229,230] Research done recently in patients with malignant melanoma focused on the effects of IFN-α on serotonin. IFN-α activates indoleamine 2,3-deoxygenase, altering the tryptophan metabolism. This leads to an increase in the production of L-kynurenine, which in turn leads to a reduction of serotonin levels (tryptophan is the metabolic precursor for serotonin). During IFN-α therapy, plasma levels of tryptophan and serotonin are reduced significantly. This decrease correlates with changes in the Montgomery Asberg Depression Rating Scale.[231,232] The onset of MDD symptoms occurs with changes in the transcription and uptake activity of the serotonin transporter.[232]

Interferon-β

Currently 2 IFN-βs are available for the treatment of multiple sclerosis. Few data are available with regard to INF-β–precipitated depression compared with IFN-α–induced depression. The incidence ranged from 20% to 33% in 2 clinical studies.[233,234] The Evidence for Interferon Dose-Effect: European-North American Comparative Efficacy (EVIDENCE) study included 677 patients who received either INF-β1a 44 μg subcutaneously 3 times in a week or INF-β1a 30 μg intramuscularly every week for 24 weeks.[235] There were no differences in depression reported in these 2 groups (17% vs 18%). The conclusion was that increasing the dose of INF-β1a was not associated with depression.

Treatment of Interferon-Induced Depression

No specific treatments are approved for depression associated with immunologic agents. Cessation of therapy helps, but remission of depressive symptoms does not always occur simultaneously. In patients with hepatitis C, SSRIs could be a good choice and are tolerated well in patients with liver disease. TCAs may increase cognitive deficits owing to their anticholinergic effects.[236] Two case reports showed benefit in patients treated with methylphenidate or venlafaxine.[237,238]

Based on the depressive symptoms, selection of a specific INF-α has been proposed. INF-αn3 is preferred in patients with suicidal tendencies; INF-α2a is suggested for patients with symptoms of depersonalization. Fewer symptoms are reported in paranoid patients when treated with INF-α2a or INF-α2b; and patients with obsessive or compulsive symptoms showed improvement when treated with INF-αn1.[239] These recommendations were based on a few studies involving small groups of patients and require further evaluation in large, randomized prospective trials.

CONCLUSION

The neurobehavioral effects of medications are relatively common and potentially life threatening. The nervous system can be affected whether the drug is targeted to treat a brain disorder or not. Sometimes the presentation follows a well-known pattern and the toxicity is relatively easy to diagnose. Other signs and symptoms may be subtle, not recognized by patients or caregivers, or ignored leading to prolonged problems and risk of more serious complications.

The world's population is aging, and this is especially true of the Baby Boom generation in the United States. Prescription medication use is prevalent in patients over the age of 65. Therefore, elderly people are more likely to present with medication-related adverse events. In a 12-month cohort study of Medicare enrollees published in 2003, the authors found that adverse drug events occurred at a rate of 50.1 per 1000 person-years, 27.6% of which were considered preventable. Forty-two percent of serious, life-threatening, or fatal adverse drug events were judged to be preventable. Cardiovascular drugs were implicated most commonly, followed by antibiotics, diuretics, nonopioid analgesics, anticoagulants, hypoglycemic agents, steroids, and opioids. Interestingly, psychopharmaceuticals were not often the culprit. (Antidepressants were associated in 3.2% of events, sedative/hypnotics in 0.6%, and antipsychotics in 0.5%.) Errors included prescribing mistakes (58.4%), monitoring errors (60.8%), and patient adherence problems (21.1%), including taking the wrong dose, continuing discontinued medications, refusal to take a medication, continuing to take medicine after the development of side effects, taking a drug despite knowing about a drug interaction, and taking another person's medication. Dispensing errors were rare (<2% of the preventable events). Prescribing errors included wrong drug or wrong therapeutic choice in 27.1%, wrong dose in 24.0%, inadequate patient education in 18.0%, and known drug interaction in 13.3%. Inadequate laboratory monitoring, delay in or failure to respond to side effects, or abnormal laboratory results were found in the monitoring stage (especially with warfarin and digoxin therapy). The authors called for enhanced surveillance and reporting systems for adverse drug events in the ambulatory setting.[240]

The now-widespread use of electronic health records and prescribing systems could theoretically help prevent adverse medication effects, with pop-up flags warning of possible allergies, interactions, and contraindications. Unfortunately, because these are generated by computer software experts and not physicians, the warnings are too numerous and usually not of clinical significance, thus training the prescribers to ignore them. Diligence continues to be the best form of prevention.

REFERENCES

1. Feldman RG. Approach to diagnosis: occupational and environmental neurotoxicology. Philadelphia: Lippincott-Raven; 1999.
2. Dobbs MR. Toxic encephalopathy. Semin Neurol 2011;31:184–93.
3. Koella WP. CNS-related (side-)effects of beta-blockers with special reference to mechanisms of action. Eur J Clin Pharmacol 1985;28(Suppl):55–63.
4. Ruha A, Levine M. Central nervous system toxicity. Emerg Med Clin North Am 2014;32:205–21.
5. Dollery CT, Emslie-Smith D, Milne MD. Guanethidine in the treatment of hypertension. Lancet 1960;3:381–7.
6. MacLeod W. Case report: severe neurologic reaction to ciprofloxacin. Can Fam Physician 2001;47:553–5.
7. Westerlund A. Central nervous system side-effects with hydrophilic and lipophilic beta-blockers. Eur J Clin Pharmacol 1985;28(Suppl):73–6.
8. Cove-Smith JR, Kirk CA. CNS-related side-effects with metoprolol and atenolol. Eur J Clin Pharmacol 1985;28(Suppl):69–72.
9. Goodwin FK, Ebert MH, Bunney WE. Mental effects of reserpine in man: a review. In: Shader RI, editor. Psychiatric complications of medical drugs. New York: Raven Press; 1972. p. 73–101.

10. Raftos J, Bauer GE, Lewis RG, et al. Clonidine in the treatment of severe hypertension. Med J Aust 1973;1:786–93.
11. Benyamin R, Trescot AM, Datta S, et al. Opioid complications and side effects. Pain Physician 2008;11(2 Suppl):S105–20.
12. Collett BJ. Opioid tolerance: the clinical perspective. Br J Anaesth 1998;81: 58–68.
13. Cepeda-Benito A, Davis KW, Harraid JH. Associative and behavioral tolerance to the analgesic effects of nicotine in rats: tail flick and paw-lick assays. Psychopharmacology (Berl) 2005;180:224–33.
14. Light AB, Torrance EG. Opiate addiction. VI: the effects of abrupt withdrawal followed by readministration of morphine in human addicts, with special reference to the composition of the blood, the circulation and the metabolism. Arch Intern Med 1929;44:1–16.
15. Ballantyne JC. Opioids for chronic pain: taking stock. Pain 2006;125:3–4.
16. Mercadante S, Villari P, Ferrera P. Burst ketamine to reverse opioid tolerance in cancer pain. J Pain Symptom Manage 2003;25:302–5.
17. Mao J, Sung B, Ji RR, et al. Neuronal apoptosis associated with morphine tolerance: evidence for an opioid-induced neurotoxic mechanism. J Neurosci 2002; 22:7650–61.
18. Mercadante S, Ferrera P, Villari P, et al. Hyperalgesia: an emerging iatrogenic syndrome. J Pain Symptom Manage 2003;26:769–75.
19. Pud D, Cohen D, Lawental E, et al. Opioids and abnormal pain perception: new evidence from a study of chronic opioid addicts and healthy subjects. Drug Alcohol Depend 2006;82:218–23.
20. Ahmedzai S. New approaches to pain control in patients with cancer. Eur J Cancer 1997;33:S8–14.
21. Reissig JE, Rybarczyk AM. Pharmacologic treatment of opioid-induced sedation in chronic pain. Ann Pharmacother 2005;39:727–31.
22. Kurz A, Sessler DI. Opioid-induced bowel dysfunction: pathophysiology and potential new therapies. Drugs 2003;63:649–71.
23. Pickworth WB, Neidert GL, Kay DC. Morphinelike arousal by methadone during sleep. Clin Pharmacol Ther 1981;30:796–804.
24. Vella-Brincat J, Macleod AD. Adverse effects of opioids on the central nervous systems of palliative care patients. J Pain Palliat Care Pharmacother 2007;21: 15–25.
25. Slatkin N, Rhiner M. Treatment of opioid-induced delirium with acetylcholinesterase inhibitors: a case report. J Pain Symptom Manage 2004;27: 268–73.
26. Hanks GW. Morphine sans Morpheus. Lancet 1995;346:652–3.
27. Fishbain DA, Cutler RB, Rosomoff HL. Are opioid-dependent/tolerant patients impaired in driving related skills? A structured evidence based review. J Pain Symptom Manage 2003;25:559–77.
28. Schliamser SE, Cars O, Norrby SR. Neurotoxicity of beta-lactam antibiotics: predisposing factors and pathogenesis. J Antimicrob Chemother 1991;27: 405–25.
29. Gutnick MJ, Prince DA. Penicillinase and the convulsant action of penicillin. Neurology 1971;21:759–64.
30. Murphy MB, Alcera LC, Gill JK, et al. The inexplicably suicidal patient. Current Psychiatry 2008;7(11):74–82.
31. Araszkiewicz A, Rybakowski JK. Hoigne's syndrome, kindling, and panic disorder. Depress Anxiety 1996-1997;4(3):139–43.

32. Sternbach H, State R. Antibiotics: neuropsychiatric effects and psychotropic interactions. Harv Rev Psychiatry 1997;5(4):214–26.
33. Lin CS, Cheng CJ, Chou CH, et al. Piperacillin/tazobactam-induced seizure rapidly reversed by high flux hemodialysis in a patient on peritoneal dialysis. Am J Med Sci 2007;333:181–4.
34. Huang WT, Hsu YJ, Chu PL, et al. Neurotoxicity associated with standard doses of piperacillin in an elderly patient with renal failure. Infection 2009;37:374–6.
35. Bischoff A, Meier C, Roth F. Gentamicin neurotoxicity (polyneuropathy – encephalopathy). Schweiz Med Wochenschr 1977;107:3–8.
36. Grill MF, Maganti RK. Neurotoxic effects associated with antibiotic use: management considerations. Br J Clin Pharmacol 2011;72(3):381–93.
37. Grill MF, Maganti R. Cephalosporin-induced neurotoxicity: clinical manifestations, potential pathogenic mechanisms, and the role of electroencephalographic monitoring. Ann Pharmacother 2008;42:1843–50.
38. Sonck J, Laureys G, Verbeelen D. The neurotoxicity and safety of treatment with cefepime in patients with renal failure. Nephrol Dial Transplant 2008;23:966–70.
39. Chow KM, Hui AC, Szeto CC. Neurotoxicity induced by beta-lactam antibiotics: from bench to bedside. Eur J Clin Microbiol Infect Dis 2005;24:649–53.
40. Sugimoto M, Uchida I, Mashimo T, et al. Evidence for the involvement of GABA(A) receptor blockage in convulsions induced by cephalosporins. Neuropharmacology 2003;45:304–14.
41. Barbhaiya RH, Knupp CA, Forgue ST, et al. Pharmacokinetics of cefepime in subjects with renal insufficiency. Clin Pharmacol Ther 1990;48:268–76.
42. Koppel BS, Hauser WA, Politis C, et al. Seizures in the critically ill: the role of imipenem. Epilepsia 2001;42:1590–3.
43. Wong VK, Wright HT, Ross LA, et al. Imipenem/cilastatin treatment of bacterial meningitis in children. Pediatr Infect Dis J 1991;10:122–5.
44. Saidinejad M, Ewald MB, Shannon MW. Transient psychosis in an immune-competent patient after oral trimethoprim-sulfamethoxazole administration. Pediatrics 2005;115:e739–41.
45. Cooper GS, Blades EW, Remler BF, et al. Central nervous system Whipple's disease: relapse during therapy with trimethoprim-sulfamethoxazole and remission with cefixime. Gastroenterology 1994;106:782–6.
46. Patey O, Lacheheb A, Dellion S, et al. A rare case of cotrimoxazole-induced eosinophilic aseptic meningitis in an HIV-infected patient. Scand J Infect Dis 1998;30:530–1.
47. Isaacson SH, Carr J, Rowan AJ. Ciprofloxacin induced complex partial status epilepticus manifesting as an acute confusional state. Neurology 1993;43:1619–21.
48. Rfidah El, Findlay CA, Beattie TJ. Reversible encephalopathy after intravenous ciprofloxacin therapy. Pediatr Nephrol 1995;9:250–1.
49. Kiangkitiwan B, Doppalapudi A, Fonder M, et al. Levofloxacin-induced delirium with psychotic features. Gen Hosp Psychiatry 2008;30:381–3.
50. De Bleecker JL, Vervaet VL, De Sarro A. Reversible orofacial dyskinesia after ofloxacin treatment. Mov Disord 2004;19:731–2.
51. Pastor P, Motinho E, Elizalde I, et al. Reversible oro-facial dyskinesia in a patient receiving ciprofloxacin hydrochloride. J Neurol 1996;243:616–7.
52. Lee CH, Cheung RT, Chan TM. Ciprofloxacin-induced oral-facial dyskinesia in a patient with normal liver and renal function. Hosp Med 2000;61:142–3.
53. Thomas RJ, Reagan DR. Association of a Tourette-like syndrome with ofloxacin. Ann Pharmacother 1996;30:138–41.

54. Akahane K, Tsutomi Y, Kimura Y, et al. Levofloxacin, an optical isomer of oflox-acin, has attenuated epileptogenic activity in mice and inhibitory potency in GABA receptor binding. Chemotherapy 1994;40:412–7.
55. Zhang LR, Wang YM, Chen BY, et al. Neurotoxicity and toxicokinetics of norflox-acin in conscious rats. Acta Pharmacol Sin 2003;24:605–9.
56. Schmitz B, Robertson M, Trimble MR. Depression and schizophrenia in epi-lepsy: social and biological risk factors. Epilepsy Res 1999;35:59–68.
57. Landolt H. Serial EEG investigations during psychotic episodes in epileptic pa-tients and during schizophrenic attacks. In: Lorentz De Haas AM, editor. Lec-tures on Epilepsy. Amsterdam: Elsevier; 1958. p. 91–133.
58. Tellenbach H. Epilepsie als ansfallsleiden und als psychose. Uber alternative Psychosen paranoider Pragung bei forcierter Normal-isierung (Landolt) des Elektroenzephalogramms spileptischer. Nervenarzt 1965;36:190–202.
59. Schmitz B. Psychiatric syndromes related to antiepileptic drugs. Epilepsia 1999; 40(Suppl 10):S65–70.
60. Gobbi G, Giovannini S, Boni A, et al. Catatonic psychosis related to forced normalization in a girl with Dravet's syndrome. Epileptic Disord 2008;10(4):325–9.
61. Turan AB, Seferoglu M, Taskapilioglu O, et al. Vulnerability of an epileptic case to psychosis: sodium valproate with lamotrigine, forced normalization, postictal psychosis or all? Neurol Sci 2012;33(5):1161–3.
62. Robertson MM, Trimble MR, Townsend HRA. Phenomenology of depression in epilepsy. Epilepsia 1987;28:364–72.
63. Brent DA. Overrepresentation of epileptics in a consecutive series of suicide at-tempters seen at a children's hospital, 1978–1983. J Am Acad Child Psychiatry 1986;25:242–6.
64. Brent DA, Crumrine PK, Varma RR, et al. Phenobarbital treatment and major depressive disorder in children with epilepsy. Pediatrics 1987;80:909–17.
65. McDanal CE, Bolman WM. Delayed idiosyncratic psychosis with diphenylhy-dantoin. JAMA 1975;231:1063.
66. Kanemoto K, Tsuji T, Kawasaki J. Reexamination of interictal psychoses based on DSM IV psychosis classification and international epilepsy classification. Epilepsia 2001;42:98–103.
67. Trimble MR, Reynolds EH. Anticonvulsant drugs and mental symptoms: a review. Psychol Med 1976;6:169–78.
68. Vossler DG, Wilensky AJ, Cawthon DF, et al. Serum and CSF glutamine levels in valproate-related hyperammonemic encephalopathy. Epilepsia 2002;43:154–9.
69. Hamer HM, Knake S, Schomburg U, et al. Valproic acid induced hyperammo-nemic encephalopathy in the presence of topiramate. Neurology 2000;54:230–2.
70. Blindauer KA, Harrington G, Morris GL, et al. Fulminant progression of demye-linating disease after valproate-induced encephalopathy. Neurology 1998;51:292–5.
71. Verrotti A, Trotta D, Morgese G, et al. Valproate-induced hyperammonemic encephalopathy. Metab Brain Dis 2002;17:367–73.
72. Rumbach L, Cremel G, Marescaux C, et al. Valproate-induced hyperammone-mia of renal origin. Biochem Pharmacol 1989;38:3963–7.
73. Bohles H, Sewell AC, Wenzel D. The effect of carnitine supplementation in valproate-induced hyperammonemia. Acta Paediatr 1996;85:446–9.
74. Raskind J, El-Chaar G. The role of carnitine supplementation during valproic acid therapy. Ann Pharmacother 2000;34:630–8.

75. Wolf P, Inoue Z, Röder-Wanner UU, et al. Psychiatric complications of absence therapy and their relation to alteration of sleep. Epilepsia 1984;25:56–9.
76. Dalby MA. Behavioral effects of carbamazepine. In: Penry JK, Daly DD, editors. Complex partial seizures and their treatment. Advances in neurology, vol. 11. New York: Raven; 1975. p. 331–43.
77. Drake ME, Peruzzi WT. Manic state with carbamazepine therapy of seizures. J Natl Med Assoc 1986;78:1105–7.
78. Sander JWAS, Hart ZM, Trimble MR, et al. Vigabatrin and psychosis. J Neurol Neurosurg Psychiatry 1991;54:435–9.
79. Thomas L, Trimble MR, Schmitz B, et al. Vigabatrin and behaviour disorders: a retrospective study. Epilepsy Res 1996;25:21–7.
80. Dulac O, Chiron D, Cusmai R, et al. Vigabatrin in childhood epilepsy. J Child Neurol 1991;6(Suppl 2):30–7.
81. Fitton A, Goa KL. Lamotrigine. Drugs 1995;50:691–713.
82. Brodie MJ, Richens A, Yuen AW. Double-blind comparison of lamotrigine and carbamazepine in newly diagnosed epilepsy. UK Lamotrigine/Carbamazepine Monotherapy trial group. Lancet 1995;345:476–9.
83. Besag FMC. Behavioural effects of the new anticonvulsants. Drug Saf 2001;24: 513–36.
84. Binnie DB. Lamotrigine. In: Engel J, Pedley TA, editors. Epilepsy. A comprehensive textbook. Philadelphia; New York: Lippincott-Raven; 1997. p. 1531–40.
85. Lombroso CT. Lamotrigine-induced tourettism. Neurology 1999;52:1191–4.
86. Lee DO, Steingard RJ, Cesena M, et al. Behavioral side effects of gabapentin in children. Epilepsia 1996;37:87–90.
87. Wolf SM, Shinnar S, Kang H, et al. Gabapentin toxicity in children manifesting as behavioral changes. Epilepsia 1996;36:1203–5.
88. Schapel G, Chadwick D. Tiagabine and non-convulsive status epilepticus. Seizure 1996;5:153–6.
89. Leppik E. Tiagabine: the safety landscape. Epilepsia 1995;36(Suppl 6): 10–3.
90. Cramer JA, Blum D, Reed M, et al, Epilepsy Impact Project Group. The influence of comorbid depression on quality of life for people with epilepsy. Epilepsy Behav 2003;4:515–21.
91. Mula M, Trimble MR, Lhatoo SD, et al. Topiramate and psychiatric adverse events in patients with epilepsy. Epilepsia 2003;44:659–63.
92. Janssen-Cilag. Topamax. Product monograph, 1996.
93. Mula M, Trimble MR, Yuen A, et al. Psychiatric adverse events during levetiracetam therapy. Neurology 2003;61:704–6.
94. Matsuura M. Epileptic psychoses and anticonvulsant drug treatment. J Neurol Neurosurg Psychiatry 1999;67:231–3.
95. Trimble MR. Neuropsychiatric consequences of pharmacotherapy. In: Engel J, Pedley TA, editors. Epilepsy. A comprehensive textbook. Philadelphia; New York: Lippincott-Raven; 1997. p. 2161–6.
96. Ketter TA, Post RM, Theodore WH. Positive and negative psychiatric effects of antiepileptic drugs in patients with seizure disorders. Neurology 1999; 53(Suppl 2):53–67.
97. Stuart FA, Segal TY, Keady S. Adverse psychological effects of corticosteroids in children and adolescents. Arch Dis Child 2005;90:500–6.
98. Brody S. Psychiatric observations in patients treated with cortisone and ACTH. Psychosom Med 1952;14:94–103.
99. Kelly WF. Psychiatric aspects of Cushing's syndrome. QJM 1996;89:543–51.

100. Loosen PT, Chambliss B, DeBold CR, et al. Psychiatric phenomenology in Cushing's disease. Pharmacopsychiatry 1992;25:192–8.
101. Devoe DJ, Miller WL, Conte FA, et al. Long-term outcome for children and adolescents following transphenoidal surgery for Cushing disease. J Clin Endocrinol Metab 1997;82:3196–202.
102. Satel SL. Mental status changes in children receiving glucocorticoids: review of the literature. Clin Pediatr 1990;29:382–8.
103. Ling MHM, Perry PJ, Tsuang MT. Side effects of corticosteroid therapy: psychiatric aspects. Arch Gen Psychiatry 1981;38:471–7.
104. Lewis DA, Smith RE. Steroid-induced psychiatric syndromes. J Affect Disord 1983;5:319–32.
105. Halper JP. Corticosteroids and behavioural disturbances. In: Lin AN, Paget SA, editors. Principles of corticosteroid therapy. London: Arnold; 2002. p. 174–201.
106. Steifel FC, Breitbart WS, Holland JC. Corticosteroids in cancer: neuropsychiatric complications. Cancer Invest 1989;7:479–91.
107. The Boston Collaborative Drug Surveillance Program. Acute adverse reactions to prednisone in relation to dosage. Clin Pharmacol Ther 1972;13:694–8.
108. Reckart MD, Eisendrath SJ. Exogenous corticosteroid effects on mood and cognition: case presentations. Int J Psychosom 1990;37:57–61.
109. Fricchione G, Ayyala M, Holmes VF. Steroid withdrawal psychiatric syndromes. Ann Clin Psychiatry 1989;1:99–108.
110. Wolkowitz OM, Reus VI, Canick J, et al. Glucocorticoid medication, memory and steroid psychosis in medical illness. Ann N Y Acad Sci 1997;823: 81–96.
111. Schacke H, Wolf-Dietrich D, Asadullah K. Mechanisms involved in the side effects of glucocorticoids. Pharmacol Ther 2002;96:23–43.
112. Wolkowitz OM. Prospective controlled studies of the behavioural and biological effects of exogenous corticosteroids. Psychoneuroendocrinology 1994;19: 233–55.
113. Sapolsky RM, McEwen BS. Down regulation of neural corticosterone receptors by corticosterone and dexamethasone. Brain Res 1985;339:161–5.
114. McEwen BS. The brain is an important target of adrenal steroid actions. A comparison of synthetic and natural steroids. Ann N Y Acad Sci 1997;823:201–13.
115. Brown ES, Rush AJ, McEwen BS. Hippocampal remodelling and damage by corticosteroids. Implications for mood disorders. Neuropsychopharmacology 1999;21:474–84.
116. Sapolsky RM, Krey LC, McEwen BS. The neuroendocrinology of stress and aging: the glucocorticoid cascade hypothesis. Endocr Rev 1986;7: 284–301.
117. Orchinik M, Carroll SS, Yi-Huey L, et al. Heterogeneity of hippocampal GABAA receptors: regulation by corticosterone. J Neurosci 2001;21:330–9.
118. Taylor SE, Garralda ME, Tudor-Williams G, et al. An organic cause of neuropsychiatric illness in adolescence. Lancet 2003;361:572.
119. Carpenter WT, Gruen PH. Cortisol's effect on human mental functioning. J Clin Psychopharmacol 1982;2:91–101.
120. Richter B, Neises G, Clar C. Glucocorticoid withdrawal schemes in chronic medical disorders: a systemic review. Endocrinol Metab Clin North Am 2002; 31:751–78.
121. Dixon RB, Christy NP. On the various forms of corticosteroid withdrawal syndrome. Am J Med 1980;68:224–30.

122. Venkatarangam SH, Kutcher SP, Notkin RM. Secondary mania with steroid withdrawal. Can J Psychiatry 1988;33:631–2.

123. Reiff J, Jost WH. Drug-induced impulse control disorders in Parkinson's disease. J Neurol 2011;258(Suppl 2):S323–7.

124. American Psychiatric Association (APA). Diagnostic and statistical manual of mental disorders. text revision. 4th edition. Washington, DC: American Psychiatric Association; 2000.

125. Avanzi M, Baratti M, Cabrini S, et al. The thrill of reckless driving in patients with Parkinson's disease: an additional behavioural phenomenon in dopamine dysregulation syndrome? Parkinsonism Relat Disord 2008;14:257–8.

126. Evans AH, Strafella AP, Weintraub D, et al. Impulsive and compulsive behaviors in Parkinson's disease. Mov Disord 2009;24:1561–70.

127. Giovannoni G, O'Sullivan JD, Turner K, et al. Hedonistic homeostatic dysregulation in patients with Parkinson's disease on dopamine replacement therapies. J Neurol Neurosurg Psychiatry 2000;68:423–8.

128. Antonini A, Cilia R. Behavioural adverse effects of dopaminergic treatments in Parkinson's disease: incidence, neurobiological basis, management and prevention. Drug Saf 2009;32:475–88.

129. Leyton M, Boileau I, Benkelfat C, et al. Amphetamine-induced increases in extracellular dopamine, drug wanting, and novelty seeking: a PET/[11C]raclopride study in healthy men. Neuropsychopharmacology 2002;27:1027–35.

130. Hariri AR, Brown SM, Williamson DE, et al. Preference for immediate over delayed rewards is associated with magnitude of ventral striatal activity. J Neurosci 2006;26:13213–7.

131. Kalivas PW, Volkow ND. The neural basis of addiction: a pathology of motivation and choice. Am J Psychiatry 2005;162:1403–13.

132. Steeves TD, Miyasaki J, Zurowski M, et al. Increased striatal dopamine release in Parkinsonian patients with pathological gambling: a [11C]raclopride PET study. Brain 2009;132:1376–85.

133. Weintraub D, Hoops S, Shea JA, et al. Validation of the questionnaire for impulsive-compulsive disorders in Parkinson's disease. Mov Disord 2009;24:1461–7.

134. Mamikonyan E, Siderowf AD, Duda JE, et al. Long-term follow-up of impulse control disorders in Parkinson's disease. Mov Disord 2008;23:75–80.

135. Wolters E, van der Werf YD, van den Heuvel OA. Parkinson's disease-related disorders in the impulsive-compulsive spectrum. J Neurol 2008;255(5):48–56.

136. Thomas A, Bonanni L, Gambi F, et al. Pathological gambling in Parkinson disease is reduced by amantadine. Ann Neurol 2010;68:400–4.

137. Lim SY, O'Sullivan SS, Kotschet K, et al. Dopamine dysregulation syndrome, impulse control disorders and punding after deep brain stimulation surgery for Parkinson's disease. J Clin Neurosci 2009;16:1148–52.

138. Mihaljevic-Peles A, Sagud M, Bozina N, et al. Pharmacogenetics and antipsychotics in the light of personalized pharmacotherapy. Psychiatr Danub 2010;22:335–7.

139. Binder EB, Holsboer F. Pharmacogenomics and antidepressant drugs. Ann Med 2006;38:82–94.

140. Wall CA, Oldenkamp C, Swintak C. Safety and efficacy pharmacogenomics in pediatric psychopharmacology. Prim Psychiatry 2010;17:53–8.

141. Russell JM, Hawkins K, Ozminkowski RJ, et al. The cost consequences of treatment-resistant depression. J Clin Psychiatry 2004;65:341–7.

142. Gershenfeld HK, Philibert RA, Boehm GW. Looking forward in geriatric anxiety and depression: implications of basic science for the future. Am J Geriatr Psychiatry 2005;13:1027–40.

143. Bryant SG, Fisher S, Kluge RM. Long-term versus short-term amitriptyline side effects as measured by a postmarketing surveillance system. J Clin Psychopharmacol 1987;7:78–82.

144. Biggs JT, Riesenberg RA, Ziegler VE. Overdosing the tricyclic overdose patient. Am J Psychiatry 1977;134:461–2.

145. Biggs JT, Spiker DG, Petit JM, et al. Tricyclic antidepressant overdose: incidence of symptoms. JAMA 1977;238:135–8.

146. Bertilsson L, Nordin C, Otani K, et al. Disposition of single oral doses of e-10-hydroxynortriptyline in healthy subjects, with some observations on pharmacodynamic effects. Clin Pharmacol Ther 1986;40:261–7.

147. Dalen P, Dahl ML, Bernal Ruiz ML, et al. 10-Hydroxylation of nortriptyline in white persons with 0, 1, 2, 3, and 13 functional CYP2D6 genes. Clin Pharmacol Ther 1998;63:444–52.

148. Morita S, Shimoda K, Someya T, et al. Steady-state plasma levels of nortriptyline and its hydroxylated metabolites in Japanese patients: impact of CYP2D6 genotype on the hydroxylation of nortriptyline. J Clin Psychopharmacol 2000;20: 141–9.

149. De Leon J, Armstrong SC, Cozza KL. Clinical guidelines for psychiatrists for the use of pharmacogenetic testing for CYP450 2D6 and CYP450 2C19. Psychosomatics 2006;47:75–85.

150. McAlpine DE, O'Kane DJ, Black JL, et al. Cytochrome P450 2D6 genotype variation and venlafaxine dosage. Mayo Clin Proc 2007;82:1065–8.

151. Pilgrim JL, Gerostamoulos D, Drummer OH. Review: pharmacogenetic aspects of the effect of cytochrome P450 polymorphisms on serotonergic drug metabolism, response, interactions, and adverse effects. Forensic Sci Med Pathol 2011;7: 162–84.

152. Pan JJ, Shen WW. Serotonin syndrome induced by low-dose venlafaxine. Ann Pharmacother 2003;37:209–11.

153. Chan AN, Gunja N, Ryan CJ. A comparison of venlafaxine and SSRIS in deliberate self-poisoning. J Med Toxicol 2010;6:116–21.

154. Blazer DG, Kessler RC, McGonagle KA, et al. The prevalence and distribution of major depression in a national community sample: the national comorbidity study. Am J Psychiatry 1994;151:979–86.

155. Rothschild AJ. Management of psychotic, treatment-resistant depression. Psychiatr Clin North Am 1996;19(2):237–52.

156. Poznic Jesic M, Jesic A, Babovic Filipovic J, et al. Extrapyramidal syndromes caused by antipsychotics. Med Pregl 2012;65(11–12):521–6.

157. Raja M. Managing antipsychotic-induced acute and tardive dystonia. Drug Saf 1998;19(1):57–72.

158. Shirzadi AA, Ghaemi SN. Side effects of atypical antipsychotics: extrapyramidal symptoms and the metabolic syndrome. Harv Rev Psychiatry 2006;14(3): 152–64.

159. van Harten Peter N, Hoek Hans W, Kahn Rene S. "Acute dystonia induced by drug treatment". In: Widiger TA, Frances AJ, Pincus HA, et al, editors. DSM-IV source book. Vol 1. Washington, DC: American Psychiatric Association; 1994. p. 623–6.

160. Casey DE. Motor and mental aspects of extrapyramidal syndromes. Int Clin Psychopharmacol 1995;10(3):105–14.

161. Lehan AF, Lieberman JA, Dixon JA, et al. Practice guideline for the treatment of schizophrenia. 2nd edition. Washington, DC: American Psychiatric Association; 2004.

162. Kamishima K, Ishigooka J, Komada Y. Long term treatment with risperidone long-acting injectable in patients with schizophrenia. Jpn J Psychiatry Neurol 2009;12:1223–44.

163. Mason MN, Johnson CE, Piasecki M. Ziprasidone-induced acute dystonia. Am J Psychiatry 2005;162(3):625–6.

164. Henderson JB, Labbate L, Worley M. A case of acute dystonia after single dose of aripiprazole in a man with cocaine dependence. Am J Addict 2007;16(3):244.

165. Thanvi B, Treadwell S. Drug induced parkinsonism: a common cause of parkinsonism in older people. Postgrad Med J 2009;85(1004):322–6.

166. Lieberman JA, Tollefson G, Tohen M, et al. Comparative efficacy and safety of atypical and conventional antipsychotic drugs in first-episode psychosis: a randomized, double-blind trial of olanzapine versus haloperidol. Am J Psychiatry 2003;160(8):1396–404.

167. Rana AQ, Chaudry ZM, Blanchet PJ. New and emerging treatments for symptomatic tardive dyskinesia. Drug Des Devel Ther 2013;7:1329–40.

168. Fenton WS, Blyler CR, Wyatt RJ, et al. Prevalence of spontaneous dyskinesia in schizophrenic and non-schizophrenic psychiatric patients. Br J Psychiatry 1997;171:265–8.

169. Casey DE. Tardive dyskinesia and atypical antipsychotic drugs. Schizophr Res 1999;35:S61–6.

170. Llorca P, Chereau I, Bayle F, et al. Tardive dyskinesias and antipsychotics: a review. Eur Psychiatry 2002;17(3):129–38.

171. Margolese HC, Chouinard G, Kolivakis TT, et al. Tardive dyskinesia in the era of typical and atypical antipsychotics. Part 2: incidence and management strategies in patients with schizophrenia. Can J Psychiatry 2005;50(11): 703–14.

172. Woods SW, Morgenstern H, Saksa JR, et al. Incidence of tardive dyskinesia with atypical versus conventional antipsychotic medications: a prospective cohort study. J Clin Psychiatry 2010;71(4):463–74.

173. Treisman GJ, Kaplan AI. Neurologic and psychiatric complications of antiretroviral agents. AIDS 2002;16:1201–15.

174. Bing EG, Burnam MA, Longshore D, et al. Psychiatric disorders and drug use among human immunodeficiency virus-infected adults in the United States. Arch Gen Psychiatry 2001;58:721–8.

175. Swindells S, Zheng J, Gendelman HE. HIV associated dementia: new insights into disease pathogenesis and therapeutic interventions. AIDS Patient Care STDS 1999;13:153–63.

176. Catalan J, Meadows J, Douzenis A. The changing patterns of mental health problems in HIV infection: the view from London, UK. AIDS Care 2000;12: 333–41.

177. Gonzalez A, Everall IP. Lest we forget: neuropsychiatry and the new generation anti-HIV Drugs. AIDS 1998;12:2365–7.

178. Harry TC, Matthews M, Salvary I. Indinavir use: associated reversible hair loss and mood disturbance. Int J STD AIDS 2000;11:474–6.

179. Everall IP, Drummond S, Catalan J. Guidelines for the prescribing of medication for mental health disorders for people with HIV infection (draft) (council report CR127). London: Royal College of Psychiatrists; 2004.

180. Foster R, Olajide D, Everall IP. Antiretroviral therapy-induced psychosis: case report and brief review of the literature. HIV Med 2003;4:139–44.
181. Lang JP, Halleguen O, Picard A, et al. Apropos of atypical melancholia with Sustiva (efavirenz). Encephale 2001;27:290–3.
182. Peyriere H, Mauboussin RI, Rouanet I, et al. Management of sudden psychiatric disorders related to efavirenz. AIDS 2001;15:1323–8.
183. Puzantian T. Central nervous system adverse effects with efavirenz: case report and review. Pharmacotherapy 2002;22:930–3.
184. Colebunders R, Verdonck K. Reply to Gonzalez and Everall: lest we forget: neuropsychiatry and the new generation anti-HIV Drugs. AIDS 1999;13:869.
185. Sanz de la Garza CL, Paoletti-Duarte S, García-Martín C, et al. Efavirenz-induced psychosis. AIDS 2001;15:1911–2.
186. Tseng AL, Fosy MM. Significant interactions with new antiretrovirals and psychotropic drugs. Ann Pharmacother 1999;33:461–73.
187. James JS. St John's wort warning: do not combine with protease inhibitors, NNRTIs. AIDS Treat News 2000;18(337):3–5.
188. Meyer JM, Marsh J, Simpson G, et al. Differential sensitivities to risperidone and olanzapine in a human immunodeficiency virus patient. Biol Psychiatry 1998;44:791–4.
189. Lera G, Zirulnik J. Pilot study with clozapine in patients with HIV-associated psychosis and drug-induced parkinsonism. Mov Disord 1999;14:128–31.
190. Antoniou T, Tseng AL. Interactions between recreational drugs and antiretroviral agents. Ann Pharmacother 2002;36:1598–613.
191. Vichaya EG, Chiu GS, Krukowski K, et al. Mechanisms of chemotherapy-induced behavioral toxicities. Front Neurosci 2015;9:131.
192. Cleeland CS, Bennett GJ, Dantzer R, et al. Are the symptoms of cancer and cancer treatment due to a shared biologic mechanism? A cytokine-immunologic model of cancer symptoms. Cancer 2003;97:2919–25.
193. Dantzer R, Heijnen CJ, Kavelaars A, et al. The neuroimmune basis of fatigue. Trends Neurosci 2014;37:39–46.
194. Miller AH, Ancoli-Israel S, Bower JE, et al. Neuroendocrine-immune mechanisms of behavioral comorbidities in patients with cancer. J Clin Oncol 2008;26:971–82.
195. Walker AK, Kavelaars A, Heijnen CJ, et al. Neuroinflammation and comorbidity of pain and depression. Pharmacol Rev 2014;66:80–101.
196. Cella D, Davis K, Breitbart W, et al. Cancer-related fatigue: prevalence of proposed diagnostic criteria in a United States sample of cancer survivors. J Clin Oncol 2001;19:3385–91.
197. Prue G, Rankin J, Allen J, et al. Cancer-related fatigue: a critical appraisal. Eur J Cancer 2006;42:846–63.
198. Berger AM, Abernethy AP, Atkinson A, et al. Cancer-related fatigue. J Natl Compr Canc Netw 2010;8:904–31.
199. Curt GA. Impact of fatigue on quality of life in oncology patients. Semin Hematol 2000;37:14–7.
200. Davis JM. Central and peripheral factors in fatigue. J Sports Sci 1995;13:S49–53.
201. Chaudhuri A, Behan PO. Fatigue and basal ganglia. J Neurol Sci 2000;179:34–42.
202. Sadler IJ, Jacobsen PB, Booth-Jones M, et al. Preliminary evaluation of a clinical syndrome approach to assessing cancer-related fatigue. J Pain Symptom Manage 2002;23:406–16.

203. Van Belle S, Paridaens R, Evers G, et al. Comparison of proposed diagnostic criteria with FACT-F and VAS for cancer-related fatigue: proposal for use as a screening tool. Support Care Cancer 2005;13:246–54.
204. Lecrubier Y. Physical components of depression and psychomotor retardation. J Clin Psychiatry 2006;67(Suppl 6):23–6.
205. Wedding U, Koch A, Röhrig B, et al. Requestioning depression in patients with cancer: contribution of somatic and affective symptoms to Beck's Depression Inventory. Ann Oncol 2007;18:1875–81.
206. Wood LJ, Nail LM, Perrin NA, et al. The cancer chemotherapy drug etoposide (VP-16) induces proinflammatory cytokine production and sickness behavior-like symptoms in a mouse model of cancer chemotherapy-related symptoms. Biol Res Nurs 2006;8:157–69.
207. Novak CM, Burghardt PR. The use of a running wheel to measure activity in rodents: relationship to energy balance, general activity, and reward. Neurosci Biobehav Rev 2012;36:1001–14.
208. Hutchinson AD, Hosking JR. Objective and subjective cognitive impairment following chemotherapy for cancer: a systematic review. Cancer Treat Rev 2012;38:926–34.
209. O'farrell E, Mackenzie J. Clearing the air: a review of our current understanding of "chemo fog". Curr Oncol Rep 2013;15:260–9.
210. Jones D, Vichaya EG, Wang XS, et al. Acute cognitive impairment in patients with multiple myeloma undergoing autologous hematopoietic stem cell transplant. Cancer 2013;119:4188–95.
211. Seretny M, Currie GL, Sena ES, et al. Incidence, prevalence, and predictors of chemotherapy-induced peripheral neuropathy: a systematic review and meta-analysis. Pain 2014;155:2461–70.
212. Wieseler-Frank J, Maier SF. Immune-to-brain communication dynamically modulates pain: physiological and pathological consequences. Brain Behav Immun 2005;19:104–11.
213. Jounai N, Kobiyama K, Takeshita F, et al. Recognition of damage-associated molecular patterns related to nucleic acids during inflammation and vaccination. Front Cell Infect Microbiol 2012;2:168.
214. Seigers R, Timmermans J, van der Horn HJ, et al. Methotrexate reduces hippocampal blood vessel density and activates microglia in rats but does not elevate central cytokine release. Behav Brain Res 2010;207:265–72.
215. Ganz PA, Kwan L, Castellon SA, et al. Cognitive complaints after breast cancer treatments: examining the relationship with neuropsychological test performance. J Natl Cancer Inst 2013;105:791–801.
216. Silverman DH, Dy CJ, Castellon SA, et al. Altered frontocortical cerebellar, and basal ganglia activity in adjuvant treated breast cancer survivors 5-10 years after chemotherapy. Breast Cancer Res Treat 2007;103(3):303–11.
217. Doctors are finding it harder to deny "chemobrain". The Virginian-Pilot October 2, 2007.
218. Whyche S. Modafinil relieves cognitive chemotherapy side effects. Psychiatric News 2007;42(15):31.
219. Matsuda T, Takayama T, Tashiro M, et al. Mild cognitive impairment after adjuvant chemotherapy in breast cancer patients–evaluation of appropriate research design and methodology to measure symptoms. Breast Cancer 2005;12(4):279–87.
220. Schaefer M, Schmidt F, Folwaczny C, et al. Adherence and mental side effects during hepatitis C treatment with interferon alfa a ribavirin in psychiatric risk groups. Hepatology 2003;34:443–51.

221. Valentine AD, Meyers CA, Kling MA, et al. Mood and cognitive side effects of interferon-a therapy. Semin Oncol 1998;25(Suppl 1):39–47.
222. Dieperink E, Willenbring M, Ho SB. Neuropsychiatric symptoms associated with hepatitis C and interferon alpha: a review. Am J Psychiatry 2000;157:867–76.
223. Janssen HLA, Brouwer JT, van der Mast RC, et al. Suicide associated with alfa interferon therapy for chronic viral hepatitis. J Hepatol 1994;21:241–3.
224. Bonaccorso S, Puzella A, Marino V, et al. Immunotherapy with interferon-alpha in patients affected by chronic hepatitis C induces an intercorrelated stimulation of the cytokine network and an increase in depressive and anxiety symptoms. Psychiatry Res 2001;105:45–55.
225. Maes M, Bonaccorso S, Marino V, et al. Treatment with interferon-alpha (INFα) of hepatitis C patients induces lower serum dipeptidyl peptidase IV activity, which is related to INFα-induced depressive and anxiety symptoms and immune activation. Mol Psychiatry 2001;6:475–80.
226. Malaguarnera M, Laurino A, di Fazio I, et al. Neuropsychiatric effects and type of INF-α in chronic hepatitis C. J Interferon Cytokine Res 2001;21:273–8.
227. Hauser P, Khosla J, Aurora H, et al. A prospective study of the incidence and open-label treatment of interferon-induced major depressive disorder in patients with hepatitis C. Mol Psychiatry 2002;7:942–7.
228. Beck A, Ward C, Mendelson M, et al. An inventory for measuring depression. Arch Gen Psychiatry 1961;4:561–71.
229. Zdilar D, Franco-Bronson K, Buchler N, et al. Hepatitis C, interferon alfa, and depression. Hepatology 2000;31:1207–11.
230. Trask PC, Esper P, Riba M, et al. Psychiatric side effects of interferon therapy: prevalence, proposed mechanisms, and future directions. J Clin Oncol 2000;18:2316–26.
231. Capuron L, Ravaud A, Neveu PJ, et al. Association between decreased serum tryptophan concentrations and depressive symptoms in cancer patients undergoing cytokine therapy. Mol Psychiatry 2002;7:468–73.
232. Bonaccorso S, Marino V, Puzella A, et al. Increased depressive ratings in patients with hepatitis C receiving interferon-a–based immunotherapy are related to interferon-a–induced changes in the serotonergic system. J Clin Psychopharmacol 2002;22:86–90.
233. Billings RF, Stein MB. Depression associated with ranitidine. Am J Psychiatry 1986;143:915–6.
234. Stocky A. Ranitidine and depression. Aust N Z J Psychiatry 1991;25:415–8.
235. The IFNB Multiple Sclerosis Study Group and The University of British Columbia MS/MRI Analysis Group. Interferon beta-1b in the treatment of multiple sclerosis: final outcome of the randomized controlled trial. Neurology 1995;45:1277–85.
236. Victoroff JI, Benson DF, Engel J, et al. Interictal depression in patients with medically intractable complex partial seizures: electroencephalography and cerebral metabolic correlates [Abstract]. Ann Neurol 1990;28:221.
237. Camacho A, Ng B. Methylphenidate for α-interferon induced depression. J Psychopharmacol 2006;20:687–9.
238. Malek-Ahmadi P, Prabhu F. Venlafaxine for treatment of interferon alfa-induced depression. Ann Pharmacother 2006;40:2075.
239. Zigante F, Bastie A, Buffet C, et al. Incidence of interferon alfa-induced depression inpatients with chronic hepatitis C. Hepatology 2002;35:978–9.
240. Gurwitz JH, Field TS, Harrold LR, et al. Incidence and preventability of adverse drug events among older persons in the ambulatory setting. JAMA 2003;289:1107–16.

Frontotemporal Dementia

Roger E. Kelley, MD*, Ramy El-Khoury, MD

KEYWORDS

- Dementia • Behavioral disturbance • Abulia • Inattention • Disinhibition • Impulsivity
- Aphasia neurodegenerative disorder

KEY POINTS

- The initial description of this disorder is attributed to Arnold Pick in 1892.
- Involvement of the dominant hemisphere is characterized by primary progressive aphasia.
- The primary manifestations of the behavioral variant, reflective of nondominant hemisphere involvement, include the following: cognitive impairment including loss of initiative with apathy, abulia reflective of this loss of initiative including impaired executive function and lack of spontaneity, impulsivity, disinhibition, oral fixation, lack of sympathy and empathy, and repetitive behavior.
- There is well-recognized heterogeneity of clinicopathologic correlations.

OVERVIEW

A major challenge in the detection of frontotemporal dementia (FTD) is the potential for subtle presentation, which can result in serious consequences for patients unless the confounding early manifestations are correctly identified.[1-3] This point is illustrated in the following 3 case presentations:

Case Presentation 1

A 56-year-old right-handed man is brought to your office accompanied by his wife of 30 years. He is an accountant who is on administrative leave from his work because of increasing errors over the past several months. He has been described as a mild-mannered salt-of-the-earth type who regularly attends church and serves as a deacon. However, over the past year, he has made suggestive comments to several of his female coworkers, which is highly atypical for him according to his wife, and began looking at porn sites on his computer. This behavior is also viewed as highly atypical. He comes across as a bit reserved initially, and his wife provides much of

Disclosures: None.
Department of Neurology, Tulane University School of Medicine, 1430 Tulane Avenue, 8065, New Orleans, LA 70112, USA
* Corresponding author.
E-mail address: rkelley2@tulane.edu

his history. Generally, he has been in excellent health outside of hypertension of several years' duration and recently placed on a statin for dyslipidemia.

He has a college education, never smoked, drinks an occasional beer or glass of wine, and has never used illicit drugs. He has no history of sexually transmitted disease and has no history of significant head trauma. There is the question of dementia affecting his maternal grandfather in his 60s as well as a maternal uncle, but the specifics are not well known. There was an interesting recollection of a great uncle, described as a religious teetotaler, who ended up being killed in a brothel under mysterious circumstances.

The general examination is unremarkable. He does not come across as overly depressed and seems to cooperate fairly well with testing, often glancing over at his wife. On neurologic testing, he is somewhat delayed in his responses, with 2 mistakes on serial 7 subtractions, difficulty reproducing a design, and scores 27 out of 30 on the mini-mental state examination. The neurologic examination is otherwise quite normal. You order routine laboratory tests along with a serum vitamin B12 and folate level and thyroid profile with all coming back normal. A computed tomography (CT) brain scan and MRI brain scan both reveal fairly prominent frontotemporal atrophy, especially on the right. An electroencephalogram (EEG) reveals some bifrontal slowing but no epileptiform activity.

Case Presentation 2

A 62-year-old right-handed woman comes to your office with her female partner. They have lived together for the past 12 years and both have worked as elementary school teachers. The patient has been noted to having some communication issues in recent months, and it is beginning to be picked up by other teachers as well as the students. She has word-finding difficulty, with speech hesitancy, and uses inappropriate word choices at times. She has complained of some reading difficulty as well, and this is of particular concern to her as she has been an avid reader.

She has been quite healthy all her life and was a marathon runner at one time as well as a state tennis champion. She has been on no medications and continues an active daily exercise program but is noticing diminished exercise tolerance in recent months. She is quite selective in her diet and has maintained a weight of 120 lb during her adult life with a height of 5 ft 3 in. However, her weight is recorded at 114 lb in your office. The patient is surprised by this, although her partner has noticed a reduction in her typically finely toned musculature over the past half year. She has never smoked, drinks a glass of wine each evening, and does not use recreational drugs. The family history is noncontributory as she is adopted.

On examination, she looks quite healthy but has some obvious speech hesitancy and the suggestion of a mild bulbar type of dysarthria at times. The general physical is quite normal. She has some difficulty with naming and repetition, although comprehension seems to be intact. Her palate elevates symmetrically, and her gag reflex is intact. Her tongue is not of full bulk with suggestion of fasciculations. There is fair rapid alternating movement of the tongue. Strength and tone seems to be normal on motor testing, with some atrophy of the shoulder muscles; scattered fasciculations are noted. She does well with cerebellar testing and with gait, and no sensory loss is noted. Deep tendon reflexes are 3+ in both biceps and triceps and 3+ to 4− at both knees with a crossed adduction response, and there are several beats of clonus at both ankles, with the Babinski response positive on both sides and with a 2+ jaw jerk.

Brain imaging reveals the suggestion of frontal lobe atrophy, more prominent on the left. Blood tests come back fine. The cervical spine MRI is normal. Electromyography reveals increased insertional activity in several muscles of the upper and lower extremities with denervation and reinnervation changes.

Case Presentation 3

This patient is a 60-year-old gentleman whose cousin has made this appointment. He is accompanied by the cousin who provides essentially all of the history. The patient was once the life of the party and had several wives in his younger years. He was a very successful car salesman and could sell ice to the Eskimos, as his cousin termed it. He was known to drink liberally in the past and was a former smoker. He was under treatment of gout and had been treated for a manic episode by a psychiatrist several years ago. He refused to take medication for this episode and was never the same, according to his cousin. A former wife tried to make contact with him recently and found him to be somewhat rambling and incoherent on the phone leading her to call the cousin to check on him.

The cousin had found the patient in a disheveled condition in his apartment. He had not been seen by neighbors for several days and typically ventured out at night to get some groceries. The apartment was in shambles with food scattered about. The patient was noted to have poor personal hygiene. He is initially quite passive and apathetic but becomes easily irritated with any attempt at questioning him. He was not cooperative in the examination. He responds, "I don't know," to most questions. The examiner makes note of facial blunting and obvious bradykinesia. No tremor is noted. There is the suggestion of resistance to passive movement versus actual rigidity during the limited motor testing that the patient allows. Strength is fairly good throughout with limited cooperation in assessment of dexterity or in cerebellar function. He walks with a somewhat stooped posture with limited arm swing. A bilateral grasp reflex and suck reflex is noted.

CASE DISCUSSION

The first case illustrates the not-uncommon presentation of the behavioral form of FTD. This gentleman demonstrates personality change, which is initially subtle but progressive. Such patients are often referred for psychiatric evaluation. However, the onset of symptoms, at this age, with no prior psychiatric history suggests the vagaries of the behavioral form of FTD. Impulsive behavior, with disinhibition, can lead to physical interactions as well as criminal activity. Pillars of the community may end up in illicit sexual relationships, which causes extreme embarrassment for the family. Recognition of the cause of such personality change is obviously of great value in determining how best to avoid such activity. On the other hand, some patients display increasing loss of initiative with apathy and are pretty much confined to a listless lifestyle based on their selective involvement by the pathologic process.

The second patient is an example of the primary progressive aphasia (PPA) form of FTD. The onset tends to be insidious and usually does not invoke acute stroke in the differential. However, an atypical subtle stroke presentation affecting the communication centers of the dominant cerebral hemisphere is a potential explanation in some patients as is a structural lesion, such as neoplasm, abscess, or subdural hematoma. This second case also illustrates the potential association of FTD and motor neuron disease.[4] This relationship has been identified with the GGCCC (G_4C_2) repeat expansion of the C9orf72 gene, which is the most common cause for familial amyotrophic lateral sclerosis (ALS), FTD, as well as ALS-FTD.[5]

In addition, to the potential overlap of ALS and FTD, one can also see features of parkinsonism with FTD.[6] The parkinsonism is typically of the akinetic-rigid type and is not generally responsive to levodopa. This type is illustrated in the third case. The overlap of FTD and parkinsonism has been linked to mutations in the gene encoding the microtubule-associated protein tau (*MAPT*; Online Mendelian Inheritance of Man [OMIM] + 157140) on chromosome 17.[7] However, not all kindreds with this familial overlap presentation have been attributed to a tauopathy with *MAPT* mutations. Certain kindreds have mutations of the gene encoding progranulin (*PGRN*; OMIM *138945), which is in close proximity to the *MAPT* location on chromosome 17.[8]

MANIFESTATION KEY POINTS

- It is the most common cause of dementia in adults less than 60 years of age.[9]
- The most common age of onset is in the sixth decade.
- Most cases of FTD are sporadic.
- Up to 10% to 15% of cases are associated with an autosomal dominant genetic mutation.[10]
- The initial manifestations are often initially reported to psychiatrists, psychologists, marriage or addiction counselors, human relations officers, or those in the legal realm reflective of the potential for aberrant behavior.[11]
- Semantic PPA type is characterized by impaired single-word comprehension and marked anomia but with fluent speech.[12]
- The nonfluent/agrammatic PPA type is characterized by limited speech production with grammatical and syntax errors.[12]
- The logopenic PPA type is characterized by intermixed fluent and nonfluent speech related to significant word-finding difficulty typically resulting in slow or delayed speech.[12]

DIFFERENTIAL DIAGNOSIS

The potential manifestations of FTD result in a bridging between psychiatric disease and other causes of dementia. The potential alternative explanations are outlined in **Box 1**.

GENOTYPIC AND PHENOTYPIC FACTORS

The phenotypic variability reflects genetic variations, which can include tau mutations, progranulin gene mutations, as well as repeat expansions (GGGCCC) of the C9orf72 gene. Three subtypes of FTD have been designated based on the type of inclusions in brain tissue.[13] These subtypes include tau protein, transactive response DNA-binding protein 43 (TDP-43), and RNA-binding protein fused in sarcoma (FUS). Such inclusions impact on the potential manifestations. Tau pathology is often associated with features of parkinsonism but typically not with ALS. On the other hand, TDP-43 and FUS are not uncommonly seen in combined FTD and ALS. In terms of frequency, roughly 50% of patients with FTD have FTD-TDP as the major pathologic subtype,[14,15] whereas FTD-tau accounts for roughly 45% of patients and FTD-FUS 5% or less.[16]

DIAGNOSTIC APPROACH KEY POINTS

- Clinicians must have a certain index of suspicion that the behavioral disturbance or communication deficit is not in the psychiatric realm but in the neurodegenerative realm.
- Atypical presentations can obviously be misleading, such as an unexpectedly young age of onset, such as in the 20s or 30s.

Box 1
Differential diagnosis of FTD

1. Previously unrecognized bipolar disorder
2. Previously unrecognized schizoaffective disorder
3. Sociopathic personality disorder
4. Alzheimer disease
5. Dementia with Lewy bodies
6. Parkinsonism-dementia complex
7. Normal pressure hydrocephalus
8. Neoplastic disease of the brain
9. Remote effect of malignancy, such as limbic encephalitis
10. Anti-N-methyl-d-aspartate receptor encephalitis
11. Human immunodeficiency virus–related dementia
12. Spinocerebellar ataxia 3 (Machado-Joseph disease)
13. Epilepsy-related encephalopathy
14. Medication-induced encephalopathy
15. Metabolic encephalopathy
16. Endocrine-related encephalopathy, for example, Hashimoto encephalopathy
17. Neurosyphilis
18. Cryptococcal meningitis
19. Herpes simplex encephalitis
20. West Nile encephalitis
21. Chronic traumatic encephalopathy
22. Vascular dementia
23. Mercury toxicity
24. Methamphetamine/phencyclidine/cocaine/psychostimulant abuse
25. Late-onset metachromatic leukodystrophy
26. Late-onset Nasu-Hakola disease
27. Late-onset Niemann-Pick disease type C
28. Adult Tay-Sachs disease
29. Adult Gaucher disease
30. Adult neuronal ceroid lipofuscinosis
31. Adult polyglucosan body disorder

- Neuroimaging is key, with the finding of atrophy of the frontal and temporal lobes on either brain CT or MRI scan of key importance.
- The potential for familial predisposition can be an important clue.
- Coexistent manifestations, such as motor neuron disease or parkinsonism, can help in putting the clinical picture in proper perspective.
- As with other dementing illness, exclusion of other potential explanations with brain imaging, blood work, and possibly EEG can be elucidating.

- Special imaging techniques, such as ^{18}fludeoxyglucose (FDG) PET scan, and new techniques, such as beta-amyloid and tau imaging PET scan as well as diffusion tensor MRI, can provide pertinent supportive or nonsupportive information.

The particular frontotemporal involvement can be demonstrated anatomically with CT brain scan or MRI brain scan as mentioned earlier (**Fig. 1**). Significant hypodensity changes in the subcortical white matter in the periventricular region on a CT brain scan or the corresponding signal hyperintensity changes on an MRI brain scan tends to reflect microvascular ischemic disease. One can readily exclude a significant component of communicating hydrocephalus on such scans as well as potential structural lesions or larger vessel cerebrovascular disease on such scans.

Cerebral PET scan with ^{18}FDG can demonstrates hypometabolism in the frontotemporal region, which will help distinguish FTD from the fairly characteristic pattern for Alzheimer disease of biparietal hypometabolism earlier on in the course of this disorder. The fluorine 18 –florbetapir PET scan allows in vivo imaging of beta-amyloid plaque deposition within the brain and can be of potential value in determining a primarily Alzheimer component to the dementia.[17] More recently, tau in vivo brain imaging with PET has become available with the potential to identify primarily tau-mediated neurodegenerative disease.[16] The potential for such advanced imaging in distinguishing one form of dementia from another was illustrated in a recent case report.[18]

Diagnostic biomarkers may also have utility in the diagnostic assessment. In Alzheimer disease, for example, there is a fairly consistent pattern of elevated total tau protein and diminished beta-amyloid-42 protein concentration in the cerebrospinal fluid.[19] It is hoped that similar biomarkers will be identified for FTD. One potential biomarker for FTD is a specific antibody for TDP-43 for patients with FTD who have a proteinopathy characterized by brain inclusions for transactive response DNA-binding protein of 43 kDA.[20]

MONITORING OF DISEASE ACTIVITY

Obviously, the expected clinical course of a neurodegenerative disease is progression. However, the natural history of FTD, reflective of the significant variability in

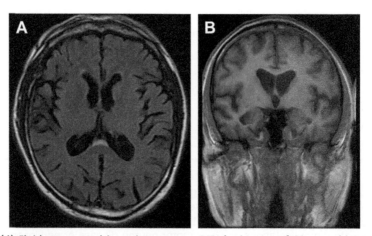

Fig. 1. (*A*) Fluid-attentuated inversion recovery MRI brain scan of 68-year-old gentleman with 5-year history of increasing difficulty with executive function, impulsivity, mood swings, and inattention, which displays frontotemporal region atrophy. (*B*) Coronal T1-weighted MRI demonstrating particular involvement of the temporal lobes.

phenotypic expression, makes accurate prognostication for patients and family members challenging at best. Unlike Alzheimer disease, whereby the progression over 6- to 12-month intervals can be fairly accurately determined by reports of family members and simple office cognitive testing, the behavioral variant of FTD can be difficult to objectively quantitate with the not-expected fluctuation. Even for the language variant of FTD, it is not at all uncommon to see fluctuation in communication ability from day to day.

Volumetric analysis of dementia with modalities such as MRI can provide quantitative measurement of tissue loss, that is, atrophy, over time. Efforts have been made to distinguish the selective atrophy of FTD from the atrophy pattern seen with Alzheimer disease.[21] In an MRI volumetric analysis of Alzheimer disease and FTD,[22] the investigators reported some differentiation of the degree of atrophy for the hippocampus and amygdale in Alzheimer disease versus FTD but not for the cingulated gyrus. There has

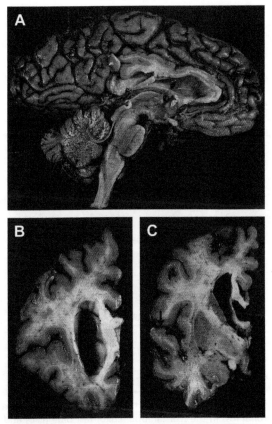

Fig. 2. Brains sections at autopsy of a man in his 30s with progressive cognitive impairment, behavioral disturbance, and parkinsonism. (*A*) Demonstrates a moderate degree of frontal and temporal lobe atrophy. (*B*) Demonstrated evidence of cortical atrophy and ventricular enlargement. (*C*) Demonstrates selective atrophy of the frontal and temporal lobe region with relative sparing of the superior temporal gyrus (*arrow*). (*From* Miller BL, Dickerson BC, Lucente DE, et al. Case records of the Massachusetts General Hospital. Case 9-2015. A 31-year-old man with progressive personality changes and progressive neurologic decline. N Engl J Med 2015;372:1158; with permission.)

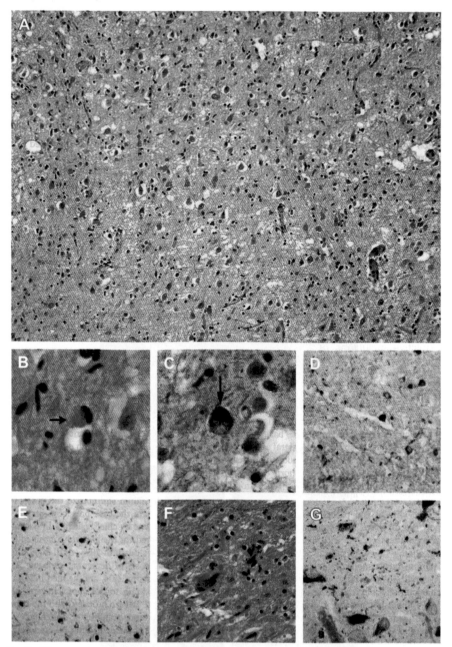

Fig. 3. Microscopic neuropathologic images of the patient in **Fig. 2**. (*A*) Stain that reveals reactive gliosis and neuronal loss in the frontal lobe (Luxol fast blue [LFB] and hematoxylin and eosin [H&E]). (*B*) Demonstration of a Pick body (*arrow*) (LFB and H&E). (*C*) Demonstration of a Pick body (Bielschowsky silver method) (*arrow*). (*D, E*) Immunohistochemical staining with phospho-specific antibodies against tau reflective of tau protein-containing inclusions. (*F*) Stain demonstrating neuronal loss in the pars compacta of the substantia nigra (LFB and H&E). (*G*) Immunohistochemical staining for PHF1 shows cytoplasmic inclusions and neuropil threads, within the substantia nigra, which contain phosphorylated tau. (*From* Miller BL, Dickerson BC, Lucente DE, et al. Case records of the Massachusetts General Hospital. Case 9-2015. A 31-year-old man with progressive personality changes and progressive neurologic decline. N Engl J Med 2015;372:1159; with permission.)

been a recent report of the potential value of longitudinal diffusion tensor imaging as a biomarker of disease activity in FTD.[23] This study was of the behavioral variant group with measurements at baseline and approximately 1.3 years later. Rates of change in fractional anisotropy and mean diffusivity suggested selective involvement over time of the pericallosal cingulate region, in the 23 patients as a whole, with *MAPT* carriers showing greatest change in the left uncinate fasciculus and sporadic and *C9orf72* carriers with the greatest change in the left uncinate fasciculus.

TREATMENT APPROACH

Addressing the underlying molecular pathology will eventually significantly impact the treatment approach.[12] There are presumably multiple pathways potentially involved, which lead to the progressive atrophic process within the frontal and temporal lobes as illustrated in **Fig. 2**. This patient was a case presentation of the case records of the Massachusetts General Hospital published in the *New England Journal of Medicine*.[11] The onset of personality change and progressive neurologic decline was at 28 years of age with death in a debilitated state, with manifestations of both dementia with behavioral disturbance as well as parkinsonism at 33 years of age. This case reflects the not-uncommon progressive impairment seen in a neurodegenerative-related dementia over a 5-year time frame. The pathology for this gentleman is illustrated in **Fig. 3**. Special staining reflected tau-based pathology, specifically tau-positive inclusions of the Pick disease subtype. This particular presentation was due to a *Gly389Arg* mutation. Unfortunately, no specific treatment is presently available for such a presentation outside of supportive care. Not uncommonly, such patients will be tried on cholinesterase inhibitors, memantine, and vitamin E supplementation, along with various mediations related to the behavioral disturbance variant.

In order to develop effective strategies against such proteinopathies, neuroscientists will need to elucidate the responsible network of RNA and protein interactions.[24] Biomarkers for specific disease identification and level of expression have significant potential in this quest.[25] Elucidation of genetic susceptibility, such as determination of low-frequency coding variants with intermediate effect size by genome-wide exom array multi-ancestral studies,[26] will also be important. An example of where such innovative research might take us, McMillan and colleagues[27] reported recently on the potential for *C9orf72* promoter hypermethylation to be potentially neuroprotective in disorders associated with inclusions of TDP-43. They surmised that such an approach could result in transcriptional silencing of mutant *C9orf72* and be a potential avenue for drug development in both FTD and ALS.

REFERENCES

1. Pick A. Über die Beziehungen der senile Hirnatrophie zur Aphasie. Prager Med Wochenschr 1892;17:165–7.
2. Gorno-Tempini ML, Hillis AE, Weintraub S, et al. Classification of primary progressive aphasia and its variants. Neurology 2011;76:1006–14.
3. Rascovsky K, Hodges JR, Knopman D, et al. Sensitivity of revised diagnostic criteria for the behavioral variant of frontotemporal dementia. Brain 2011;134: 2456–77.
4. Majounie E, Renton AE, Mok K, et al. Frequency of the C9orf72 hexanucleotide repeat expansion in patients with amyotrophic lateral sclerosis and frontotemporal dementia: a cross-sectional study. Lancet Neurol 2012;11:323–30.

5. Cruts M, Gijselnick I, Van Langenhove T, et al. Current insights into the C9orf72 repeat expansion diseases of the FTLD/ALS spectrum. Trends Neurosci 2013; 36:450–9.
6. Boeve BF, Hutton M. Refining frontotemporal dementia with parkinsonism linked to chromosome 17. Arch Neurol 2008;65:460–4.
7. Pickering-Brown SM, Baker M, Gass J, et al. Mutations in progranulin explain atypical phenotypes with variants in MAPT. Brain 2006;129:3124–6.
8. Rosenberg RN. Progranulin and tau gene mutations both as cause for dementia; 17q21 finally defined. Arch Neurol 2007;64:18–9.
9. Knopman DS, Petersen RC, Edland SD, et al. The incidence of frontotemporal lobar dementia in Rochester, Minnesota 1990 through 1994. Neurology 2004; 62:506–8.
10. Seelaar H, Kamphorst W, Rosso SM, et al. Distinct genetic forms of frontotemporal dementia. Neurology 2008;71:1220–6.
11. Miller BL, Dickerson BC, Lucente DE, et al. Case records of the Massachusetts General Hospital. Case 9-2015. A 31-year-old man with progressive personality changes and progressive neurologic decline. N Engl J Med 2015;372:1151–62.
12. Harris JM, Jones M. Pathology in primary progressive aphasia syndromes. Curr Neurol Neurosci Rep 2014;14:466–74.
13. Sieben A, Van Langehove T, Engelborghs S, et al. The genetics and neuropathology of frontotemporal lobar degeneration. Acta Neuropathol 2012;124: 353–72.
14. Neumann M, Sampathu DM, Kwong LK, et al. Ubiquitinated TDP-43 in frontotemporal lobar degeneration and amyotrophic lateral sclerosis. Science 2006;314: 130–3.
15. Irwin DJ, Cairns NJ, Grossman M, et al. Frontotemporal lobar degeneration: defining phenotypic diversity through personalized medicine. Acta Neuropathol 2015;129:469–91.
16. Mitsis EM, Bender HA, Kostakoglu L, et al. A consecutive case series experience with [18 F] florbetapir PET imaging in an urban dementia center: impact on quality of life, decision making, and disposition. Mol Neurodegener 2014;9:10.
17. Xia CF, Arteaga J, Chen G, et al. [^{18}F]T807, a novel tau positron emission tomography imaging agent for Alzheimer's disease. Alzheimers Dement 2013;9:666–76.
18. Mitsis EM, Riggio S, Kostakoglu L, et al. Tauopathy PET and amyloid PET in the diagnosis of chronic traumatic encephalopathies: studies of a retired NFL player and a man with FTD with severe head injury. Transl Psychiatry 2014;4:1–8.
19. Frankfort SV, Tulner LR, van Campen JP, et al. Amyloid beta protein and tau in the cerebrospinal fluid and plasma as biomarkers for dementia: a review of recent literature. Curr Clin Pharmacol 2008;3:123–31.
20. Goossens J, Vanmechelen E, Trojanowski JQ, et al. TDP-43 as a possible biomarker for frontotemporal lobar degeneration: a systematic review of existing antibodies. Acta Neuropathol Commun 2015;3:1–8.
21. Bocti C, Rockel C, Roy P, et al. Differential topography of Alzheimer's disease and frontotemporal dementia: an MRI volumetric analysis from Sunnybrook dementia study. Brain Cogn 2004;54:151–3.
22. Varghese T, Kumari S, Mathuranath PS. Volumetric analysis of regional atrophy for the differential diagnosis of AD and FTD. Int J Comp App 2013;62:43–8.
23. Mahoney CJ, Simpson IJ, Nicholas JM, et al. Longitudinal diffusion tensor imaging in frontotemporal dementia. Ann Neurol 2015;77:33–46.
24. Fontana F, Siva K, Denti MA. A network of RNA and protein interactions in fronto temporal dementia. Front Mol Neurosci 2015;8:1–30.

25. Grossman M. Biomarkers in primary progressive aphasias. Aphasiology 2014;28: 922–40.
26. Chen JA, Wang Q, Davis-Turak J, et al. A multiancestral genome-wide exome array study of Alzheimer's disease, frontotemporal dementia, and progressive supranuclear palsy. JAMA Neurol 2015;72:414–22.
27. McMillan CT, Russ J, Wood EW, et al. *C9orf72* promoter hypermethylation is neuroprotective. Neuroimaging and neuropathologic evidence. Neurology 2015;84: 1622–30.

Treatment of Cognitive Deficits in Epilepsy

Beth A. Leeman-Markowski, MD, MA, MMSc[a],*, Steven C. Schachter, MD[b]

KEYWORDS

- Epilepsy • Seizures • Cognition • Memory • Attention • Language
- Executive function • Neuropsychological

KEY POINTS

- Cognitive deficits in epilepsy are common, often affecting multiple domains and impairing quality of life.
- Attaining better seizure control may improve cognition.
- The older anticonvulsants (i.e. phenobarbital) typically cause greater cognitive side effects than newer medications.
- Treatment of co-morbid depression is essential. Selective serotonin reuptake inhibitors are first-line agents.
- Cognitive rehabilitation is beneficial in selected patients.

INTRODUCTION

Cognitive deficits in epilepsy are common in the setting of newly diagnosed epilepsy, as well as in patients with long-standing seizures.[1–5] Deficits may affect multiple cognitive domains, including memory, attention, executive function, and language.[3] The etiology is typically multifactorial, with impairments secondary to ongoing seizures, interictal epileptiform discharges (IEDs), the underlying epilepsy syndrome, structural lesions, treatment effects, genetic influences, and psychosocial issues. Treatment for cognitive deficits in patients with epilepsy is individualized, based upon identification of the contributing factors. Management may involve alteration of the anticonvulsant regimen,

Disclosures: None.

To be published in: Neurobehavioral Manifestations of Neurological Diseases: Diagnosis and Treatment, Neurologic Clinics of North America, edited by Drs Alireza Minagar, Glenn Finney, and Kenneth M. Heilman.

[a] Department of Neurology, Emory University, 101 Woodruff Circle, Suite 6000, Atlanta, GA 30322, USA; [b] Department of Neurology, Beth Israel Deaconess Medical Center, Massachusetts General Hospital – CIMIT, Harvard Medical School, 165 Cambridge Street, Suite 702, Boston, MA 02114, USA

* Corresponding author.

E-mail address: beth.a.leeman@emory.edu

suppression of interictal discharges, treatment of underlying psychiatric disorders, cognitive rehabilitation, and in the setting of epilepsy surgery, attempts to predict and prevent postoperative cognitive decline. These methods will be discussed in this article, along with experimental approaches, including use of acetylcholinesterase inhibitors, stimulants, N-methyl-D-aspartate (NMDA)-receptor antagonists, herbal supplementation, and brain stimulation.

DIAGNOSIS

Cognitive deficits may be subtle in many patients, yet disabling in others. In highly functioning patients, even mild deficits may be impairing. In some cases, however, cognitive dysfunction may go unnoticed or unreported. Witt and colleagues[5] found that 28.7% and 25.1% of subjects with newly diagnosed epilepsy reported inattention and memory problems, respectively. In contrast, objective neuropsychological testing demonstrated attentional and executive dysfunction in 49.4% of subjects and memory deficits in 47.8% of subjects. Detailed neuropsychological testing also revealed that even patients with benign epilepsy syndromes, such as benign rolandic epilepsy[6,7] and juvenile myoclonic epilepsy (JME)[8] can have cognitive sequelae across multiple domains. Such cases underscore the importance of formal neuropsychological testing in the diagnosis of cognitive impairment.

The National Institute of Neurological Disorders and Stroke (NINDS) Common Data Elements[9] suggest several domains to be tested, in addition to recommended measures for assessment (**Table 1**). Most epilepsy centers have a preferred battery to be administered routinely pre- and postoperatively and in the setting of cognitive complaints. Results can then be compared with published normative values obtained in control populations matched for demographic variables such as sex and age.

Specific tests vary with respect to sensitivity, specificity, reliability, and validity. In general, the sensitivity of neuropsychological testing is limited, in that some patients may report cognitive deficits that are not detected upon formal testing. Memory impairment in patients with epilepsy, for example, may not be identified using existing measures of 30- to 40-minute delayed recall. Eliciting memory deficits may necessitate delayed testing at hours to weeks to detect accelerated long-term forgetting.[10] Detecting nonverbal impairments may also be challenging, as visuospatial functions are less strongly lateralized than verbal functions.[11,12] At present, no cognitive tests can specifically assess nondominant temporal function.

Computerized testing methods have gained popularity given their ease and efficiency of administration, cost-effectiveness, and accessibility. These batteries may be useful for objective screening in the setting of subjective cognitive complaints, repeated measures, coregistration with electroencephalogram (EEG) data, and intraoperative testing. In the future, mobile devices may be used to assess cognitive function outside of the hospital or clinic setting. Further data are needed, however, regarding sensitivity and specificity with respect to epilepsy-related variables and the assessment of individual patients. In most cases, current computerized testing packages should not replace traditional detailed neuropsychological evaluations.[13]

The patterns of deficits on standard neuropsychological testing generally reflect dysfunction of the underlying epileptogenic brain regions. Greater impairments on testing correlate with the severity of hippocampal atrophy,[14,15] as well as longer duration of the seizure disorder,[16] earlier age of onset,[17] greater seizure frequency,[18] and lower quality of life.[19] Repeated testing is sensitive to changes in function over time, allowing the clinician to track the response to treatment.

Table 1
Neuropsychological testing. Recommendations per the National Institute of Neurological Disorders and Stroke Common Data Elements

Cognitive Domain	Recommended Test Batteries	Anatomic Correlates
Verbal memory	• Rey auditory verbal learning test • California verbal learning test-2 • Selective reminding test	Dominant temporal lobe
Spatial memory[a]	• Wechsler memory scale visual reproduction • Rey-Osterrieth complex figure test • Brief visuospatial memory test–revised • Nonverbal selective reminding test	Nondominant temporal lobe
Naming	Boston naming test	Dominant temporal and inferior parietal lobes, insula, putamen
Verbal IQ (VIQ) and Performance IQ (PIQ)	• Wechsler adult intelligence test-fourth edition • Wechsler abbreviated scale of intelligence	Multiple brain regions assessed; VIQ and PIQ generally reflect dominant and nondominant hemisphere function, respectively, but significant overlap prevents diagnostic use in individual patients
Frontal/executive function	• Wisconsin card sorting • Trails A and B • Digit span	Frontal lobe (cortical and subcortical), especially prefrontal; limbic structures, nondominant hemisphere

[a] No test was recommended; however, the scales listed were noted as measures to consider.
From National Institute of Neurological Disorders and Stroke. NINDS Common Data Elements. 2010. Available at: http://www.commondataelements.ninds.nih.gov/Epilepsy.aspx#tab=Data_Standards. Accessed August 24, 2014.

TREATMENT OF COGNITIVE DEFICITS IN EPILEPSY
Optimizing Seizure Control

Seizure-related factors may impact cognition, including

1. Seizure type. In children, primary or secondary generalized seizures may pose more risk than simple or complex partial seizures.[17,20]
2. Seizure syndrome. Idiopathic generalized epilepsy syndromes typically carry a better cognitive prognosis than epilepsy caused by focal lesions, hereditary metabolic syndromes, or neurodegenerative disorders.
3. Etiology. The specific etiology of the epilepsy syndrome is also significant. Patients with hippocampal sclerosis, for example, may have more diffuse impairments than patients with temporal lobe epilepsy (TLE) from other causes.[21]
4. Location of seizure onset. In focal-onset epilepsy, specific patterns of deficits may reflect the localization of seizure onset. Frontal lobe epilepsy, for example, may be associated with impaired motor coordination and response inhibition.[22] Patients

with TLE may exhibit material-specific deficits, reflecting the lateralization of the epileptogenic zone. Patients with dominant hemisphere TLE are at risk for verbal memory loss, while those with nondominant hemisphere TLE may have nonverbal memory dysfunction.[23,24] Patients with generalized epileptic syndromes may also have deficits that suggest a region with a greater burden of epileptiform or ictal discharges, as in the verbal auditory agnosia and language regression seen with temporal or parieto-occipital EEG paroxysms in Landau-Kleffner syndrome.

5. Acute ictal effects. Cognition may be disrupted before (preictal), during (ictal), or after a seizure (postictal), often with specific deficits reflecting the site of seizure onset. Although relatively uncommon, seizures may manifest solely or primarily as cognitive dysfunction. This phenomenon may be seen, for example, with ictal aphasia caused by dominant temporal or temporoparietal seizures[25,26] or transient epileptic amnesia in the setting of unilateral or bilateral temporal lobe seizures.[27] Limited data regarding postictal cognition have demonstrated a return to baseline memory function within 30 minutes to 1 hour after reorientation from temporal lobe seizures,[28] although the precise time course varied based upon seizure lateralization and the type of stimuli.

As seizure frequency correlates with impaired cognition,[18] attaining improved seizure control would be an important initial step in treating cognitive deficits. Better seizure control was associated with beneficial cognitive effects of levetiracetam.[29]

Minimizing Antiepileptic Drug Adverse Effects

Cognitive dysfunction may also result as an adverse effect of antiepileptic drug (AED) use. The goal of AED therapy is to control seizures while minimizing adverse effects. Using slower titration rates, lowering dosages, maintaining lower blood levels, and minimizing polypharmacy, when possible, may lessen negative cognitive effects.

The type of anticonvulsant must also be considered. In general, the older AEDs, particularly benzodiazepines and barbiturates, have more cognitive clouding effects than newer agents. Carbamazepine, phenytoin, and valproate have moderate impairing effects as well. These older agents have been shown to cause objective deficits in response inhibition, verbal fluency, attention and vigilance, psychomotor speed, P3 potentials, sensory discrimination, and memory, as well as subjective confusion and memory loss.[30–33] In the setting of cognitive dysfunction, the clinician may consider dosage reduction or use of alternative agents, if possible.

Data regarding the new generation of AEDs are mixed. Overall, the newer AEDs are believed to cause fewer cognitive adverse effects than older drugs, with the exceptions of topiramate and zonisamide. Topiramate and zonisamide have consistently demonstrated associations with dysfunction across multiple domains, with language deficits being most common. Nearly 50% of patients taking zonisamide report mild cognitive complaints,[34] with objective deficits in verbal intelligence,[35] verbal learning,[34,36] delayed verbal and nonverbal memory,[34,36] and verbal fluency.[34] Topiramate has been shown to impair IQ, verbal comprehension, verbal and nonverbal memory, verbal and nonverbal fluency, response inhibition, working memory, attention, processing and psychomotor speed, visuospatial skills, naming, and problem solving.[35,37–42] Up to 50% of patients report anomia or other expressive difficulties with topiramate.[39–41,43] Effects of zonisamide[34–36] and topiramate,[35,41,43] however, are typically reversible with dosage reduction or drug discontinuation.

Levetiracetam is unique in that it is considered to be a nootropic or cognition-enhancing AED. Subjective improvement was reported in 58% of patients, and objective improvement was noted in 23% to 29% of patients on measures of executive function, memory, fluency, comprehension, and visuospatial skills after 6 months of treatment.[29] Levetiracetam also had beneficial effects on verbal and visual attention, psychomotor speed, and subjective alertness.[44,45] Levetiracetam may be a preferred agent in the setting of epilepsy and cognitive dysfunction in patients without comorbid depression, although longer-term studies are needed.

Preventing Postoperative Deficits

In approximately 30% of patients, seizures are refractory to medication. In selected medically refractory patients, surgical resection offers a greater likelihood of seizure freedom than continued medication trials. Anterior temporal lobectomy (ATL), the most common surgical procedure performed, may result in freedom from seizures that impair awareness in approximately 60% of patients.[46] In some cases, resection yields improved cognitive function. Stroup and colleagues[47] noted that 3% of dominant and 7% of nondominant ATL patients had postoperative improvement of verbal memory, while others have suggested improvement in up to 25% of patients.[48–50] The underlying mechanism likely relates to the removal of nociferous tissue, allowing the remaining healthy tissue to function uninterrupted.

More often, however, there is a risk for postoperative cognitive deficits. Of particular concern are the effects of dominant hemisphere ATL, in which postresection verbal memory decline may be evident in up to 60% of patients.[47,51] The deficits are severe in an estimated 21% of patients.[52] Visuospatial deficits following nondominant temporal resections, in contrast, are more variable and likely to resolve over time. A number of techniques may be used to determine the risk of postoperative impairment (**Table 2**). In general, tests that suggest functional tissue will be removed, or indicate that the remaining tissue would be unable to support cognitive function, imply greater risks of postoperative dysfunction. The goal is to tailor the resection or use alternative surgical approaches to minimize effects on cognition, when possible.

Given the possibility of postoperative decline, there is a desire to develop alternative surgical approaches and implantable devices to minimize risk (**Table 3**). These approaches must balance the odds of seizure freedom with the risks to cognition. Although techniques such as selective amygdalo-hippocampectomy may limit the amount of tissue removed, with seizure control comparable to more extensive resections, damage to neighboring structures and white matter tracts during surgery may still lead to postoperative cognitive deficits. Device implantations, in contrast, may spare cognitive function, but are less likely to lead to seizure freedom. These factors must be considered individually for each patient.

Interictal Discharge Suppression

IEDs are evident on electroencephalography in an estimated 90% of patients with epilepsy.[71] They appear as intermittent spike and sharp wave discharges and result from the synchronous firing of hyperexcitable neurons. IEDs, by definition, are not seizures and do not evolve into seizures. They are considered only to be markers of epilepsy, and IEDs alone are not typically targeted with medications. An increasing amount of data, however, suggest that both focal and generalized IEDs disrupt cognitive function, a process termed transient cognitive impairment (TCI). IEDs have been associated with poorer performance on tests of intelligence,[69,70,72] memory,[72–78] motor speed and target detection,[79–86] and continuous visual–motor performance.[87]

Several AEDs have been shown to suppress IEDs, including lamotrigine,[88] levetiracetam,[89,90] valproic acid,[91] and topiramate.[92] It is unknown, however, whether pharmacologic suppression of the discharges would improve cognition. The data

Table 2
Tests used to assess the cognitive risks of surgical resection

Test	Indication of Good Prognosis	Risk Factor for Poor Prognosis
Preoperative EEG	Abnormalities restricted to the epileptogenic region	Bilateral abnormalities
Structural MRI	Abnormal-appearing hippocampus on the side of ATL	• Normal-appearing hippocampus on the side of ATL • Abnormal MRI findings other than unilateral mesial temporal sclerosis in TLE
Neuropsychological testing	Impaired function of regions implicated in epileptogenesis	• Normal performance • Impaired function of regions not implicated in epileptogenesis
Wada testing	Intact performance following anesthetic injections ipsilateral to the seizure focus	• Impaired memory following anesthetic injections ipsilateral to the seizure focus in TLE • Aphasia following anesthetic injections ipsilateral to the seizure focus • Intact performance following anesthetic injections contralateral to the seizure focus
Functional MRI[a]	Task-related blood oxygenation level dependent (BOLD) signal increases lie outside of to-be-resected tissue	Task-related BOLD signal increases within to-be-resected tissue
Cortical mapping	Normal performance with direct cortical stimulation of to-be-resected tissue	Direct cortical stimulation disrupts language, motor, sensory, or memory function in to-be-resected tissue

[a] At present, the clinical utility of fMRI is limited, and Wada testing remains the gold standard for language lateralization.

regarding the effects of IED suppression on cognition are limited to small trials and case series. Mixed results with use of valproic acid[91,93] highlight the need to balance treatment of TCI with the negative cognitive effects of the AED itself, increased doses and blood levels, and polypharmacy. Preliminary studies with the new generation of AEDs (eg, levetiracetam, lamotrigine), however, suggest that IED suppression is associated with improvements in behavior[88] and memory,[89] as well as better performance across a broad battery of neuropsychological tests.[94] A trial of discharge suppression may be warranted in patients with frequent IEDs and cognitive impairment, to be determined on an individual basis.

Treatment of Depression

Depression is more prevalent in the setting of epilepsy than in the general population, affecting 10% to 20% of patients with well-controlled seizures and 20% to 60% of patients with refractory epilepsy.[95,96] Depression can lead to objective impairments of attention, intelligence, language, visuoperceptual ability, psychomotor speed, memory, and executive function,[97] as well as subjective memory, attention, and language complaints.[98] Timely diagnosis and treatment are essential, as improvement in mood has been associated with improved cognitive function.[99,100]

Iatrogenic effects should be addressed as the initial step in management of comorbid depression and epilepsy. When possible, the use of AEDs with negative effects on mood (primidone, phenobarbital, topiramate, vigabatrin, tiagabine, felbamate, gabapentin, levetiracetam, and zonisamide) should be avoided in patients with depression. Epilepsy treatments with mood-stabilizing effects (carbamazepine, lamotrigine, valproic acid, and vagus nerve stimulation) or agents with possible positive mood-enhancing effects (rufinamide, lacosamide, ezogabine, perampanel, and clobazam) may be considered in this population. Conversely, recent reduction or cessation of mood-enhancing treatments may also contribute to depression. The addition of an enzyme-inducing AED may increase clearance of coadministered antidepressants, leading to breakthrough depressive symptoms, as well.

For patients with peri-ictal depression, improved seizure control may be the only necessary treatment. When alteration of the AED regimen is impossible or ineffective, antidepressant medications may be used. For patients with resistant peri-ictal depression, interictal major depressive disorder, persistent depressive disorder, or interictal dysphoric disorder, antidepressant treatment is indicated. Selective serotonin reuptake inhibitors (SSRIs) are considered first-line agents in adults and children. Citalopram and escitalopram are typically favored because of their lack of hepatic enzyme effects. Clinicians may refer to the Epilepsy Foundation's Mood Disorders Initiative recommendations regarding treatment of depression in adults with epilepsy (**Fig. 1**).[101] Similar recommendations have been proposed by the Canadian Network for Mood and Anxiety Treatments (CANMAT), although CANMAT guidelines differ in that lamotrigine, folate supplementation, and vagus nerve stimulator (VNS) implantation are included as possible treatments for depression. In the setting of bipolar disorder, psychotic features, suicidal ideation, or symptoms refractory to two antidepressant trials, referral to a psychiatrist is advisable.[102]

The goal of treatment is complete symptom remission, as any residual symptoms of depression increase the risk of relapse. The International League Against Epilepsy (ILAE) consensus guidelines recommend continuation of treatment for 6 months after recovery from the initial episode and for at least 2 years after recovery from any subsequent episodes.[103] Three or more periods of depression, residual symptoms, suicidality, psychosis, or an otherwise severe episode indicate the need for long-term treatment.

Depression remains undertreated in patients with epilepsy. Wiegartz and colleagues[104] found, for example, that 38% of epilepsy patients with a lifetime history of major depressive disorder (MDD) had never received treatment. This may be due to various factors, including a lack of screening by health care practitioners,[105] difficulty in diagnosis due to atypical symptoms or confounding drug adverse effects, and the misconception that all anticonvulsants significantly lower the seizure threshold. The reality is that medications with substantial risk are few, although it is prudent to avoid bupropion, maprotiline, clomipramine, and amoxapine because of their potential for seizure exacerbation.[106] SSRIs, however, are unlikely to worsen seizure frequency or severity and are generally effective for depressive symptoms.

Cognitive Rehabilitation

Cognitive rehabilitation programs may employ a variety of techniques.[107] Methods for improving memory and attentional function commonly include direct retraining (ie, completion of computerized tasks) and use of compensatory strategies, both external (eg, calendars, alarms, daily routines) and internal (eg, semantic associations, mental imagery, reducing task complexity). Improvements in verbal memory have been noted with deep processing, use of cues, and self-generated elaboration or encoding strategies in patients with localization-related epilepsy.[108,109] Koorenhof and colleagues[99]

Table 3
Alternative approaches for the treatment of medically refractory epilepsy

Treatment Method	Mechanism of Effect	Rate of Seizure Freedom	Cognitive Outcomes
Surgical procedures			
Selective amygdalo-hippocampectomy (SAH)	Removes mesial temporal structures, while lateral temporal neocortex remains intact	70.6% of ATL vs 78.1% of SAH patients at 1 y[53]	Overall trend for better cognitive outcomes than with ATL; slight decline (nonsignificant [NS]) in verbal memory after left-sided resection, improvement in verbal memory after right-sided resection, improved IQ at 1 y[53]
Multiple hippocampal transections	Transects the pyramidal layer of the hippocampus, without resection of tissue and leaving fibers subserving memory intact	• 82% at >1 y[54] • 67.6% at 1–7.8 y[55] • 94.7% at 2–5 y[56]	• No change in IQ, spatial memory, or verbal memory at 6-mo follow-up[54] • No adverse effects on verbal or nonverbal memory at 6–12 mo follow-up, with right-sided procedures leading to improvements in verbal memory[55] • Verbal memory improved in 7/9 patients and was unchanged in 2 of 9 patients at 3–6 mo Nonverbal memory improved in 4 of 9 patients, slightly deteriorated in 2 of 9 patients, and was unchanged in 3 of 9 patients[56]
Radiofrequency amygdalohippocampectomy	Radiofrequency ablation of tissue	75.5% at 2 y[57]	Improvements in measures of memory, attention, and IQ at 2-y follow-up[57]
Gamma knife radiosurgery	Focuses gamma radiation to create lesions restricted to the amygdala, anterior hippocampus, and parahippocampal gyrus	• 67% seizure-free for the prior 12 mo at 3-y follow-up (high dose: 76.9%; low dose: 58.8%)[58] • 65% at 2 y (range 33%–77% across study sites)[59]	• Verbal memory impairment in 25% of patients with dominant radiosurgeries and 7% of patients with nondominant radiosurgeries at 1- and 2-y follow-up. Significant improvements in 16% of patients with dominant radiosurgeries and 7% of patients with nondominant radiosurgeries[58] • No declines in visual or verbal memory at 2-y follow-up, with 20% experiencing improvement[59]

Stereotactic laser amygdalo-hippocampotomy (SLAH)	MRI-guided insertion of a laser fiber into the region of seizure onset, which uses heat to cause tissue destruction; preserves white matter pathways and neocortex	63% at $\geq$ 1 y (75% if mesial temporal sclerosis [MTS]+)[60]	• No declines in face and object naming and facial recognition at 6 mo[61] • Beneficial effects on memory[60,a]
Devices			
Vagus nerve stimulators (VNS)	Stimulates the left vagus nerve with programmable pulse generator	0.5% in patients with partial-onset seizures at 3 m with high stimulation[62]	• No overall adverse or beneficial effects • Initial positive effect of high stimulation on IQ at 5 m was not sustained at 9.75 m[63]
Responsive neurostimulation (RNS)	Detects when a seizure occurs and delivers electrical stimulation to abort the event via electrodes implanted within the seizure onset zone	9% over most recent 3 m period, 2 y after implant[64]	• Improvements in verbal functioning, visuospatial ability, cognitive flexibility, and memory at 1- and 2-y follow-up[64,65] • No declines in naming or verbal memory with hippocampal or extrahippocampal RNS at 1- and 2-y follow-up[66] • Naming improvement with neocortical (particularly frontal) RNS; smaller beneficial effect on verbal memory with medial temporal and temporal lobe RNS at 1- and 2-y follow-up[67]
Deep brain stimulation (DBS) of the anterior nucleus	Stimulation via electrodes placed within the anterior nucleus of the thalamus	10.1% of patients randomized seizure-free for at least 6 m at 5-y follow-up[68]	• No cognitive effects at 2-y follow-up[69] • Improvements in verbal fluency and verbal delayed recall; no changes in IQ, psychomotor speed, attention, or executive function at mean of 16-mo follow-up[70] • Improvements in attention, executive function, subjective cognitive function. 6.4% reported device-related subjective memory loss at 5 y[68]

[a] Time of postoperative testing unknown.

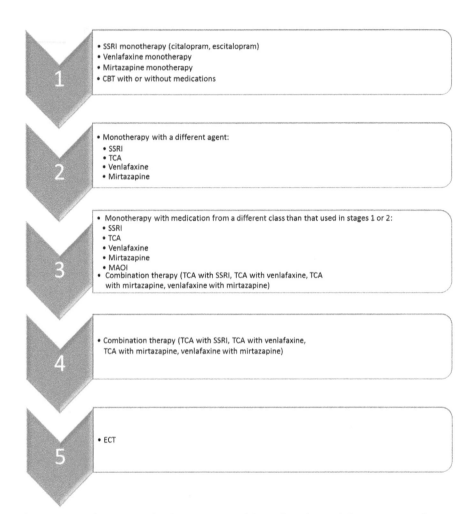

Fig. 1. Stages of treatment for depression in adults with epilepsy. If the patient is refractory to a given treatment, the next stage of management should be initiated. TCAs are contra-indicated in children, however, due to the risk of seizure exacerbation. CBT, cognitive behavioral therapy; ECT, electroconvulsive therapy; MAOI, monoamine oxidase inhibitor; SSRI, selective serotonin reuptake inhibitor; TCA, tricyclic antidepressant. (*Adapted from* Barry JJ, Ettinger AB, Friel P, et al. Consensus statement: the evaluation and treatment of people with epilepsy and affective disorders. Epilepsy Behav 2008;13(Suppl 1):S1–29.)

also demonstrated benefits in verbal learning and recall with the use of external and internal strategies (eg, mental imagery, elaboration, and computer-based training) when administered either pre- or postoperatively in patients with left TLE.

These techniques, however, suffer from two primary limitations. First, patients often have only partial compensation. Benefits of verbal memory rehabilitation are particularly limited in left TLE patients after ATL, who are likely the most in need of treatment for verbal memory deficits.[110,111] Second, training on a given set of tasks does not necessarily translate to other activities. Engelberts and colleagues,[112] for example, attained improvements on objective and subjective measures of attention using direct retraining with computerized tasks and compensatory strategies in patients with localization-related epilepsy. The benefits, however, did not extend to tests of attention not directly related to the training program.

Nevertheless, cognitive rehabilitation remains the primary modality available for the treatment of cognitive deficits in epilepsy and may be useful in selected patients. When providing a rehabilitation program, a holistic approach may be more helpful than selective interventions.[107] In addition, the goals of rehabilitation should be individualized, small, concrete, and reflect the patient's interests (ie, returning to work).

INVESTIGATIONAL TREATMENTS
Acetylcholinesterase Inhibitors

Animal models have demonstrated that hippocampal cholinergic transmission is reduced in epilepsy, as in Alzheimer's disease. This finding suggests that acetylcholinesterase inhibitors used for the treatment of Alzheimer's disease might improve memory function in patients with epilepsy.[113] Although a pilot study found improved verbal short-term memory after 3 months of open-label treatment with donepezil,[114] a randomized, double-blind, placebo-controlled crossover trial showed no effect of donepezil on verbal delayed recall.[115] Galantamine also failed to demonstrate significant effects on verbal and nonverbal memory in patients with epilepsy.[116] These largely negative findings, combined with a possible risk of seizure exacerbation,[114] have limited investigation into use of these agents.

Methylphenidate

The effectiveness of methylphenidate for the treatment of attention deficit hyperactivity disorder (ADHD) suggests a possible role for this drug in the treatment of epilepsy-related cognitive dysfunction. Much of the research in this area examines treatment of ADHD in the setting of pediatric epilepsy, with a particular focus on the possible potential of methylphenidate to exacerbate seizures. The prescribing information for methylphenidate warns of a lowered seizure threshold, particularly in patients with a history of seizures or EEG abnormalities, and recommends cessation of the drug in the setting of seizures. Overall, however, an increased risk of seizures has not been clearly demonstrated in the literature.[117–120]

Multiple studies in children with epilepsy and ADHD found improved attention and impulsivity with use of the drug,[121–126] with no effect on seizure frequency in the vast majority of patients. Methylphenidate was also effective in a small sample of adults with epilepsy and ADHD, with no changes in seizure frequency or severity.[127] One study to date assessed the open-label use of methylphenidate in adults without ADHD who had cognitive deficits related to focal-onset epilepsy and AED use.[128] Attention, memory, spatial processing, information processing speed, and overall measures of cognition were improved after treatment, with 1 of 8 patients having increased seizure frequency.

Methylphenidate may provide a reasonable option for the treatment of cognitive impairments in patients with well-controlled epilepsy. Clinicians may also consider a pretreatment EEG to evaluate the risk of seizure exacerbation.[129] Further research is needed, however, with larger samples, patients with more frequent seizures, varying seizure types, and long-term use.

N-methyl-D-aspartate Receptor Antagonists

The agonist action of glutamate at N-methyl-D-aspartate (NMDA) receptors within the hippocampus is a key component in the pathway of glutamate-mediated excitotoxicity, which leads to hippocampal sclerosis and memory dysfunction. It follows that NMDA receptor antagonists may act to preserve hippocampal structure and function.

NMDA antagonists have shown promising results with respect to learning and memory in animal models of epilepsy.[130–132] In humans, the NMDA antagonist memantine is used for the treatment of moderate to severe Alzheimer's disease,[133–135] but it is unknown whether this agent would be of benefit in patients with epilepsy-related cognitive dysfunction. A randomized, double-blind, placebo-controlled study of the effects of memantine on memory function in patients with localization-related epilepsy is ongoing (Leeman-Markowski et al, unpublished data, 2015). If beneficial, this would provide a much-needed treatment option with a more favorable safety profile than cholinergic medications.

Vinpocetine

Vinpocetine is an herbal supplement derived from the lesser periwinkle (Vinca minor). This compound inhibits Ca+2/calmodulin-dependent phosphodiesterase (PDE) type 1,[136] which prevents the breakdown of cAMP to 5′-AMP, maintaining activation of cyclic AMP response element-binding protein (CREB) and protein kinases implicated in memory formation and synaptic plasticity. Trials suggesting a benefit in human memory were conducted in young healthy volunteers.[137–139] Improvements in the Clinical Global Index (CGI) were also noted in subjects with cognitive impairment due to vascular, Alzheimer's, mixed (vascular and Alzheimer's disease), and other dementias.[140–143] Only one published study to date, limited by an unblinded and uncontrolled design, has evaluated the use of vinpocetine in subjects with epilepsy-related cognitive impairment.[144] In this trial, vinpocetine was shown to improve attention and memory in patients with cognitive deficits caused by epilepsy or dementia, with a greater benefit in epilepsy patients. A randomized double-blind, single-dose, placebo-controlled crossover study in subjects with localization-related epilepsy and healthy controls, followed by an open-label extension in epilepsy patients, is ongoing, and will assess the effects of vinpocetine on memory, attention, executive function, and psychomotor speed (Meador and colleagues, unpublished data). The anticonvulsant properties of vinpocetine demonstrated in animal models[145–150] and people with epilepsy[151,152] make this agent an attractive candidate for study.

Brain Stimulation for Cognitive Enhancement

Trials have evaluated the potential cognition-enhancing effects of deep brain stimulation (DBS) in patients with TLE, using a variety of stimulation sites and parameters. Not surprisingly, such studies have demonstrated variable results. Initial data regarding stimulation of the fornix and entorhinal cortex have been encouraging with respect to delayed verbal recall[153] and spatial recall,[154] respectively. In contrast, hippocampal stimulation has not been found to significantly enhance memory,[155,156] and may impair memory formation in some patients.[157] Clearly, effects of DBS will depend upon location, stimulation parameters, and underlying structural abnormalities, among other factors.[158] Brain stimulation techniques for improvement of cognitive function remain an active area of investigation, with large-scale multicenter clinical trials underway.

SUMMARY

Cognitive deficits are common in the setting of epilepsy and can negatively impact daily functioning. Multiple domains may be impaired, including memory, attention, executive function, and language, with the diagnosis based upon detailed neuropsychological testing. Cognitive dysfunction in epilepsy is typically multifactorial, often reflecting the effects of ongoing seizures, treatment adverse effects, frequent interictal discharges, and comorbid psychiatric disorders. Treatment should address these underlying etiologies. Although cognitive rehabilitation remains the standard treatment modality and may be useful in some patients, this strategy fails to address the underlying mechanisms, and benefits are limited. Several therapies, however, are currently under investigation, including acetylcholinesterase inhibitors, methylphenidate, memantine, vinpocetine, and deep brain stimulation, with some encouraging preliminary results. Research in this area is of great clinical importance, as effective treatments for cognitive dysfunction in epilepsy may have a significant impact on quality of life, employability, or need for assistance with activities of daily living in this patient population.

REFERENCES

1. Aikiä M, Salmenperä T, Partanen K, et al. Verbal memory in newly diagnosed patients and patients with chronic left temporal lobe epilepsy. Epilepsy Behav 2001;2(1):20–7.
2. Pulliainen V, Kuikka P, Jokelainen M. Motor and cognitive functions in newly diagnosed adult seizure patients before antiepileptic medication. Acta Neurol Scand 2000;101(2):73–8. Available at: http://www.ncbi.nlm.nih.gov/pubmed/10685851. Accessed November 30, 2014.
3. Taylor J, Kolamunnage-Dona R, Marson AG, et al. Patients with epilepsy: cognitively compromised before the start of antiepileptic drug treatment? Epilepsia 2010;51(1):48–56.
4. Jokeit H, Ebner A. Effects of chronic epilepsy on intellectual functions. Prog Brain Res 2002;135:455–63.
5. Witt J-A, Helmstaedter C. Should cognition be screened in new-onset epilepsies? A study in 247 untreated patients. J Neurol 2012;259(8):1727–31.
6. Northcott E, Connolly AM, Berroya A, et al. The neuropsychological and language profile of children with benign rolandic epilepsy. Epilepsia 2005;46(6):924–30.
7. Baglietto MG, Battaglia FM, Nobili L, et al. Neuropsychological disorders related to interictal epileptic discharges during sleep in benign epilepsy of childhood with centrotemporal or Rolandic spikes. Dev Med Child Neurol 2001;43(6):407–12. Available at: http://www.ncbi.nlm.nih.gov/pubmed/11409830. Accessed May 26, 2015.
8. Pascalicchio TF, de Araujo Filho GM, da Silva Noffs MH, et al. Neuropsychological profile of patients with juvenile myoclonic epilepsy: a controlled study of 50 patients. Epilepsy Behav 2007;10(2):263–7.
9. National Institute of Neurological Disorders and Stroke. NINDS Common Data Elements. 2010. Available at: http://www.commondataelements.ninds.nih.gov/Epilepsy.aspx#tab=Data_Standards. Accessed August 24, 2014.
10. Elliott G, Isaac CL, Muhlert N. Measuring forgetting: a critical review of accelerated long-term forgetting studies. Cortex 2014;54:16–32.
11. Lee TMC, Yip JTH, Jones-Gotman M. Memory deficits after resection from left or right anterior temporal lobe in humans: a meta-analytic review. Epilepsia 2002;43(3):283–91. Available at: http://www.ncbi.nlm.nih.gov/pubmed/11906514. Accessed January 4, 2015.
12. Glikmann-Johnston Y, Saling MM, Chen J, et al. Structural and functional correlates of unilateral mesial temporal lobe spatial memory impairment. Brain 2008;131(Pt 11):3006–18.
13. Witt J-A, Alpherts W, Helmstaedter C. Computerized neuropsychological testing in epilepsy: overview of available tools. Seizure 2013;22(6):416–23.

14. Kilpatrick C, Murrie V, Cook M, et al. Degree of left hippocampal atrophy correlates with severity of neuropsychological deficits. Seizure 1997;6(3):213–8. Available at: http://www.ncbi.nlm.nih.gov/pubmed/9203250. Accessed May 26, 2015.

15. Baxendale SA, van Paesschen W, Thompson PJ, et al. The relationship between quantitative MRI and neuropsychological functioning in temporal lobe epilepsy. Epilepsia 1998;39(2):158–66. Available at: http://www.ncbi.nlm.nih.gov/pubmed/9577995. Accessed May 26, 2015.

16. Jokeit H, Ebner A. Long term effects of refractory temporal lobe epilepsy on cognitive abilities: a cross sectional study. J Neurol Neurosurg Psychiatry 1999;67:44–50.

17. O'Leary DS, Lovell MR, Sackellares JC, et al. Effects of age of onset of partial and generalized seizures on neuropsychological performance in children. J Nerv Ment Dis 1983;171(10):624–9. Available at: http://www.ncbi.nlm.nih.gov/pubmed/6413648. Accessed May 26, 2015.

18. Dikmen S, Matthews CG. Effect of major motor seizure frequency upon cognitive-intellectual functions in adults. Epilepsia 1977;18(1):21–9. Available at: http://www.ncbi.nlm.nih.gov/pubmed/404137. Accessed May 26, 2015.

19. Meneses RF, Pais-Ribeiro JL, da Silva AM, et al. Neuropsychological predictors of quality of life in focal epilepsy. Seizure 2009;18(5):313–9.

20. Mandelbaum DE, Burack GD. The effect of seizure type and medication on cognitive and behavioral functioning in children with idiopathic epilepsy. Dev Med Child Neurol 1997;39(11):731–5. Available at: http://www.ncbi.nlm.nih.gov/pubmed/9393886. Accessed May 27, 2015.

21. York MK, Rettig GM, Grossman RG, et al. Seizure control and cognitive outcome after temporal lobectomy: a comparison of classic Ammon's horn sclerosis, atypical mesial temporal sclerosis, and tumoral pathologies. Epilepsia 2003; 44(3):387–98.

22. Helmstaedter C, Kemper B, Elger CE. Neuropsychological aspects of frontal lobe epilepsy. Neuropsychologia 1996;34(5):399–406.

23. Meador KJ. Cognitive outcomes and predictive factors in epilepsy. Neurology 2002;58(8 Suppl 5):S21–6. Available at: http://www.ncbi.nlm.nih.gov/pubmed/11971129. Accessed January 3, 2015.

24. Barr WB. Examining the right temporal lobe's role in nonverbal memory. Brain Cogn 1997;35(1):26–41.

25. Grimes DA, Guberman A. De novo aphasic status epilepticus. Epilepsia 1997; 38(8):945–9. Available at: http://www.ncbi.nlm.nih.gov/pubmed/9579898. Accessed June 21, 2015.

26. Sadiq SB, Hussain SA, Norton JW. Ictal aphasia: an unusual presentation of temporal lobe seizures. Epilepsy Behav 2012;23(4):500–2.

27. Butler CR, Zeman A. The causes and consequences of transient epileptic amnesia. Behav Neurol 2011;24(4):299–305.

28. Helmstaedter C, Elger CE, Lendt M. Postictal courses of cognitive deficits in focal epilepsies. Epilepsia 1994;35(5):1073–8. Available at: http://www.ncbi.nlm.nih.gov/pubmed/7925154. Accessed May 27, 2015.

29. Helmstaedter C, Witt J-A. The effects of levetiracetam on cognition: a non-interventional surveillance study. Epilepsy Behav 2008;13(4):642–9.

30. Meador KJ, Loring DW, Huh K, et al. Comparative cognitive effects of anticonvulsants. Neurology 1990;40(3 Pt 1):391–4. Available at: http://www.ncbi.nlm.nih.gov/pubmed/2314578. Accessed March 23, 2015.

31. Meador KJ, Loring DW, Allen ME, et al. Comparative cognitive effects of carbamazepine and phenytoin in healthy adults. Neurology 1991;41(10):1537–40.

Available at: http://www.ncbi.nlm.nih.gov/pubmed/1922792. Accessed March 23, 2015.

32. Meador KJ, Loring DW, Moore EE, et al. Comparative cognitive effects of phenobarbital, phenytoin, and valproate in healthy adults. Neurology 1995;45(8): 1494–9. Available at: http://www.ncbi.nlm.nih.gov/pubmed/7644047. Accessed March 23, 2015.

33. Hindmarch I, Trick L, Ridout F. A double-blind, placebo- and positive-internal-controlled (alprazolam) investigation of the cognitive and psychomotor profile of pregabalin in healthy volunteers. Psychopharmacology (Berl) 2005;183(2): 133–43.

34. Park S-P, Hwang Y-H, Lee H-W, et al. Long-term cognitive and mood effects of zonisamide monotherapy in epilepsy patients. Epilepsy Behav 2008;12(1): 102–8.

35. Ojemann LM, Ojemann GA, Dodrill CB, et al. Language disturbances as side effects of topiramate and zonisamide therapy. Epilepsy Behav 2001;2(6): 579–84.

36. Berent S, Sackellares JC, Giordani B, et al. Zonisamide (CI-912) and cognition: results from preliminary study. Epilepsia 1987;28(1):61–7. Available at: http://www.ncbi.nlm.nih.gov/pubmed/3098556. Accessed March 23, 2015.

37. Martin R, Kuzniecky R, Ho S, et al. Cognitive effects of topiramate, gabapentin, and lamotrigine in healthy young adults. Neurology 1999;52(2):321–7. Available at: http://www.ncbi.nlm.nih.gov/pubmed/9932951. Accessed March 23, 2015.

38. Meador KJ, Loring DW, Vahle VJ, et al. Cognitive and behavioral effects of lamotrigine and topiramate in healthy volunteers. Neurology 2005;64(12):2108–14.

39. Reife R, Pledger G, Wu SC. Topiramate as add-on therapy: pooled analysis of randomized controlled trials in adults. Epilepsia 2000;41(Suppl 1):S66–71. Available at: http://www.ncbi.nlm.nih.gov/pubmed/10768304. Accessed March 23, 2015.

40. Meador KJ, Loring DW, Hulihan JF, et al. Differential cognitive and behavioral effects of topiramate and valproate. Neurology 2003;60(9):1483–8. Available at: http://www.ncbi.nlm.nih.gov/pubmed/12743236. Accessed March 23, 2015.

41. Lee S, Sziklas V, Andermann F, et al. The effects of adjunctive topiramate on cognitive function in patients with epilepsy. Epilepsia 2003;44(3):339–47. Available at: http://www.ncbi.nlm.nih.gov/pubmed/12614389. Accessed March 23, 2015.

42. Burton LA, Harden C. Effect of topiramate on attention. Epilepsy Res 1997;27(1): 29–32. Available at: http://www.ncbi.nlm.nih.gov/pubmed/9169288. Accessed March 23, 2015.

43. Thompson PJ, Baxendale SA, Duncan JS, et al. Effects of topiramate on cognitive function. J Neurol Neurosurg Psychiatry 2000;69(5):636–41. Available at: http://www.pubmedcentral.nih.gov/articlerender.fcgi?artid=1763392&tool=pmcentrez&rendertype=abstract. Accessed March 23, 2015.

44. Koo DL, Hwang KJ, Kim D, et al. Effects of levetiracetam monotherapy on the cognitive function of epilepsy patients. Eur Neurol 2013;70(1–2):88–94.

45. Ciesielski A-S, Samson S, Steinhoff BJ. Neuropsychological and psychiatric impact of add-on titration of pregabalin versus levetiracetam: a comparative short-term study. Epilepsy Behav 2006;9(3):424–31.

46. Wiebe S, Blume WT, Girvin JP, et al. A randomized, controlled trial of surgery for temporal-lobe epilepsy. N Engl J Med 2001;345(5):311–8.

47. Stroup E, Langfitt J, Berg M, et al. Predicting verbal memory decline following anterior temporal lobectomy (ATL). Neurology 2003;60(8):1266–73.

Available at: http://www.ncbi.nlm.nih.gov/pubmed/12707428. Accessed March 11, 2015.

48. Leijten FSS, Alpherts WCJ, Van Huffelen AC, et al. The effects on cognitive performance of tailored resection in surgery for nonlesional mesiotemporal lobe epilepsy. Epilepsia 2005;46(3):431–9.

49. Cukiert A, Buratini JA, Machado E, et al. Seizure-related outcome after cortico-amygdalohippocampectomy in patients with refractory temporal lobe epilepsy and mesial temporal sclerosis evaluated by magnetic resonance imaging alone. Neurosurg Focus 2002;13(4):ecp2. Available at: http://www.ncbi.nlm.nih.gov/pubmed/15771407. Accessed March 12, 2015.

50. Sanyal SK, Chandra PS, Gupta S, et al. Memory and intelligence outcome following surgery for intractable temporal lobe epilepsy: relationship to seizure outcome and evaluation using a customized neuropsychological battery. Epilepsy Behav 2005;6(2):147–55.

51. Paglioli E, Palmini A, Paglioli E, et al. Survival analysis of the surgical outcome of temporal lobe epilepsy due to hippocampal sclerosis. Epilepsia 2004;45(11): 1383–91.

52. Ivnik RJ, Sharbrough FW, Laws ER. Anterior temporal lobectomy for the control of partial complex seizures: information for counseling patients. Mayo Clin Proc 1988;63(8):783–93. Available at: http://www.ncbi.nlm.nih.gov/pubmed/ 3398596. Accessed March 12, 2015.

53. Morino M, Uda T, Naito K, et al. Comparison of neuropsychological outcomes after selective amygdalohippocampectomy versus anterior temporal lobectomy. Epilepsy Behav 2006;9(1):95–100.

54. Shimizu H, Kawai K, Sunaga S, et al. Hippocampal transection for treatment of left temporal lobe epilepsy with preservation of verbal memory. J Clin Neurosci 2006;13(3):322–8.

55. Uda T, Morino M, Ito H, et al. Transsylvian hippocampal transection for mesial temporal lobe epilepsy: surgical indications, procedure, and postoperative seizure and memory outcomes. J Neurosurg 2013;119(5):1098–104.

56. Patil AA, Andrews R. Long term follow-up after multiple hippocampal transection (MHT). Seizure 2013;22(9):731–4.

57. Malikova H, Kramska L, Vojtech Z, et al. Stereotactic radiofrequency amygdalo-hippocampectomy: two years of good neuropsychological outcomes. Epilepsy Res 2013;106(3):423–32.

58. Barbaro NM, Quigg M, Broshek DK, et al. A multicenter, prospective pilot study of gamma knife radiosurgery for mesial temporal lobe epilepsy: seizure response, adverse events, and verbal memory. Ann Neurol 2009;65(2): 167–75.

59. Régis J, Rey M, Bartolomei F, et al. Gamma knife surgery in mesial temporal lobe epilepsy: a prospective multicenter study. Epilepsia 2004;45(5):504–15.

60. Gross RE, Mahmoudi B, Riley JP. Less is more: novel less-invasive surgical techniques for mesial temporal lobe epilepsy that minimize cognitive impairment. Curr Opin Neurol 2015;28(2):182–91.

61. Drane DL, Loring DW, Voets NL, et al. Better object recognition and naming outcome with MRI-guided stereotactic laser amygdalohippocampotomy for temporal lobe epilepsy. Epilepsia 2015;56(1):101–13.

62. Handforth A, DeGiorgio CM, Schachter SC, et al. Vagus nerve stimulation therapy for partial-onset seizures: a randomized active-control trial. Neurology 1998; 51(1):48–55. Available at: http://www.ncbi.nlm.nih.gov/pubmed/9674777. Accessed May 15, 2015.

63. Klinkenberg S, van den Bosch CNCJ, Majoie HJM, et al. Behavioural and cognitive effects during vagus nerve stimulation in children with intractable epilepsy—a randomized controlled trial. Eur J Paediatr Neurol 2013;17(1):82–90.

64. Morrell MJ. Responsive cortical stimulation for the treatment of medically intractable partial epilepsy. Neurology 2011;77(13):1295–304.

65. Heck CN, King-Stephens D, Massey AD, et al. Two-year seizure reduction in adults with medically intractable partial onset epilepsy treated with responsive neurostimulation: final results of the RNS System Pivotal trial. Epilepsia 2014; 55(3):432–41.

66. Loring DW, Kapur R, Meador K, et al. Long-term memory and language outcomes with responsive cortical stimulation do not differ by stimulation localization. American epilepsy society annual Meeting. Seattle, December 5–9, 2014.

67. Loring DW, Kapur R, Meador K, et al. Long-term memory and language outcomes with responsive cortical stimulation do not differ by stimulation localization. Platform Presentation, American Epilepsy Society Annual Meeting. Seattle, December 5–9, 2014.

68. Salanova V, Witt T, Worth R, et al. Long-term efficacy and safety of thalamic stimulation for drug-resistant partial epilepsy. Neurology 2015;84(10):1017–25.

69. Fisher R, Salanova V, Witt T, et al. Electrical stimulation of the anterior nucleus of thalamus for treatment of refractory epilepsy. Epilepsia 2010;51(5):899–908.

70. Oh Y-S, Kim HJ, Lee KJ, et al. Cognitive improvement after long-term electrical stimulation of bilateral anterior thalamic nucleus in refractory epilepsy patients. Seizure 2012;21(3):183–7.

71. Binnie CD, Stefan H. Modern electroencephalography: its role in epilepsy management. Clin Neurophysiol 1999;110(10):1671–97. Available at: http://www.ncbi.nlm.nih.gov/pubmed/10574283. Accessed May 28, 2015.

72. Hovey HB, Kooi KA. Transient disturbances of thought processes and epilepsy. AMA Arch Neurol Psychiatry 1955;74(3):287–91. Available at: http://www.ncbi.nlm.nih.gov/pubmed/13248285. Accessed March 4, 2015.

73. Dodrill CB, Wilkus RJ. Relationships between intelligence and electroencephalographic epileptiform activity in adult epileptics. Neurology 1976;26(6 Pt 1): 525–31. Available at: http://www.ncbi.nlm.nih.gov/pubmed/819859. Accessed March 4, 2015.

74. Kooi KA, Hovey HB. Alterations in mental function and paroxysmal cerebral activity. AMA Arch Neurol Psychiatry 1957;78(3):264–71. Available at: http://www.ncbi.nlm.nih.gov/pubmed/13457501. Accessed March 4, 2015.

75. Wilkus RJ, Dodrill CB. Neuropsychological correlates of the electroencephalogram in epileptics: I. Topographic distribution and average rate of epileptiform activity. Epilepsia 1976;17(1):89–100. Available at: http://www.ncbi.nlm.nih.gov/pubmed/817896. Accessed May 28, 2015.

76. Aarts JH, Binnie CD, Smit AM, et al. Selective cognitive impairment during focal and generalized epileptiform EEG activity. Brain 1984;107(Pt 1):293–308. Available at: http://www.ncbi.nlm.nih.gov/pubmed/6421454. Accessed January 3, 2015.

77. Mameniskiene R, Jatuzis D, Kaubrys G, et al. The decay of memory between delayed and long-term recall in patients with temporal lobe epilepsy. Epilepsy Behav 2006;8(1):278–88.

78. Kleen JK, Scott RC, Holmes GL, et al. Hippocampal interictal epileptiform activity disrupts cognition in humans. Neurology 2013;81(1):18–24.

79. Tromp SC, Weber JW, Aldenkamp AP, et al. Relative influence of epileptic seizures and of epilepsy syndrome on cognitive function. J Child Neurol 2003;

18(6):407–12. Available at: http://www.ncbi.nlm.nih.gov/pubmed/12886976. Accessed January 3, 2015.

80. Shewmon DA, Erwin RJ. The effect of focal interictal spikes on perception and reaction time. I. General considerations. Electroencephalogr Clin Neurophysiol 1988;69(4):319–37. Available at: http://www.ncbi.nlm.nih.gov/pubmed/2450731. Accessed March 4, 2015.

81. Shewmon DA, Erwin RJ. The effect of focal interictal spikes on perception and reaction time. II. Neuroanatomic specificity. Electroencephalogr Clin Neurophysiol 1988;69(4):338–52. Available at: http://www.ncbi.nlm.nih.gov/pubmed/2450732. Accessed March 4, 2015.

82. Tizard B, Margerison JH. The relationship between generalized paroxysmal E.E.G. discharges and various test situations in two epileptic patients. J Neurol Neurosurg Psychiatry 1963;26:308–13. Available at: http://www.pubmedcentral.nih.gov/articlerender.fcgi?artid=495588&tool=pmcentrez&rendertype=abstract. Accessed March 4, 2015.

83. Browne TR, Penry JK, Proter RJ, et al. Responsiveness before, during, and after spike-wave paroxysms. Neurology 1974;24(7):659–65. Available at: http://www.ncbi.nlm.nih.gov/pubmed/4858089. Accessed May 28, 2015.

84. Sellden U. Psychotechnical performance related to paroxysmal discharges in EEG. Clin Electroencephal 1971;2(1):18–27.

85. Schwab R. Reaction time in petit mal epilepsy. Res Publ Assoc Res Nerv Ment Dis 1947;26:339–41.

86. Tizard B, Margerison JH. Psychological functions during wave-spike discharge. Br J Soc Clin Psychol 1963;3:6–15.

87. Goode DJ, Penry JK, Dreifuss FE. Effects of paroxysmal spike-wave on continuous visual-motor performance. Epilepsia 1970;11(3):241–54. Available at: http://www.ncbi.nlm.nih.gov/pubmed/5276416. Accessed March 4, 2015.

88. Pressler RM, Robinson RO, Wilson GA, et al. Treatment of interictal epileptiform discharges can improve behavior in children with behavioral problems and epilepsy. J Pediatr 2005;146(1):112–7.

89. Mintz M, Legoff D, Scornaienchi J, et al. The underrecognized epilepsy spectrum: the effects of levetiracetam on neuropsychological functioning in relation to subclinical spike production. J Child Neurol 2009;24(7):807–15.

90. Gallagher MJ, Eisenman LN, Brown KM, et al. Levetiracetam reduces spike-wave density and duration during continuous EEG monitoring in patients with idiopathic generalized epilepsy. Epilepsia 2004;45(1):90–1. Available at: http://www.ncbi.nlm.nih.gov/pubmed/14692914. Accessed March 4, 2015.

91. Binnie CD. Significance and management of transitory cognitive impairment due to subclinical EEG discharges in children. Brain Dev 1993;15(1):23–30. Available at: http://www.ncbi.nlm.nih.gov/pubmed/8338208. Accessed May 28, 2015.

92. Placidi F, Tombini M, Romigi A, et al. Topiramate: effect on EEG interictal abnormalities and background activity in patients affected by focal epilepsy. Epilepsy Res 2004;58(1):43–52.

93. Ronen GM, Richards JE, Cunningham C, et al. Can sodium valproate improve learning in children with epileptiform bursts but without clinical seizures? Dev Med Child Neurol 2000;42(11):751–5. Available at: http://www.ncbi.nlm.nih.gov/pubmed/11104347. Accessed May 31, 2015.

94. Leeman BA, Moo LR, Leveroni CL, et al. Cognitive effects of treatment of focal interictal discharges with levetiracetam [abstract]. Epilepsia 2008;49(Suppl 7):136–7.

95. Mendez MF, Cummings JL, Benson DF. Depression in epilepsy. Significance and phenomenology. Arch Neurol 1986;43(8):766–70. Available at: http://www. ncbi.nlm.nih.gov/pubmed/3729756. Accessed May 30, 2015.

96. Tellez-Zenteno JF, Patten SB, Jetté N, et al. Psychiatric comorbidity in epilepsy: a population-based analysis. Epilepsia 2007;48(12):2336–44.

97. Paradiso S, Hermann BP, Blumer D, et al. Impact of depressed mood on neuropsychological status in temporal lobe epilepsy. J Neurol Neurosurg Psychiatry 2001; 70(2):180–5. Available at: http://www.pubmedcentral.nih.gov/articlerender.fcgi? artid=1737223&tool=pmcentrez&rendertype=abstract. Accessed May 31, 2015.

98. Cramer JA, Blum D, Reed M, et al. The influence of comorbid depression on quality of life for people with epilepsy. Epilepsy Behav 2003;4(5):515–21. Available at: http://www.ncbi.nlm.nih.gov/pubmed/14527494. Accessed May 31, 2015.

99. Koorenhof L, Baxendale S, Smith N, et al. Memory rehabilitation and brain training for surgical temporal lobe epilepsy patients: a preliminary report. Seizure 2012;21(3):178–82.

100. Sackeim HA, Keilp JG, Rush AJ, et al. The effects of vagus nerve stimulation on cognitive performance in patients with treatment-resistant depression. Neuropsychiatry Neuropsychol Behav Neurol 2001;14(1):53–62. Available at: http:// www.ncbi.nlm.nih.gov/pubmed/11234909. Accessed May 31, 2015.

101. Barry JJ, Ettinger AB, Friel P, et al. Consensus statement: the evaluation and treatment of people with epilepsy and affective disorders. Epilepsy Behav 2008;13(Suppl 1):S1–29.

102. De Oliveira GNM, Kummer A, Salgado JV, et al. Psychiatric disorders in temporal lobe epilepsy: an overview from a tertiary service in Brazil. Seizure 2010; 19(8):479–84.

103. Kerr MP, Mensah S, Besag F, et al. International consensus clinical practice statements for the treatment of neuropsychiatric conditions associated with epilepsy. Epilepsia 2011;52(11):2133–8.

104. Wiegartz P, Seidenberg M, Woodard A, et al. Co-morbid psychiatric disorder in chronic epilepsy: recognition and etiology of depression. Neurology 1999;53(5 Suppl 2):S3–8. Available at: http://www.ncbi.nlm.nih.gov/pubmed/10496228. Accessed May 31, 2015.

105. Gilliam FG, Santos J, Vahle V, et al. Depression in epilepsy: ignoring clinical expression of neuronal network dysfunction? Epilepsia 2004;45(Suppl 2): 28–33.

106. Pisani F, Spina E, Oteri G. Antidepressant drugs and seizure susceptibility: from in vitro data to clinical practice. Epilepsia 1999;40(Suppl 1):S48–56. Available at: http://www.ncbi.nlm.nih.gov/pubmed/10609604. Accessed May 31, 2015.

107. Farina E, Raglio A, Giovagnoli AR. Cognitive rehabilitation in epilepsy: an evidence-based review. Epilepsy Res 2015;109C:210–8.

108. Bresson C, Lespinet-Najib V, Rougier A, et al. Verbal memory compensation: application to left and right temporal lobe epileptic patients. Brain Lang 2007; 102(1):13–21.

109. Schefft BK, Dulay MF, Fargo JD, et al. The use of self-generation procedures facilitates verbal memory in individuals with seizure disorders. Epilepsy Behav 2008;13(1):162–8.

110. Jones MK. Imagery as a mnemonic aid after left temporal lobectomy: Contrast between material-specific and generalized memory disorders. Neuropsychologia 1974;12(1):21–30.

111. Helmstaedter C, Loer B, Wohlfahrt R, et al. The effects of cognitive rehabilitation on memory outcome after temporal lobe epilepsy surgery. Epilepsy Behav 2008; 12(3):402–9.

112. Engelberts NHJ, Klein M, Ade HJ, et al. The effectiveness of cognitive rehabilitation for attention deficits in focal seizures: a randomized controlled study. Epilepsia 2002;43(6):587–95.

113. Mishra A, Goel RK. Adjuvant anticholinesterase therapy for the management of epilepsy-induced memory deficit: a critical pre-clinical study. Basic Clin Pharmacol Toxicol 2014;115(6):512–7.

114. Fisher RS, Bortz JJ, Blum DE, et al. A pilot study of donepezil for memory problems in epilepsy. Epilepsy Behav 2001;2(4):330–4.

115. Hamberger MJ, Palmese CA, Scarmeas N, et al. A randomized, double-blind, placebo-controlled trial of donepezil to improve memory in epilepsy. Epilepsia 2007;48(7):1283–91.

116. Griffith HR, Martin R, Andrews S, et al. The safety and tolerability of galantamine in patients with epilepsy and memory difficulties. Epilepsy Behav 2008;13(2): 376–80.

117. Torres AR, Whitney J, Gonzalez-Heydrich J. Attention-deficit/hyperactivity disorder in pediatric patients with epilepsy: review of pharmacological treatment. Epilepsy Behav 2008;12(2):217–33.

118. Baptista-Neto L, Dodds A, Rao S, et al. An expert opinion on methylphenidate treatment for attention deficit hyperactivity disorder in pediatric patients with epilepsy. Expert Opin Investig Drugs 2008;17(1):77–84.

119. Koneski JAS, Casella EB. Attention deficit and hyperactivity disorder in people with epilepsy: diagnosis and implications to the treatment. Arq Neuropsiquiatr 2010; 68(1):107–14. Available at: http://www.ncbi.nlm.nih.gov/pubmed/20339664. Accessed May 31, 2015.

120. McBride MC, Wang DD, Torres CF. Methylphenidate in therapeutic doses does not lower seizure threshold. Ann Neurol 1986;20:428.

121. Semrud-Clikeman M, Wical B. Components of attention in children with complex partial seizures with and without ADHD. Epilepsia 1999;40(2):211–5. Available at: http://www.ncbi.nlm.nih.gov/pubmed/9952269. Accessed January 5, 2015.

122. Yoo HK, Park S, Wang H-R, et al. Effect of methylphenidate on the quality of life in children with epilepsy and attention deficit hyperactivity disorder: and open-label study using an osmotic-controlled release oral delivery system. Epileptic Disord 2009;11(4):301–8.

123. Gucuyener K, Erdemoglu AK, Senol S, et al. Use of methylphenidate for attention-deficit hyperactivity disorder in patients with epilepsy or electroencephalographic abnormalities. J Child Neurol 2003;18(2):109–12. Available at: http://www.ncbi.nlm.nih.gov/pubmed/12693777. Accessed January 4, 2015.

124. Feldman H, Crumrine P, Handen BL, et al. Methylphenidate in children with seizures and attention-deficit disorder. Am J Dis Child 1989;143(9):1081–6. Available at: http://www.ncbi.nlm.nih.gov/pubmed/2672786. Accessed January 4, 2015.

125. Finck S, Metz-Lutz MN, Becache E, et al. Attention-deficit hyperactivity disorder in epileptic children: a new indication for methylphenidate? [abstract]. Ann Neurol 1995;38:520.

126. Gross-Tsur V, Manor O, van der Meere J. Epilepsy and attention deficit hyperactivity disorder: is methylphenidate safe and effective? J Pediatr 1997;130(4): 670–4.

127. Van der Feltz-Cornelis CM, Aldenkamp AP. Effectiveness and safety of methylphenidate in adult attention deficit hyperactivity disorder in patients with epilepsy: an open treatment trial. Epilepsy Behav 2006;8(3):659–62.

128. Moore JL, McAuley JW, Long L, et al. An evaluation of the effects of methylphenidate on outcomes in adult epilepsy patients. Epilepsy Behav 2002;3(1):92–5. Available at: http://www.ncbi.nlm.nih.gov/pubmed/12609358. Accessed January 4, 2015.

129. Hemmer SA, Pasternak JF, Zecker SG, et al. Stimulant therapy and seizure risk in children with ADHD. Pediatr Neurol 2001;24(2):99–102. Available at: http://www.ncbi.nlm.nih.gov/pubmed/11275457. Accessed January 5, 2015.

130. Kelsey JE, Sanderson KL, Frye CA. Perforant path stimulation in rats produces seizures, loss of hippocampal neurons, and a deficit in spatial mapping which are reduced by prior MK-801. Behav Brain Res 2000;107(1–2):59–69. Available at: http://www.ncbi.nlm.nih.gov/pubmed/10628730. Accessed January 4, 2015.

131. De Groot DM, Bierman EP, Bruijnzeel PL, et al. Beneficial effects of TCP on soman intoxication in guinea pigs: seizures, brain damage and learning behaviour. J Appl Toxicol 2001;21(Suppl 1):S57–65. Available at: http://www.ncbi.nlm.nih.gov/pubmed/11920922. Accessed December 8, 2014.

132. Jia L-J, Wang W-P, Li Z-P, et al. Memantine attenuates the impairment of spatial learning and memory of pentylenetetrazol-kindled rats. Neurol Sci 2011;32(4):609–13.

133. Tariot PN, Farlow MR, Grossberg GT, et al. Memantine treatment in patients with moderate to severe Alzheimer disease already receiving donepezil: a randomized controlled trial. JAMA 2004;291(3):317–24.

134. Reisberg B, Doody R, Stöffler A, et al. Memantine in moderate-to-severe Alzheimer's disease. N Engl J Med 2003;348(14):1333–41.

135. Reisberg B, Doody R, Stöffler A, et al. A 24-week open-label extension study of memantine in moderate to severe Alzheimer disease. Arch Neurol 2006;63(1):49–54.

136. Beavo JA. Cyclic nucleotide phosphodiesterases: functional implications of multiple isoforms. Physiol Rev 1995;75(4):725–48. Available at: http://www.ncbi.nlm.nih.gov/pubmed/7480160. Accessed January 10, 2015.

137. Subhan Z, Hindmarch I. Psychopharmacological effects of vinpocetine in normal healthy volunteers. Eur J Clin Pharmacol 1985;28(5):567–71. Available at: http://www.ncbi.nlm.nih.gov/pubmed/3899677. Accessed January 10, 2015.

138. Bhatti JZ, Hindmarch I. Vinpocetine effects on cognitive impairments produced by flunitrazepam. Int Clin Psychopharmacol 1987;2(4):325–31. Available at: http://www.ncbi.nlm.nih.gov/pubmed/3693872. Accessed January 10, 2015.

139. Coleston DM, Hindmarch I. Possible memory-enhancing properties of vinpocetine. Drug Dev Res 1988;14(3–4):191–3.

140. Szatmari SZ, Whitehouse PJ. Vinpocetine for cognitive impairment and dementia. Cochrane Database Syst Rev 2003;(1):CD003119.

141. Blaha L, Erzigkeit H, Adamczyk A, et al. Clinical evidence of the effectiveness of vinpocetine in the treatment of organic psychosyndrome. Hum Psychopharmacol Clin Exp 1989;4(2):103–11.

142. Hindmarch I, Fuchs HH, Erzigkeit H. Efficacy and tolerance of vinpocetine in ambulant patients suffering from mild to moderate organic psychosyndromes. Int Clin Psychopharmacol 1991;6(1):31–43. Available at: http://www.ncbi.nlm.nih.gov/pubmed/2071888. Accessed January 10, 2015.

143. Fenzl E, Apecechea M, Schaltenbrand R, et al. Long-term study concerning tolerance and efficacy of vinpocetine in elderly patients suffering from a mild

to moderate organic psychosyndrome. In: Bes A, Cahn J, Cahn R, editors. Senile dementias: early detection. London: John Libby Eurotext; 1986. p. 580–5.

144. Ogunrin A. Effect of vinpocetine (Cognitol™) on cognitive performances of a Nigerian population. Ann Med Health Sci Res 2014;4(4):654–61.

145. Molnár P, Erdö SL. Vinpocetine is as potent as phenytoin to block voltage-gated Na+ channels in rat cortical neurons. Eur J Pharmacol 1995;273(3):303–6. Available at: http://www.ncbi.nlm.nih.gov/pubmed/7737339. Accessed January 10, 2015.

146. Sitges M, Nekrassov V. Vinpocetine prevents 4-aminopyridine-induced changes in the EEG, the auditory brainstem responses and hearing. Clin Neurophysiol 2004;115(12):2711–7.

147. Sitges M, Chiu LM, Guarneros A, et al. Effects of carbamazepine, phenytoin, lamotrigine, oxcarbazepine, topiramate and vinpocetine on Na+ channel-mediated release of [3H]glutamate in hippocampal nerve endings. Neuropharmacology 2007;52(2):598–605.

148. Nekrassov V, Sitges M. Vinpocetine inhibits the epileptic cortical activity and auditory alterations induced by pentylenetetrazole in the guinea pig in vivo. Epilepsy Res 2004;60(1):63–71.

149. Nekrassov V, Sitges M. Additive effects of antiepileptic drugs and pentylenetetrazole on hearing. Neurosci Lett 2006;406(3):276–80.

150. Nekrassov V, Sitges M. Comparison of acute, chronic and post-treatment effects of carbamazepine and vinpocetine on hearing loss and seizures induced by 4-aminopyridine. Clin Neurophysiol 2008;119(11):2608–14.

151. Dutov AA, Gal'tvanitsa GA, Volkova VA, et al. Cavinton in the prevention of the convulsive syndrome in children after birth injury. Zh Nevropatol Psikhiatr Im S S Korsakova 1991;91(8):21–2 [in Russian] Available at: http://www.ncbi.nlm.nih.gov/pubmed/1661506. Accessed January 10, 2015.

152. Dutov AA, Tolpyshev BA, Petrov AP, et al. Use of cavinton in epilepsy. Zh Nevropatol Psikhiatr Im S S Korsakova 1986;86(6):850–5 [in Russian] Available at: http://www.ncbi.nlm.nih.gov/pubmed/3751419. Accessed January 10, 2015.

153. Koubeissi MZ, Kahriman E, Syed TU, et al. Low-frequency electrical stimulation of a fiber tract in temporal lobe epilepsy. Ann Neurol 2013;74(2):223–31.

154. Suthana N, Haneef Z, Stern J, et al. Memory enhancement and deep-brain stimulation of the entorhinal area. N Engl J Med 2012;366(6):502–10.

155. Fell J, Staresina BP, Do Lam AT, et al. Memory modulation by weak synchronous deep brain stimulation: a pilot study. Brain Stimul 2013;6(3):270–3.

156. Vonck K, Sprengers M, Carrette E, et al. A decade of experience with deep brain stimulation for patients with refractory medial temporal lobe epilepsy. Int J Neural Syst 2013;23(1):1250034.

157. Boëx C, Seeck M, Vulliémoz S, et al. Chronic deep brain stimulation in mesial temporal lobe epilepsy. Seizure 2011;20(6):485–90.

158. Suthana N, Fried I. Deep brain stimulation for enhancement of learning and memory. Neuroimage 2014;3(Pt 85):996–1002.

Stroke and Behavior

Victor W. Mark, MD[a,b,c],*

KEYWORDS

- Cognition • Stroke • Rehabilitation • Activities of daily living • Recovery

KEY POINTS

- The clinician who manages stroke survivors must be aware of the variety of associated behavioral changes, methods of simple assessment, and management options.
- Behavioral changes assessed at bedside or in the clinic in response to verbal command cannot be assumed to represent the patient's spontaneous conduct in the home setting.
- Dissociations between activities in these settings can occur, particularly with respect to whether they are performed spontaneously and adequately.
- Behavioral changes after stroke may result from direct damage to brain parenchyma or may emerge from interactions with the environment in relation to sustained neurologic deficit.
- Post-stroke behavioral changes tend to improve in severity, but may qualitatively change, while others may continually worsen.

Videos of various behavioral changes caused by stroke accompany this article at http://www.neurologic.theclinics.com/

"Stroke" is the clinical term for a sustained neurologic deficit arising from abrupt focal vascular injury (ischemic or hemorrhagic) within the brain parenchyma. Behavioral changes commonly follow and are often disabling. The character of the behavioral changes is often determined by the part of the brain that has been directly injured, which reflects the anatomic concentration of many functions. For example, the most severe language disorders almost invariably follow left rather than right hemisphere stroke, at least in right-handed adults. Disturbances of visual perception arise primarily from stroke in the back of the brain rather than the front. In contrast, other post-stroke disorders can arise from damage to any of a multitude of locations. For example, disordered self-regulatory ability (executive function), apathy (loss of interest

Disclosures: None.
[a] Department of Physical Medicine and Rehabilitation, University of Alabama at Birmingham, 1720 2nd Avenue South, SRC 190, Birmingham, AL 35294-7330, USA; [b] Department of Neurology, University of Alabama at Birmingham, AL, USA; [c] Department of Psychology, University of Alabama at Birmingham, AL, USA
* Department of Physical Medicine and Rehabilitation, University of Alabama at Birmingham, 1720 2nd Avenue South, SRC 190, Birmingham, AL 35294-7330.
E-mail address: vwmark@uabmc.edu

and initiative), or unilateral spatial neglect can follow stroke from widely different anatomic sites.[1–5] This diversity may reflect the organization of the brain for these functions along extensive, widely distributed neuronal networks.[6]

Because the behavioral changes that follow stroke can be exceedingly diverse, clinicians who treat stroke patients should make every effort to recognize these phenomena. Moreover, an average of 20% of acute strokes may have cognitive changes that evade routine evaluation, resulting in so-called silent infarcts (or covert infarcts)[7] that might be recognized by more careful cognitive evaluation. This review orients clinicians to the most common behavioral changes and notes some uncommon and often overlooked behavioral manifestations. In this way, the clinician may become sensitized to still other behavioral effects that may be encountered in practice but that are not covered herein. This review also helps to prepare the clinician to (1) interpret for patients and their caregivers these behavioral changes and how they may affect everyday activities and (2) guide management. As will be shown, some behavioral changes have only limited disabling effects, or have not been shown (so far) directly to affect self-care abilities, but nonetheless may be biomarkers of disability.

EPIDEMIOLOGY

Based on worldwide disease surveys, stroke is the commonest neurologic disorder, with an annual incidence of 183 per 100,000 individuals.[8] Although stroke can occur at any age, even in childhood, advanced age is a leading risk factor for stroke, as are also conditions associated with cardiovascular disease (smoking, diabetes, and hypertension).[9] The advancing average age of the general population will increase stroke prevalence over the coming decades.

GENERAL FEATURES OF STROKE

Because the brain's vascular supply and its control over movement and sensation are lateralized, stroke that follows injury to a single blood vessel characteristically results in lateralized disturbances of movement or sensation. In contrast, stroke that follows concurrent vascular injury to both sides of the brain (eg, after multiple cardiac emboli, medial frontal aneurysmal rupture with vasospasm, or occlusion of an anomalous artery) may result in bilateral disturbances.[10,11] However, most behavioral effects of stroke, even after a solitary lesion, do not have lateralized effects.

One factor that governs the severity of the neurologic deficits of stroke, compared with other focal brain illnesses, is its sudden onset. Various neurologic diseases can permanently disrupt a focal region of once-healthy tissue. But for a given amount of lost parenchyma, the effects of stroke are much more severe than of slowly growing brain tumors.[12,13] This difference is believed to reflect that neuroplastic reorganization in response to injury can proceed only at a slow rate.

Such reorganization, however, does eventually come to aid the damaging effects of stroke. After short-term neurologic improvement by way of revascularization from collateral vessels and resolution of cerebral edema or hemorrhage,[14] neurologic impairments that follow stroke in most instances improve over weeks to months.[15,16] This reflects the effects of such neuroplastic changes, despite permanent focal tissue loss as well as concurrent acceleration of cerebral atrophy.[17]

Recovery of neurologic impairment after a stroke (which is assessed by measuring performance capacity, or maximal ability, to verbal command) is not tied closely to improvement in activities of daily living.[18,19] Thus, for example, complete and enduring paralysis on 1 side of the body may still allow recovery of self-care abilities through learning compensatory techniques with the other side of the body.[20] In a similar manner, aphasic stroke patients with markedly impaired comprehension or expression can nonetheless sometimes resume employment through adapting their activities.[21] This implies that assessing neurologic impairment (eg, with the National Institutes of Health [NIH] Stroke Scale or routine bedside examination) should not be used to predict functional ability or recovery after stroke.

CAVEATS ABOUT THE EVIDENCE FOR BEHAVIORAL CHANGES THAT FOLLOW STROKE

The caregiver of a stroke patient will often be impressed, or even burdened, by the behavioral changes that follow. But, nonetheless, it is not well-understood how best to evaluate them and whether such evaluations capture real-world effects. Because of limited time, resources, or perhaps even understanding, clinicians and investigators largely restrict their behavioral evaluations to the controlled environment of the clinic or laboratory, using tests and materials that are contrived to simulate daily living activities, but that nonetheless fall short of presenting the demands of the outside world. Moreover, performance is generally evaluated in response to the examiner's prompting ("on command"), yet much of real life occurs spontaneously, without prompting, and in a much more familiar environment. This article highlights the marked differences in behavior that can occur between laboratory and home settings. Despite this dissociation, however, contemporary research to a large extent uncritically assumes that findings under such artificial conditions can be extrapolated to predict real-life conduct, without evidence.

Another caution is that behavioral studies of stroke primarily assess its acute effects. However, as will be shown, the severity as well as the quality of behavioral effects of stroke may considerably change over the long run. One should also recognize that many of the behavioral studies of stroke have followed adults from industrialized societies who were formally well-educated and whose native language was nontonal (ie, languages in which a word's meaning is not affected by its intonation).[22] The behavioral changes after stroke among individuals who fall outside of these characteristics—for example, from rural China—are less well understood. Some findings suggest that, after left hemisphere damage, aphasic native Chinese speakers are more impaired in tone production during speech (which is crucial for interpreting individual word meanings in that language) than patients who had grown up learning a nontonal language.[23] Low educational attainment has been associated with worse severity of a multitude of cognitive deficits after stroke[24] as well as with altered hemispheric recruitment for language.[25] Recent evidence suggests that illiterates have different white matter structure than literates who speak the same language,[26] which could bear upon responses to stroke.

It should come as no surprise that markedly impaired speech comprehension is widely used to exclude patients from stroke studies that involve nonverbal cognitive tests. Hence, developing a general understanding for the consequences of stroke on nonverbal abilities commonly omits a sizable portion of the stroke population, about 20% altogether, based on recent studies.[27,28] Yet, comprehension-challenged individuals can comply with certain cognitive tests if one can accommodate their processing deficits. For example, although impaired speech comprehension has often led a priori to excluding stroke patients from being given the cancellation (target marking) test to assess spatial attention,[29–33] such individuals actually can be tested after careful, gentle demonstration of the procedure.[34]

Finally, the field of clinical behavioral science is hamstrung by inconsistency for what operations that specific cognitive tests are supposed to assess. For example, the Token Test[35] is widely used to index speech comprehension,[36] and hence it is a mainstay of aphasia evaluation. However, the test is as much sensitive to deficits of speech production as it is to comprehension, thus raising question for what it is actually measuring.[37] The Trail Making Test version B is a widely used and validated measure of executive control,[38] and yet elsewhere it has been used to study "attention,"[39] even when other tests are included specifically to assess "executive control" in the same subjects.[40] Inconsistency in reporting what cognitive tests are measuring specifically is commonplace in clinical behavioral research, at least in part because cognitive tests do not purely enlist 1 function.

In short, the field of clinical behavioral science suffers from the lack of consideration for the effects of test conditions on the generalization of findings, minimal inclusion of individuals from diverse cultural or educational backgrounds or with impaired speech comprehension, limited understanding of how pathologic behavior may change over time, and inconsistency for what specific tests are supposed to assess. Nonetheless, many patterns of behavioral change stand out after a stroke. This article summarizes these patterns; however, one must recognize that considerable neuroplastic reorganization of the field itself is due.

BEHAVIORAL CHANGES AFTER PEDIATRIC STROKE

In the United States, the incidence of stroke in children is 4 to 6 per 100,000.[9] Strokes in children are much more often hemorrhagic than in adults. The low incidence of stroke in children probably contributes to there being limited research on pediatric behavioral outcomes. The limited research may underlie inconsistency in the reported incidence of cognitive deficits after a pediatric stroke.[41] According to 1 study, the laterality of stroke in children affects the character of cognitive deficits, similar to adults. Thus, language deficits prevail after left hemisphere stroke and visuospatial deficits after right hemisphere stroke.[42] Executive functions are reported to be minimally affected when compared with age-similar healthy children.[43]

POST-STROKE BEHAVIORAL CHANGES IN ADULTS: GENERAL COMMENTS

Surveys of the incidence of cognitive disorders after a stroke yield varying results. As many as 72% of acute stroke patients may show cognitive impairment relative to healthy individuals; this may diminish to about 30% by 3 months after stroke onset.[44] However, despite an initial improvement in cognitive function in the first year, continued cognitive decline may occur in stroke patients when seen 1 year later, particularly with respect to memory and executive function, despite the absence of further stroke.[45–47] Multiple reasons may underlie behavioral changes after stroke: direct injury to brain areas involved with cognitive processing, secondary effects of behavioral changes provoked by adjustment to the stroke (eg, anxiety, depression, sleep disturbance), or a stroke may bring to clinical attention preexisting behavioral changes associated with long-standing but previously unnoticed cerebrovascular disease.[48]

Understanding the best ways to evaluate cognitive changes after stroke is a priority for clinicians.[49] However, despite a plethora of published cognitive assessments to date, it has been difficult to develop tests that are optimally sensitive to cognitive deficits while keeping the time required for assessment to a comfortable amount. This limitation is particularly of concern given the vulnerability of brain-impaired patients to fatigue associated with prolonged assessment, and the susceptibility of persons with stroke to fatigue even in the absence of major noncognitive neurologic deficit.[50]

Several evaluation screens are available that may be given in fewer than 30 minutes to broadly sample cognitive abilities. Although the Mini-Mental State Examination[51] is the most widely used such evaluation, it was not intended to evaluate stroke, is biased toward evaluating linguistic deficits at the expense of detecting nonlinguistic difficulties, and is insensitive to executive dysfunction.[52] Among the other competing brief assessments, the Montreal Cognitive Assessment[53] best meets the shortcomings of the Mini-Mental State Examination for evaluating common deficits that follow stroke,[54] is more sensitive to mild cognitive impairment,[55] and has been rapidly gaining acceptance as a tool for screening or triage for stroke studies. It requires about 15 minutes to administer for stroke patients, and is freely available for download online (available from www.mocatest.org).

The following sections describe characteristics mainly of the most widely discussed subtypes of cognitive disorders that can follow stroke. For the most part, they are arranged in descending order according to their frequency of coverage in published clinical studies,[56] except that we start by reviewing disturbances of executive functions because of their primacy for regulating other functions.

EXECUTIVE FUNCTIONS

This very broad category refers to processes that regulate other functions, in the same way that a company's executive controls subsidiary operations (eg, marketing, hiring, promotion, production, support services) without directly being involved with them. Although there is not complete agreement on what these processes are, the consensus supports that executive functions involve planning (which requires abstraction), initiation, staying mindful of task objectives (working memory), prioritizing goals, sequencing activities for specific goals, and inhibiting attention to irrelevant stimuli (minimizing distraction).[57,58] Executive dysfunction has become increasingly recognized as a leading predictor of limited functional recovery after a stroke.[58–70] It is thus unsurprising that executive control is vital to functional recovery after stroke, particularly in rehabilitation, where the patient must confront and cope with novel environments, personnel, training regimens, cacophonous gyms, and compromised function. Although prototypically held to reflect "frontal" disturbance, executive dyscontrol can also follow lesions to posterior cerebral areas[67,71–73] or reflect effects of diffuse cerebrovascular damage.[68,74–76] The precise incidence of executive dyscontrol after acute stroke is uncertain, owing in part to differences in test methods, but it is apparently very common, with figures as high as 50% to 75% having been reported.[77–79] In 1 epidemiologic survey, executive function led other cognitive disturbances for its susceptibility to accelerated decline years after stroke onset.[47]

Nonetheless, despite the preeminence of executive dyscontrol for post-stroke functional recovery, executive assessments in stroke studies have been hindered either because they often involve lengthy, laborious procedures[77,80] or require patients to understand complex instructions or give spoken responses. These latter linguistic requirements commonly end up excluding a large number of aphasic patients from executive function studies.[61,62,77,81–89]

Executive disturbances after stroke can include lack of spontaneity, distractibility, performing multistep operations in the wrong order, failure to inhibit behaviors that are inappropriate to a situation (eg, laughing while attending a funeral), or performing actions repeatedly for a goal or in response to stimulation, but needlessly (perseveration; Videos 1 and 2). "Recurrent perseveration" is a subtype of perseveration that is common in aphasia.[90] In this disorder, patients uncritically repeat a response that they had provided to a previous question, but now when given a new question, for which the response is inappropriate.

The clinician may briefly screen executive disturbance by asking the patient to list as many unique animals as possible in 60 seconds (a test of semantic fluency). A reasonable cutoff score for impairment is less than 12 unique animals.[91] Although such disturbances can be vivid once they are identified in a patient, they are often unrecognized by both patients and caregivers alike before diagnosis, particularly if they occur without other neurologic disorders, because they greatly overlap commonly recognized "personality disorders" or aspects of aging, such as irritability or absent-mindedness. Treatment of executive dysfunction has not been well-developed. Bromocriptine occasionally can improve speech initiation after a stroke,[92] but its efficacy has been inconsistent. Modafinil has been reported to improve initiation and rehabilitation participation after intracerebral hemorrhage.[93]

LANGUAGE

In a review that ranked reports of post-stroke cognitive disturbances by their frequency of publication, aphasia was one of the leaders.[56] This ranking is unsurprising, considering that language is the most distinctively human of overt behaviors, essential to social interaction and cooperation. The modern neurologic evaluation of language disorders originated with the seminal investigations of the 19th-century European aphasiologists Paul Broca and Marc Dax that associated acute aphasia with left hemisphere disease.[94] These observations inspired developing the scientific field of behavioral neurology, which owed itself to the striking ability of aphasia to seize the concern of clinical investigators, more so than other behavioral disorders.

Aphasia is the disruption of spoken symbolic information, either in its interpretation or expression. In most instances stroke disrupts both processes,[95] albeit to a variable extent from 1 patient to the next. Commonly, disruption of written communication[96] or other forms of symbolic communication (eg, sign language[97]) are affected as well (**Fig. 1**). Aphasia must be distinguished from speech dysarthria, mutism, aphonia (inability to vocalize), and hearing loss, which do not selectively affect the symbolic aspects of speech. The jumbled speech of some patients with aphasia can resemble psychosis,[98] until one notes that aphasic speech does not dwell on a particular theme or delusion, such as persecution (Video 3).

Although there are many classification schemes for aphasia, the easiest as well as the most reliable distinction is to classify aphasia as either fluent or nonfluent.[99] Fluent aphasia retains a fairly normal flow of speech output, mostly uninterrupted. Nonfluent aphasia is denoted by effortful, halting speech, or minimal production at all.

Aphasia occurs in about one-third of acute stroke patients and predicts worse survival than in nonaphasic stroke patients.[28] This may be because aphasia is a biomarker for advanced cardiovascular disease or its typically afflicting older patients,[100] rather than representing a direct effect of aphasia. By 6 months after stroke onset, aphasia may improve in more than one-half of patients and completely resolve in about 38%.[101]

As is well known, aphasia primarily results from left hemisphere injury. Rarely, classic aphasic disorders follow right hemisphere stroke, which is called crossed aphasia (see **Fig. 1**, Video 4). More often, the linguistic impairments that follow right hemisphere stroke are subtle and difficult to recognize, including the patient having impaired interpretation of the social signals in discourse (such as failing to notice when another individual wants to end discussion), misunderstanding ambiguity, and meandering topics during speech expression.[102] Research on the communication impairments of right hemisphere stroke has been minimal, owing in part to difficulties with devising reliable assessments, and the finding that patients who are tested under

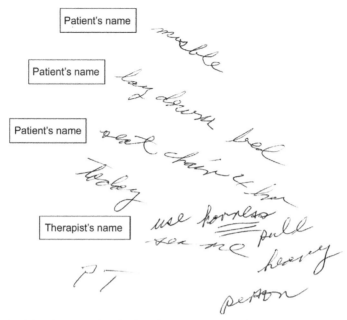

Fig. 1. Handwriting in crossed aphasia. This patient in Video 4 was premorbidly right-handed and had a right hemisphere stroke that resulted in left hemiplegia and a classic Broca aphasia, with halting, effortful replies that left out parts of speech (agrammatism). Most patients with Broca aphasia have right hemiplegia after left hemisphere stroke, which disrupts handwriting if they are right-handed. When this patient was asked to write answers to questions about her activities, her responses with her dominant hand showed excellent pen control but agrammatism that mirrored her speech. This rare example of motorically well-controlled handwriting in aphasia thus shows that aphasia is a central disorder of language processing that can affect different channels of communication in parallel. (The patient's and therapist's names have been masked in this sample.)

contrived situations in the laboratory often are less impaired (if at all) during spontaneous discourse.

The assessment and treatment for aphasia is best left to a speech–language pathologist, but the general clinician can easily test basic language functions over a few minutes to diagnose aphasia. The common operations that can be tested include speech comprehension (such as answering yes or no questions, where the examiner knows the answer; pointing to objects in the room on command), repetition of words, phrases, or sentences ("No ifs, ands, or buts" having strong sensitivity), naming objects that are presented (eg, watch, thumb), and listening for whether the patient has normal sentence composition during conversation (thus evaluating grammar). It should be noted, however, that language in the aphasic patient can fluctuate and even deteriorate over several minutes of assessment, which may lead to failure to appreciate the patient's best linguistic capabilities.[103,104] Allowing rest periods after a few minutes may help to restore the patient to improved performance.

Although aphasia usually improves to less severe forms, it is remarkable that the character of the aphasic disturbance may itself change during an individual's recovery. Thus, for example, global aphasia (typified by markedly impoverished speech comprehension and production) may change to Wernicke aphasia (fluent but nonsensical speech and poor comprehension); Broca aphasia (good comprehension, poor speech production) may resolve to anomic aphasia (good comprehension and fluency, but with word-finding difficulties).[105] Thus, in recovery, nonfluent aphasia often gives way to fluent aphasia. In contrast, one does not find fluent aphasia changing to nonfluent aphasia.

Despite severe disturbances of comprehension, aphasic patients may nonetheless respond well to therapists through relying on less affected nonlinguistic routes of communication. Thus, for example, aphasic individuals often can understand emotional facial gestures,[106] along with gross limb gestures (eg, beckoning a patient to approach), and emotional intonation.[107]

Few speech therapies have much of an evidence basis behind them. Several promising and aggressively investigated approaches include Melodic Intonation Therapy (which progressively shapes the patient over a few weeks from singing to speaking short phrases while the patient rhythmically taps)[108] and various medications (piracetam, donepezil, memantine, galantamine) or forms of noninvasive brain stimulation (transcranial magnetic stimulation, transcranial direct current stimulation).[109,110] A major limitation to these studies is the failure to evaluate effects on real-life language. An approach to evaluating the effects of aphasia therapy on real-life behaviors has come from the emerging intervention termed Constraint-Induced Aphasia Therapy (CIAT), for which there have been multiple small trials.[111] This approach is intended to improve spontaneous speech in aphasic patients who have become inhibited in their speaking because of reduced communicative efficacy or increased speaking effort. A recent pilot study of CIAT found significant improvement on a self-report measure of real-world speech (the Verbal Activity Log) that had been validated against objectively measured speech that had been digitally recorded in the home.[112] For unclear reasons, the treatment can also benefit speech comprehension,[111] even though this aspect is not trained directly.

Disturbances in using and interpreting speech intonation may also follow stroke. This disturbance is termed aprosodia and may grossly be classified into 2 kinds: affective aprosodia, which is the disturbed interpretation or expression of emotional tone in speech,[113] and linguistic aprosodia, the disturbance of nonemotional tone, for example, the conveyance of emphasis ("!") or interrogation ("?") in a sentence.[114] In such disorders, the problem is not with word selection or sentence construction, but rather with determining the speaker's social perspective (Is he angry?) or need for information (Is she asking a question?). Aprosodia is not associated with damage to 1 particular brain area or side.[115] Testing for aprosodia is again complicated by the reliance on contrived situations that may not represent ordinary conditions for discourse.[116]

Apraxia of speech can also follow stroke. This disturbance involves the inconsistent production of speech sounds (particularly consonants, depending on whether they are initial vs later in a word)[117] and is considered a deficit of planning speech movements. This inconsistency thus differs from speech dysarthria. Associated difficulties include slowed rate of speech and abnormal rhythm and intonation. The disorder often is found with concurrent nonfluent aphasia. Reliable diagnosis and treatment have not been well-developed; its incidence in stroke is undetermined.

ATTENTION

Deficits of attention have been reported even more often than language disorders after a stroke. Attention is the process of enhancing detection of a signal or stimulus from the environment, to the point where it can then be acted upon. Inattention may either be lateralized or nonlateralized with respect to the environment.

The lateralized deficit is termed unilateral spatial neglect (neglect for short) and is a topic of intense research. This interest may be in part because the disorder, like aphasia, is easily noticed. The patient with acute severe neglect consistently gazes toward the side of hemispheric damage (Vulpian sign[118]), in the absence of oculomotor palsy. When patients with acute neglect combined with hemiplegia are asked to clap their hands, often they wave only the relatively good hand toward the body midline repeatedly without accommodating the lack of movement ability in the other hand. This action has become known as the Eastchester clapping sign, or in effect, the appearance of "1-handed clapping."[119] General action initiation is decreased, as is affective speech prosody. There is a general decrease in exploring toward the contralateral side of space, which can be improved with cueing toward that direction (eg, by flashing lights to 1 side).[120] Often patients are unaware of their difficulties, or may even deny either their attentional deficit or associated unilateral limb paralysis (anosognosia).[121] The persistence of such difficulties can hamper activities of daily living, extending to locomotion (including car or wheelchair navigation), eating, grooming, reading, and protecting the paralyzed limbs from injury during transfers between bed and chair. Neglect, therefore, can pertain to one's own body as well to the environment beyond the body. Unilateral spatial neglect may even occur in one's imagination, for example, when describing a familiar space that is out of view, such as a distant plaza.[122] Unfortunately, some patients may show neglect on some tests but not on others, for unclear reasons, and hence to thoroughly screen for neglect, multiple tests may be needed.[123]

Therapists frequently observe that patients with unilateral neglect are much more impaired with recovery of basic activities of daily living than are patients with other cognitive or noncognitive neurologic disorders, and they also exhibit poor carryover of what they have learned from day to day. The finding of acute neglect is often associated with long-term dependency.[124]

Neglect must be distinguished from other overt unilateral neurologic disturbances such as somatosensory loss (hemianesthesia), hemiparesis, and hemianopia. The unilateral deficits of somatosensory or visual awareness, or voluntary limb movement, can be overcome in neglect by prompting, which is not so with these other disorders. Although neglect is most often considered a disturbance of lateralized perception or action initiation, patients may also show reduced spontaneity of contralateral limb movement that can be improved by cueing, a disturbance that is termed motor neglect (Video 5).[125]

In its acute presentation, neglect is about equally common after left versus right hemisphere damage,[126] but generally right unilateral neglect is milder and resolves more rapidly. Neglect is almost invariably opposite the side of hemispheric injury rather than on the same side of injury. Neglect can be easily assessed by the clinician, either through observing the patient's spontaneous behavior at the bedside (eg, noticing whether the patient symmetrically explores the environment to either side), or formally through simple pen-and-paper exercises. One of the easiest is to present a roughly 20-cm horizontal line centered on a sheet of paper that is centered in front of the patient's midline and have the patient mark the line's midpoint. Another exercise that requires not much more effort is to provide a sheet of paper that is covered with about 20 toothpick-size lines of differing orientations across the page, and have the patient cross them out until he or she believes to have gotten them all (the cancellation test). Neglect will be manifest by a unilateral concentration of the lines left unmarked. It is striking how patients in this situation will believe that they have found all of the lines, yet lack the incentive to carefully explore all around the edges of the page to check their work and ensure completion.

Drawing exercises can not only demonstrate neglect but other deficits as well, including continuous perseveration that is poorly monitored or inhibited by the patient (**Fig. 2**). Less often, neglect has been identified in the other 2 dimensions of space in relation to the patient, thus either far versus near the patient (radial neglect),[127] or above or below eye level (vertical or altitudinal neglect).[128] Combined forms of multi-dimensional neglect can also occur, so-called diagonal neglect.[129] But because humans commonly operate in a horizontally aligned visual ellipsoid of space that is centered at eye level and navigate mostly on 1 level rather than traverse stairs or climb trees, the horizontal (ie, right vs left) rather than the radial or vertical aspects of neglect most often are noticed.

Neglect is very common after acute stroke, occurring in about one-half of all patients.[130] The incidence then quickly diminishes, such that by about 3 months the proportion of stroke patients with neglect is about 30%.[131] Nonetheless, it is possible that standard neglect assessments may underestimate its occurrence. For example, with the kinds of assessments on contrived everyday activities that occupational therapists may use (eg, requesting the patient to self-groom or find one's way in a wheelchair), neglect may appear despite its absence or only minimal manifestation on standard pen-and-paper assessments.[132,133]

Experimental treatments for neglect abound, but none has been shown to benefit spontaneous everyday activities of daily living outside of the clinic consistently. Currently, considerable attention is paid to an intriguing manipulation of lateralized exploration and action, which is termed prism adaptation. In this approach, patients with left unilateral neglect wear prismatic eyewear that shifts the view toward the right, while they practice reaching with the right hand in front of themselves for 10 to 15 minutes. After removal of the lenses, the gaze spontaneously becomes biased toward the left for a while—the adaptation effect—and performance on standard pen-and-paper tests improves. However, carryover to spontaneous activities of daily living outside of the clinic has been found so far in just 1 study, based on a self-report survey.[134] Unfortunately, this author's requests to review the survey tool went unanswered, and so its validity for everyday functional abilities is unclear.

A limitation to research on the daily living implications of neglect is that frequently accompanying behavioral deficits are often overlooked. Already indicated was the

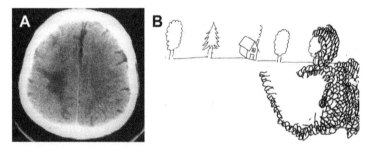

Fig. 2. Left unilateral spatial neglect and perseveration during figure copying. (*A*) Computed tomography scan indicating acute right frontal infarction. (*B*) Copy result. The patient was asked to copy the provided scene in the space below it without a time limit. This took about 20 minutes. Note (1) excessive reproduction of the loops of the tree outline, (2) the "closing in" phenomenon (inability to disengage from the original drawing, even though he was instructed to copy in the space below), and (3) neglect of the other figures in the drawing. When asked why he drew excessively, the patient replied he did not know. As a result, this shows poor error monitoring.

condition of limited insight into either neglect itself or associated hemiparesis, termed anosognosia. Anosognosia for hemiparesis may occur in one-third of acute stroke patients, but it remains in very few patients by 6 months. Even if the patient can acknowledge having neglect, this may not be sufficient to overcome the disturbance (one may call this "lip service"). A case study of the esteemed Italian film director Federico Fellini showed that he mocked his neglect in his stroke inpatient cartoon drawings, yet he failed to overcome the disorder.[135]

Patients with neglect are also susceptible to nonlateralized deficits of attention, including impaired sustaining of attention (or vigilance) over several minutes and slowed response times.[136] As shown in **Fig. 2**, impoverished error monitoring can also occur, in the form of disinhibited action execution (perseveration) without correction. The finding that acute neglect may be a biomarker for chronic disability or impaired nonlateralized visuospatial processing even in the absence of demonstrable neglect[124,137] suggests that it may not be neglect per se that is most disabling, but rather an associated general inattention disorder. Unfortunately, there has been little investigation into nonspatial attentional deficits, their effect on daily living activities, epidemiology, and natural history, let alone controlled trials of rehabilitation.

MEMORY

Memory deficits are commonly evaluated in the stroke literature.[56] When referring to memory here, we are not including the "working memory" that was indicated to be an executive function (ie, remaining constantly mindful of a fact or task requirement), but rather the process of either learning information or reconstituting it whenever necessary without staying mindful of it (episodic memory). Impaired memory may occur in about 11% of acute stroke patients.[138] Minor infarcts of the thalamus may result in memory impairment among patients without overt neurologic disruption.[7] Unlike most cognitive disorders, verbal memory may continually worsen over the years after a stroke, relative to healthy individuals of the same age.[46] Routine tests of orientation and asking the patient to recall 3 unrelated words both immediately and after a few minutes' delay are conventional brief clinical assessments of memory.

Rehabilitation for amnesia is not very advanced and has been little tried in stroke. In the neurologically healthy elderly, the ACTIVE study observed that after 5 to 6 weeks of a total of 10 to 12 hours of verbal episodic memory training, there was no improvement in episodic memory, but daily living activities showed less decline over the several years of follow-up in contrast with the untreated control group.[139] Whether such training effects can extend to stroke patients has not been evaluated.

EMOTION

Stroke can provoke a great variety of emotional changes. Diagnosing and treating these can lead to improved management and reduce suffering. Some authoritative work suggests that post-stroke emotional changes follow a sequence rather than occurring all at once.[140] Initial changes may include the "catastrophic reaction," pseudobulbar affect, and sadness, whereas frank depression emerges only after a few weeks.

The catastrophic reaction refers to short-term marked irritability, anger, anxiety, or sadness when prompted to perform a task within the first few days of stroke onset.[141] Patients with acute fluent aphasia with poor speech comprehension (Wernicke aphasia) may display marked agitation.[98,142] After recovery from the aphasia, Ross[142] found that patients reported that they had felt terrified, yet they believed that they could comprehend speech ordinarily despite clinical observations to the contrary.

Ross[143] suggested that this marked reaction may have arisen acutely because emotional processing in such cases was conducted primarily by the unlesioned right hemisphere, which some research has suggested mediates primarily negative (or "primary") emotions.

True depression follows in the weeks after stroke onset. Bogousslavsky[140] recommends reserving the term for the combination of sad mood, lack of initiative, steady state rather than cyclic emotional changes, lowered self-esteem, and feelings of guilt, particularly after patients have interacted with the complex world outside of the intensive care unit. Post-stroke depression is exceedingly common, ranging from 40% to 60% of patients, depending on the sample.[144,145] The relationship between stroke and depression is bidirectional: depression itself is a risk factor for subsequent stroke, including fatal stroke, for unclear reasons.[9] Post-stroke depression carries with it an increased risk of suicidal ideation, particularly in the first 2 years.[146] Depression is also a biomarker for general cognitive impairment[147,148] and impaired activities of daily living.[149]

Some research suggests that anterior circulation stroke is associated particularly with depression, which suggests a possible neurobiological etiology.[150,151] However, discerning the etiology for post-stroke depression is complicated by the reliance on verbal report for testing, which may lead to its underdiagnosis in aphasia that involves impaired comprehension.[152] In addition, adjustment to the effects of stroke on social life and loss of vocation may be inextricably involved with the onset of depression.[152]

Although any of several depression screens may be used for stroke, the most sensitive is reported to be the Zung Self-Rated Depression Scale.[153] However, simply asking a patient, "Do you often feel sad or depressed?" is nearly as effective as using an established scale.[154]

Fortunately, conventional antidepressant medications are efficacious for post-stroke depression.[155] Improvement in depression is associated with improved self-care skills.[149]

A disorder somewhat related to depression is post-stroke fatigue, which can occur with post-stroke depression[140] or occur in other post-stroke conditions. This too develops relatively late after stroke onset.[50,140] Although "fatigue" may describe several different conditions (eg, muscular tiredness after repeated movement attempts; performance decline over repeated procedures), in this instance we refer to the condition of declining cognitive ability that is associated with the feeling of physical or mental strain, which can corrupt even simple routine activities.[140] Post-stroke fatigue may be found in the absence of pronounced neurologic deficits and is associated with failure to return to employment.[50] It tends to be a chronic disorder. This poorly evaluated disorder has a reported prevalence ranging from 23% to 75%; treatment has not been well-studied.[156]

Pseudobulbar affect (**Fig. 3**, Video 6) is the currently preferred term for disinhibited crying or laughter that does not match the patient's mood. The condition has a large number of synonyms, including emotionalism, emotional incontinence, pathologic affect, pathologic laughter and crying (or crying and laughter), and pseudobulbar palsy. The condition has not been studied comprehensively. Its prevalence after stroke has been reported to range from 18% to 58%.[157] The condition can be readily misdiagnosed as depression, with which it may co-occur. Stress can aggravate the pathologic display of affect. Numerous mood-stabilizing medications can control the condition (eg, nortriptyline, sertraline, citalopram).[158] However, in the United States the only medication with government approval for this condition is the combination of dextromethorphan and low-dose quinidine (Nuedexta).[158]

The attitude of the stroke patient toward the paralyzed arm may be affected. Fisher[159] has observed informally that patients with right hemiplegia and global (or

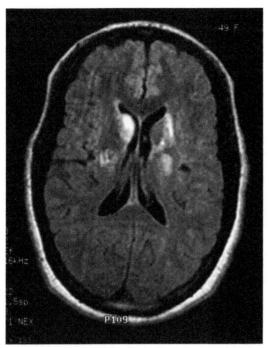

Fig. 3. Fluid-attenuated inversion recovery axial MRI scan of a patient who sustained pseudobulbar affect (Video 6) from simultaneous bilateral subcortical infarctions.

severe) aphasia may reach over with the left hand and repeatedly mobilize the limp arm in the first few hours after stroke onset. In contrast, patients with left hemiplegia after stroke are more apt to demonstrate marked hatred for the arm, a condition that is called misoplegia.[160]

Apathy refers to the combination of lack of goal-directed behaviors and diminished interest and concern. The incidence of post-stroke apathy is 20% to 25%.[161,162] The condition does not occur invariably with depression, but it does place patients at high risk for depression[4] and suicidal ideation.[163] Apathy is little investigated. Treatments with reported efficacy, but meriting further study, include dopamine agonists, methylphenidate,[4] or cognitive therapy.[164]

Diminished empathy may also follow stroke. Empathy refers to the ability to adopt the perspective of another individual with concern for that person's goals. The study of empathy is a newly emerging focus in post-stroke behavioral changes. According to a recent study, about one-half of the caregivers of patients recovering from right hemisphere stroke regarded the patients' loss of empathy as one of their greatest stressors.[165] Reduced empathy is also associated with a lack of understanding sarcasm, one aspect involved with interpreting another individual's behavior[166] and that pertains to the effects of right hemisphere stroke on language abilities that was discussed. Treatment for reduced empathy has yet to be developed for stroke. Developing treatment strategies may be difficult owing to the lack of insight into their own limitations that nonempathic stroke patients may have.[165] Hence, it remains to be demonstrated whether patients with reduced empathy would willingly participate in studies or adhere to treatment.

MOVEMENT

The behavioral regulation of movement, particularly limb movement, can be much affected by stroke. As noted, patients may manifest unilateral motor neglect, which is 1 kind of spontaneous lack of limb movement that can be improved by the examiner's prompting. Another cause is learned nonuse.[167] The difference between motor neglect and learned nonuse is that the former is considered to be based on a form of inattention, whereas the latter does not have an attentional basis but rather is hypothesized to emerge from the combination of the inability of the partially paretic limb to perform routine self-care activities and the simultaneous compensation for such activities by the opposite, better functioning arm (**Fig. 4**, Video 7). Thus, learned nonuse is behaviorally conditioned by the circumstances of chronic hemiparesis, leading to the persisting inhibition of spontaneous limb use for everyday activities, whereas motor neglect is not hypothesized to result from experience with the inhibiting effects of movement inadequacy. However, no test so far has been developed that can distinguish between these disturbances. Learned nonuse can be assessed with a self-report scale and guided interview that is called the Motor Activity Log, which has been shown to be correlated with spontaneous limb activity in the home as assessed by objective wrist accelerometry.[168]

Learned nonuse of hemiparesis, as diagnosed by a low score on the Motor Activity Log and the simultaneous ability to lift a small object with the paretic hand when prompted, can be ameliorated with an intensive counterconditioning physical and behavioral training program called Constraint-Induced Movement therapy,[169] which provided the basis for CIAT for aphasia that was described. Numerous randomized,

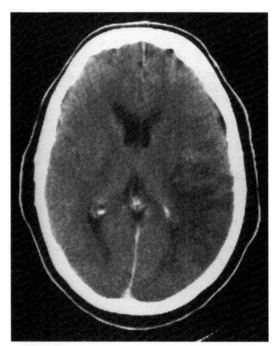

Fig. 4. Computed tomography scan of the patient in Videos 7 and 14 demonstrating an extensive left parietooccipital infarction. The lesion minimally affected the corticospinal tract and thus avoided causing severe weakness of the right hand.

controlled trials have supported the efficacy of Constraint-Induced Movement therapy.[170] It has been suggested that motor neglect could also respond to this treatment,[125] but no trials have thus far been conducted.

These disorders of motor neglect and learned nonuse of hemiparesis share the capability of motor improvement with verbal prompting. The inverse relationship can also occur—the inhibition of movement after prompting. This can occur as a form of automatic-voluntary dissociation that, despite its recognition in the 19th century,[171,172] remains a seldom investigated phenomenon. The difference in action completion depends on the extent of attention paid by the patient. For example, in the Foix–Chavany–Marie syndrome,[173] also termed the anterior opercular syndrome,[174] stroke patients may be unable to perform oral movements upon command, yet show normal movements in a more familiar context (which demands less attention), such as when presented food or in response to an emotional stimulus[175] (**Fig. 5**, Videos 8 and 9). A limb version of such automatic-voluntary dissociation has been proposed, termed exo-evoked akinesia, but has seldom been reported clinically.[176,177] Videos 10 and 11 and **Fig. 6** are of a stroke patient evaluated by the author that seems to qualify as such a presentation.

A different kind of exo-evoked akinesia may be seen in functional movement disorder, alternately termed conversion disorder or psychogenic neurologic disorder. This disorder can manifest as a movement failure when the patient attends to the affected limb or is commanded to move it, but improves with distraction (Videos 12 and 13). The disorder is commonly believed to result from unmet emotional support needs, "converting" such needs to an overt neurologic disturbance such as hemiparesis, owing to the societal stigma of psychiatric disturbances. Uncovering the contributing source of distress can be difficult, however.[178] Standard neurologic workup for stroke-like manifestations is generally negative. Nonetheless, in rare instances psychogenic neurologic illness can coexist with the neuroimaging confirmation of stroke (**Fig. 7**).[179] Consequently, the suspicion of psychogenic illness should not automatically exclude investigating for underlying structural nervous system disease. Treatments for

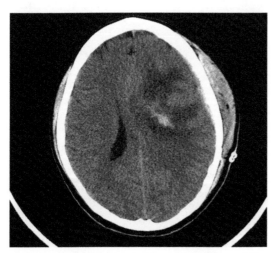

Fig. 5. Anterior opercular syndrome. Computed tomography scan of the patient in Videos 8 and 9, demonstrating an acute subcortical left frontal lobar hemorrhage in the bed of a testicular metastasis.

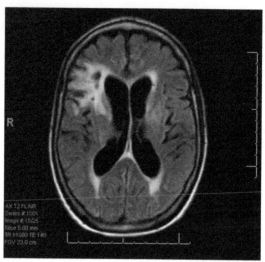

Fig. 6. Exo-evoked akinesia. Fluid-attenuated inversion recovery MRI scan of the patient in Videos 10 and 11 demonstrating multiple bilateral cerebral infarctions along with extensive white matter hyperintensities consistent with chronic cerebrovascular disease.

psychogenic illness are still being developed, but current opinion suggests that multidisciplinary rehabilitation may be beneficial.[180] These techniques would include providing to the patient the diagnosis of "functional movement disorder" to convey there is an actual disorder that is not imaginary or faked and that deserves treatment,

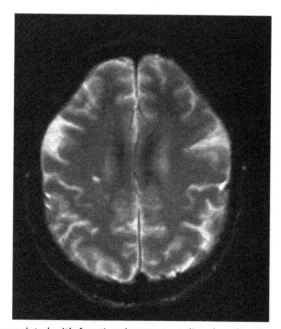

Fig. 7. MRI scan associated with functional movement disorder of patient in Videos 12 and 13. A small right subparietal infarct was found in this man who complained of left hemiparesis that improved with distraction.

but that is not accounted for by structural imaging findings. The therapeutic process should include demonstrating to the patient that motor control can improve with distraction.

A frequently described behavioral motor disturbance after stroke is termed ideo-motor apraxia (or apraxia for short). This disorder is the failure to competently generate the movements that are specific to tool use or gestures, despite the retention of suf-ficient movement capability to perform nonspecific movements and comprehension of the task requirements. Apraxia thus reflects a specific deficit in the regeneration of learned, culture-specific behavior, or skill, in contrast with limb movements that occur cross-culturally and develop from less training (eg, self-grooming, walking, infant car-rying). Although apraxia seems to be a form of memory failure (ie, an inability to recreate learned activities), the term is applied when investigators consider the retrieval failure to be specific to movement production rather than reflecting part of a more general memory disorder.

Ideomotor apraxia is most often reported with respect to upper extremity function, less so for oral movements (eg, soda straw use or blowing out a match),[95] and even less for leg use (eg, kicking a ball, stamping out a cigarette).[181] The incidence of post-stroke apraxia in 1 series was reported to be 6% to 7%.[182] Assessing apraxia most often involves requesting the patient to simulate movements that are used for specific tools (eg, hammer, screwdriver) or to imitate the examiner's use of such im-plements. Less often are actual objects used, and observing movement production on spontaneous real-life activities is rare in apraxia studies.

Apraxia is regarded widely as important to stroke care because it is a biomarker for impaired functional recovery.[183] This relationship has inspired efforts to rehabilitate apraxia through various training programs, and there is some evidence that such training can improve performance of simulated daily living activities in the clinical setting.[184] Unfortunately, to date it is unknown whether such training can carry over to improving spontaneous activities in the real-world setting. Indeed, many reports indi-cate a dissociation between intact spontaneous real-life manual activities and impov-erished performance on artificial tests of apraxia (Video 14),[185–188] and thus apraxia seems to be yet another instance of automatic-voluntary dissociation that was described. This dissociation suggests that the current clinical evaluation for apraxia falls far short in illuminating pathways to benefit functional recovery after stroke.

Alien hand syndrome is a most peculiar motor consequence of stroke. This mostly unilateral disorder involves the release of seemingly purposeful activities by 1 hand without the patient's consciously intending them, as if an alternate personality were guiding them. "Alien hand" is the more widely used term, but "anarchic hand" has been reasonably proposed to distinguish the unwanted basis for the activity[189] from the estrangement of limb ownership that can emerge in other disorders (eg, somato-paraphrenia).[190] Although various subtypes have been described, the 2 most often re-ported are frontal alien hand and callosal alien hand, named for the brain regions that are characteristically affected.[191] Frontal alien hand involves the disinhibited grabbing of objects that are within reaching distance. Often it is then hard for the patient to release the object. Callosal alien hand involves 1 hand obstructing, repeating, or un-doing the actions of the other hand that is under voluntary control (**Fig. 8**, Video 15). For example, a callosal alien hand may counteract blouse unbuttoning by the other hand.[192] Alien hand in either form may be frustrating, humiliating, or even dangerous, such as when grasping a hot object[189] or driving a car.[193] Despite a plethora of case reports, the epidemiology of alien hand has been little studied because it is scarce (or scarcely recognized); it accounted for less than 1% of stroke patients in 1 series.[194] Accordingly, treatment approaches have not been developed from clinical trials.

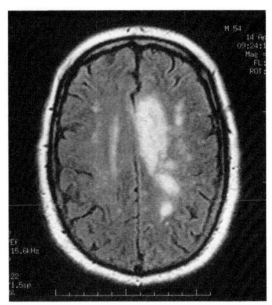

Fig. 8. MRI of patient with right callosal alien hand (Video 15), showing left callosal infarction.

SENSATION

Cognitive disturbances that are associated with altered sensory processing are not unusual after stroke, but are underrepresented relative to the foregoing disorders probably for a few reasons. (1) Because these disorders mostly arise from damage to posterior parts of the cerebrum, they often occur without much effect on motor control and therefore are less likely to warrant inpatient rehabilitation. (2) It is not unusual for patients with these disturbances to be unaware of these problems (the condition of anosognosia).

The commonly used term to address disturbances of altered perception is agnosia, from Greek for "lack of knowing." Disordered visual processing commonly follows lesions in the posterior artery distribution. Post-stroke visual impairments may be chronic in 20% of patients.[9] Patients with hemianopia (loss of visual awareness—at least for stationary objects—to 1 side) frequently are initially unaware of this loss, which has been termed "hemianopic hemiagnosia."[31] Often such patients, if they lack pronounced cognitive disorders, can readily discover their visual field limitation through interacting with the environment or through clinical education. In response, they may learn to compensate for visual loss by increasing their head or eye movements to 1 side. However, a large proportion of such patients exhibit highly disorganized visual exploration, even in their preserved visual field for unclear reasons, and are vulnerable to accidents at busy traffic intersections or in other cluttered environments.[71,133,195] Simple coaching and practice or formal oculomotor training may help to ameliorate this difficulty, although randomized controlled trials are lacking.

Seldom seen after stroke is the inability to recognize objects despite being capable of making elementary judgments about their properties. For example, in visual agnosia patients may be unable to identify familiar objects but can report their size and shape (**Fig. 9**). Similarly, patients with auditory agnosia can point to sounds and describe some of their properties (eg, "clicking" when listening to a thumb moving along a

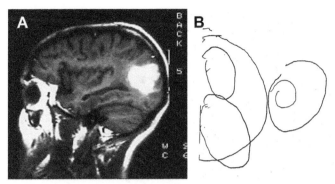

Fig. 9. Visual agnosia. This patient was unable to recognize objects that were shown to him despite being able to look at them; he had normal speech comprehension. (*A*) Fluid-attenuated inversion recovery MRI scan showing left parietooccipital infarction that was responsible. (*B*) Result of being asked to copy an adhesive tape dispenser that was put before him. Note substantial disorganization of execution, but with retention of the basic idea that the dispenser has a round shape.

pocket comb) without being able to specify the object responsible. A similar disturbance attends the rarely reported instance of tactile agnosia (Video 16).

A peculiar but little studied disorder involves the difficulty that stroke patients may have with connecting familiar percepts or concepts to each other. In particular, research by De Renzi and colleagues[196] observed that stroke patients, particularly with aphasia, were unable to color in line drawings of familiar objects with the expected colors (eg, banana → yellow). Instead, they significantly often chose unexpected colors, even though color blindness was excluded. This, accordingly, is termed color association disorder. The present author evaluated this behavior in stroke patients at his institution in an unpublished study, using a modification of the De Renzi approach by presenting multiple familiar objects in a single plausible outdoor scene (**Fig. 10**). The results in the aphasic patients vividly verified this phenomenon, while a right hemisphere stroke patient without aphasia instead perseverated with just a couple of colors.

Although such a disorder would seem to have little clinical relevance, the study that De Renzi and colleagues conducted noted that aphasic patients may also be prone to other abnormalities of percept matching, namely inability to match sounds that they heard to the most likely object in a picture array (eg, meow → cat). They also could not properly simulate object use when they were shown objects (eg, swing the arm when shown a hammer). The latter is a standard assessment of apraxia. The real-life implications of such difficulties when measured under laboratory conditions is not yet clear, but suggest a fundamental difficulty with abstraction.

Hallucinations can also follow stroke, most often the visual kind. These may take the form of simple geometric shapes, complex objects, or uncontrollable reexperiencing of objects that had just been viewed (palinopsia, or visual perseveration).[197] These disturbances are uncommon in stroke series.[194]

Still other visual disturbances for which the clinician should be aware include alexia (the inability to interpret writing or print despite being able to see it), achromatopsia (loss of color vision from brain injury), and prosopagnosia (disabled recognition of familiar faces).[198] The management of alexia suffers from the lack of well-controlled clinical trials.[199] Reports of post-stroke prosopagnosia have been limited to case reports, with some evidence that practice can improve face recognition.[200] The auditory

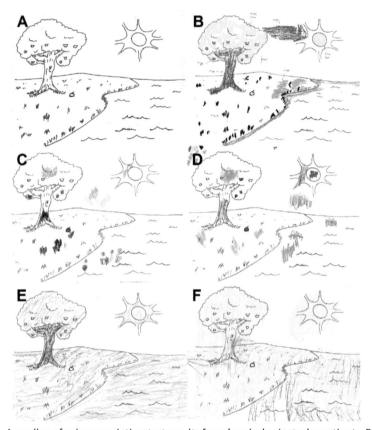

Fig. 10. A medley of color association test results from hemispheric stroke patients. Each patient was given 8 crayons of the basic colors and asked to color in the objects according to what would be appropriate. They had shown already that they were able to sort clothespins of 3 different colors (pink, green, or blue) according to color, thus demonstrating intact color discrimination. (*A*) Original black-and-white drawing that was presented to the patients. (*B*) Result from a patient with aphasia. (*C, D*) Results from another aphasic patient, 2 months apart. Note improved second attempt. (*E*) Result from another aphasic patient. (*F*) Result from a patient with right hemisphere stroke and no aphasia. Despite being given the 8 crayons, he chose only 2 colors and perseverated in his coloring, outside of the boundaries of the objects.

analog of prosopagnosia—the impaired ability to recognize familiar voices—is termed phonagnosia[201] and has been reported in stroke, but has been little studied.

ACKNOWLEDGMENTS

The author thanks Hannah Ronan-Daniell, BFA, for preparing the illustrations.

SUPPLEMENTARY DATA

Supplementary data related to this article can be found online at http://dx.doi.org/10.1016/j.ncl.2015.08.009.

REFERENCES

1. Robinson H, Calamia M, Gläscher J, et al. Neuroanatomical correlates of executive functions: a neuropsychological approach using the EXAMINER battery. J Int Neuropsychol Soc 2014;20:52–63.
2. Park KC, Yoon SS, Rhee HY. Executive dysfunction associated with stroke in the posterior cerebral artery territory. J Clin Neurosci 2011;18:203–8.
3. Vokaer M, Bier J, Elincx S, et al. The cerebellum may be directly involved in cognitive functions. Neurology 2002;58:967–70.
4. van Dalen JW, Moll van Charante EP, Nederkoorn PJ, et al. Poststroke apathy [review]. Stroke 2013;44:851–60.
5. Karnath HO, Rorden C. The anatomy of spatial neglect [review]. Neuropsychologia 2012;50:1010–7.
6. Mesulam MM. Large-scale neurocognitive networks and distributed processing for attention, language, and memory. Ann Neurol 1990;28:597–613.
7. Vermeer SE, Longstreth WT, Koudstaal PJ. Silent brain infarcts: a systematic review. Lancet Neurol 2007;6:611–9.
8. Hirtz D, Thurman DJ, Gwinn-Hardy K, et al. How common are the "common" neurologic disorders? Neurology 2007;68:326–37.
9. Mozaffarian D, Benjamin EJ, Go AS, et al. Heart disease and stroke statistics—2015 update: a report from the American Heart Association. Circulation 2015; 131:e29–322.
10. Kumral E, Bayulkem G, Evyapan D, et al. Spectrum of anterior cerebral artery territory infarction: clinical and MRI findings. Eur J Neurol 2002;9:615–24.
11. Menezes BF, Cheserem B, Kandasamy J, et al. Acute bilateral anterior circulation stroke due to anomalous cerebral vasculature: a case report. J Med Case Rep 2008;2:188.
12. Anderson SW, Damasio H, Tranel D. Neuropsychological impairments associated with lesions caused by tumor or stroke. Arch Neurol 1990;47:397–405.
13. Desmurget M, Bonnetblanc F, Duffau H. Contrasting acute and slow-growing lesions: a new door to brain plasticity [review]. Brain 2007;130:898–914.
14. Aminoff MJ, Greenberg DA, Simon RP. Clinical neurology. 9th edition. New York: McGraw-Hill Medical; 2015.
15. Twitchell TE. The restoration of motor function following hemiplegia in man. Brain 1951;74:443–80.
16. Hochstenbach JB, den Otter R, Mulder TW. Cognitive recovery after stroke: a 2-year follow-up. Arch Phys Med Rehabil 2003;84:1499–504.
17. Seghier ML, Ramsden S, Lim L, et al. Gradual lesion expansion and brain shrinkage years after stroke. Stroke 2014;45:877–9.
18. Roth EJ, Heinemann AW, Lovell LL, et al. Impairment and disability: their relation during stroke rehabilitation. Arch Phys Med Rehabil 1998;79:329–35.
19. Duncan PW, Lai SM, Keighley J. Defining post-stroke recovery: implications for design and interpretation of drug trials. Neuropharmacology 2000;39:835–41.
20. Duncan PW, Goldstein LB, Matchar D, et al. Measurement of motor recovery after stroke. Outcome assessment and sample size requirements. Stroke 1992;23: 1084–9.
21. Carriero MR, Faglia L, Vignolo LA. Resumption of gainful employment in aphasics: preliminary findings. Cortex 1987;26:667–72.
22. Lecours AR, Basso A, Moraschini S, et al. Where is the speech area, and who has seen it?. In: Caplan D, Lecours AR, Smith A, editors. Biological perspectives on language. Cambridge (MA): MIT Press; 1984. p. 220–46.

23. Packard JL. Tone production deficits in nonfluent aphasic Chinese speech. Brain Lang 1986;29:212–23.

24. Ojala-Oksala J, Jokinen H, Kopsi V, et al. Educational history is an independent predictor of cognitive deficits and long-term survival in postacute patients with mild to moderate ischemic stroke. Stroke 2012;43:2931–5.

25. Lecours AR, Mehler J, Parente MA, et al. Illiteracy and brain damage. 3. A contribution to the study of speech and language disorders in illiterates with unilateral brain damage (initial testing). Neuropsychologia 1988;26: 575–89.

26. Thiebaut de Schotten M, Cohen L, Amemiya E, et al. Learning to read improves the structure of the arcuate fasciculus. Cereb Cortex 2014;24:989–95.

27. Kauhanen ML, Korpelainen J, Hiltunen P, et al. Aphasia, depression, and non-verbal cognitive impairment in ischaemic stroke. Cerebrovasc Dis 2000;10:455–61.

28. Laska AC, Hellblom A, Murray V, et al. Aphasia in acute stroke and relation to outcome. J Intern Med 2001;249:413–22.

29. Reinvang I, Sundet K. The validity of functional assessment with neuropsychological tests in aphasic stroke patients. Scand J Psychol 1985;26:208–18.

30. Tatemichi TK, Desmond DW, Stern Y, et al. Cognitive impairment after stroke: frequency, patterns, and relationship to functional abilities. J Neurol Neurosurg Psychiatry 1994;57:202–7.

31. Celesia GG, Brigell MG, Vaphiades MS. Hemianopic hemiagnosia. Neurology 1997;49:88–97.

32. Price CI, Curless RH, Rodgers H. Can stroke patients use visual analogue scales? Stroke 1999;30:1357–61.

33. Beis JM, Keller C, Morin N, et al. Right spatial neglect after left hemisphere stroke: qualitative and quantitative study. Neurology 2004;63:1600–5.

34. Suchan J, Karnath HO. Spatial orienting by left hemisphere language areas: a relict from the past? Brain 2011;134:3059–70.

35. De Renzi E, Vignolo LA. The Token Test: a sensitive test to detect receptive disturbances in aphasics. Brain 1962;85:665–78.

36. Paci M, Lorenzini C, Fioravanti E, et al. Reliability of the 36-item version of the Token Test in patients with poststroke aphasia [Epub ahead of print]. Top Stroke Rehabil 2015.

37. Cohen R, Kelter S. Cognitive impairment of aphasics in a colour-to-picture matching task. Cortex 1979;15:235–45.

38. Arbuthnott K, Frank J. Trail making test, Part B as a measure of executive control: validation using a set-switching paradigm. J Clin Exp Neuropsychol 2000; 22:518–28.

39. Hochstenbach J, Mulder T, van Limbeek J, et al. Cognitive decline following stroke: a comprehensive study of cognitive decline following stroke. J Clin Exp Neuropsychol 1998;20:503–17.

40. Rasquin SMC, Welter J, van Heugten CM. Course of cognitive functioning during stroke rehabilitation. Neuropsychol Rehabil 2013;23:811–23.

41. Hajek CA, Yeates KO, Anderson V, et al. Cognitive outcomes following arterial ischemic stroke in infants and children. J Child Neurol 2014;29:887–94.

42. Kolk A, Talvik T. Cognitive outcome of children with early-onset hemiparesis. J Child Neurol 2000;5:581–7.

43. Kolk A, Ennok M, Laugesaar R, et al. Long-term cognitive outcomes after pediatric stroke. Pediatr Neurol 2011;44:101–9.

44. Hurford R, Charidimou A, Fox Z, et al. Domain-specific trends in cognitive impairment after acute ischaemic stroke. J Neurol 2013;260:237–41.

45. Sachdev PS, Brodaty H, Valenzuela MJ, et al. Progression of cognitive impairment in stroke patients. Neurology 2004;63:1618–23.
46. Sachdev PS, Lipnicki DM, Crawford JD, et al. Progression of cognitive impairment in stroke/TIA patients over 3 years. J Neurol Neurosurg Psychiatry 2014; 85:1324–30.
47. Levine DA, Galecki AT, Langa KM, et al. Trajectory of cognitive decline after incident stroke. JAMA 2015;314:41–51.
48. van Dijk EJ, de Leeuw FE. Recovery after stroke: more than just walking and talking again. *If you don't look for it, you won't find it* [commentary]. Eur J Neurol 2012;19:189–90.
49. Pollock A, St George B, Fenton M, et al. Top 10 research priorities relating to life after stroke - consensus from stroke survivors, caregivers, and health professionals. Int J Stroke 2014;9:313–20.
50. Radman N, Staub F, Aboulafia-Brakha T, et al. Poststroke fatigue following minor infarcts. A prospective study. Neurology 2012;79:1422–7.
51. Folstein MF, Folstein SE, McHugh PR. "Mini-Mental State". A practical method for grading the cognitive state of patients for the clinician. J Psychiatr Res 1975;12:189–98.
52. Nys GMS, van Zandvoort MJE, de Kort PLM, et al. Restrictions of the Mini-Mental State Examination in acute stroke. Arch Clin Neuropsychol 2005;20:623–9.
53. Nasreddine ZS, Phillips NA, Bédirian V, et al. The Montreal Cognitive Assessment, MoCA: a brief screening tool for mild cognitive impairment. J Am Geriatr Soc 2005;53:695–9.
54. Van Heugten CM, Walton L, Hentschel U. Can we forget the Mini-Mental State Examination? A systematic review of the validity of cognitive screening instruments within one month after stroke. Clin Rehabil 2015;29:694–704.
55. Aggarwal A, Kean E. Comparison of the Folstein Mini Mental State Examination (MMSE) to the Montreal Cognitive Assessment (MoCA) as a cognitive screening tool in an inpatient rehabilitation setting. Neurosci Med 2010;1:39–42.
56. Mark VW. Acute versus chronic functional aspects of unilateral spatial neglect. Front Biosci 2003;8:E172–89.
57. Keil K, Kaszniak AW. Examining executive function in individuals with brain injury: a review. Aphasiology 2002;16:305–35.
58. Leśniak M, Bak T, Czepiel W, et al. Frequency and prognostic value of cognitive disorders in stroke patients. Dement Geriatr Cogn Disord 2008;26: 356–63.
59. Hayes S, Donnellan C, Stokes E. Associations between executive function and physical function poststroke: a pilot study. Physiotherapy 2013;99:165–71.
60. Påhlman U, Sävborg M, Tarkowski E. Cognitive dysfunction and physical activity after stroke: the Gothenburg Cognitive Stroke Study in the elderly. J Stroke Cerebrovasc Dis 2012;21:652–8.
61. Godefroy O, Azouvi P, Robert P, et al. Dysexecutive syndrome: diagnostic criteria and validation study. Ann Neurol 2010;68:855–64.
62. Barker-Collo S, Feigin VL, Parag V, et al. Auckland Stroke Outcomes Study. Part 2: cognition and functional outcomes 5 years poststroke. Neurology 2010;75: 1608–16.
63. Ownsworth T, Shum D. Relationship between executive functions and productivity outcomes following stroke. Disabil Rehabil 2008;30:531–40.
64. Claesson L, Lindén T, Skoog I, et al. Cognitive impairment after stroke—impact on activities of daily living and costs of care for elderly people. Cerebrovasc Dis 2005;19:102–9.

65. Galski T, Bruno RL, Zorowitz R, et al. Predicting length of stay, functional outcome, and aftercare in the rehabilitation of stroke patients. The dominant role of higher-order cognition. Stroke 1993;24:1794–800.

66. Pohjasvaara T, Leskela M, Vataja R, et al. Post-stroke depression, executive dysfunction and functional outcome. Eur J Neurol 2002;9:269–75.

67. Tant MLM, Brouwer WH, Cornelissen FW, et al. Driving and visuospatial performance in people with hemianopia. Neuropsychol Rehabil 2002;12: 419–37.

68. Mok VCT, Wong A, Lam WWM, et al. Cognitive impairment and functional outcome after stroke associated with small vessel disease. J Neurol Neurosurg Psychiatry 2004;75:560–6.

69. Mark VW, Woods AJ, Mennemeier M, et al. Cognitive assessment for CI therapy in the outpatient clinic. NeuroRehabilitation 2006;21:139–46.

70. Park YH, Jang J, Park SY, et al. Executive function as a strong predictor of recovery from disability in patients with acute stroke: a preliminary study. J Stroke Cerebrovasc Dis 2015;24:554–61.

71. Zihl J. Visual scanning behavior in patients with homonymous hemianopia. Neuropsychologia 1995;33:287–303.

72. Pisella L, Berberovic N, Mattingley JB. Impaired working memory for location but not for colour or shape in visual neglect: a comparison of parietal and non-parietal lesions. Cortex 2004;40:379–90.

73. Duffau H. The "frontal syndrome" revisited: lessons from electrostimulation studies [review]. Cortex 2012;48:120–31

74. Wolfe N, Babikian VL, Linn RT, et al. Are multiple cerebral infarcts synergistic? Arch Neurol 1994;51:211–5.

75. Ruchinskas RA, Giuliano AJ. Motor perseveration in geriatric medical patients. Arch Clin Neuropsychol 2003;18:455–61.

76. Vataja R, Pohjasvaara T, Mäntylä R, et al. MRI correlates of executive dysfunction in patients with ischaemic stroke. Eur J Neurol 2003;10:625–31.

77. Zinn S, Bosworth HB, Hoenig HM, et al. Executive function deficits in acute stroke. Arch Phys Med Rehabil 2007;88:173–80.

78. Barbee A, White D. Executive dysfunction immediately post mild-stroke [abstract]. Arch Phys Med Rehabil 2012;93:E11.

79. Chung CSY, Pollock A, Campbell T, et al. Cognitive rehabilitation for executive dysfunction in adults with stroke or other adult non-progressive acquired brain damage [review]. Cochrane Database Syst Rev 2013;(4):CD008391.

80. Phillips LH. Do "frontal tests" measure executive function? Issues of assessment and evidence from fluency tests. In: Rabbitt P, editor. Methodology of frontal and executive function. Hove (United Kingdom): Psychology Press; 1997. p. 191–213.

81. Brownsett SLE, Warren JE, Geranmayeh F, et al. Cognitive control and its impact on recovery from aphasic stroke. Brain 2014;137:242–54.

82. Kopp B, Rösser N, Tabeling S, et al. Disorganized behavior on Link's cube test is sensitive to right hemispheric frontal lobe damage in stroke patients. Front Hum Neurosci 2014;8:79.

83. Lange G, Waked W, Kirshblum S, et al. Organizational strategy influence on visual memory performance after stroke: cortical/subcortical and left/right hemisphere contrasts. Arch Phys Med Rehabil 2000;81:89–94.

84. Leeds L, Meara RJ, Woods R, et al. A comparison of the new executive functioning domains of the CAMCOG-R with existing tests of executive function in elderly stroke survivors. Age Ageing 2001;30:251–4.

85. Ballard C, Rowan E, Stephens S, et al. Prospective follow-up study between 3 and 15 months after stroke. Improvements and decline in cognitive function among dementia-free stroke survivors >75 years of age. Stroke 2003;34:2440–4.
86. Stephens S, Kenny RA, Rowan E, et al. Neuropsychological characteristics of mild vascular cognitive impairment and dementia after stroke. Int J Geriatr Psychiatry 2004;19:1053–7.
87. Nys GMS, van Zandvoort MJE, de Kort PLM, et al. The prognostic value of domain-specific cognitive abilities in acute first-ever stroke. Neurology 2005; 64:821–7.
88. Hoffmann M, Schmitt F. Metacognition in stroke: bedside assessment and relation to location, size, and stroke severity. Experimental studies. Cogn Behav Neurol 2006;19:85–94.
89. Allen CM, Martin RC, Martin N. Relations between short-term memory deficits, semantic processing, and executive function. Aphasiology 2012;26:428–61.
90. Sandson J, Albert ML. Perseveration in behavioral neurology. Neurology 1987; 37:1736–41.
91. Duff Canning SJ, Leach L, Stuss D, et al. Diagnostic utility of abbreviated fluency measures in Alzheimer disease and vascular dementia. Neurology 2004;62:556–62.
92. Raymer AM. Treatment of adynamia in aphasia [review]. Front Biosci 2003;8: s845–51.
93. Sugden SG, Bourgeois JA. Modafinil monotherapy in poststroke depression. Psychosomatics 2004;45:80–1.
94. Clarac F, Barbara JG, Broussolle E, et al. Figures and institutions of the neurological sciences in Paris from 1800 to 1950. Introduction and Part I: neuroanatomy. Rev Neurol (Paris) 2012;168:2–14.
95. Kimura D, Watson N. The relation between oral movement control and speech. Brain Lang 1989;37:565–90.
96. Alexander MP, Fischette MR, Fischer RS. Crossed aphasias can be mirror image or anomalous. Brain 1989;112:953–73.
97. Hickok G, Bellugi U, Klima E. The neurobiology of sign language and its implications for the neural basis of language. Nature 1996;381:699–702.
98. Sambunaris A, Hyde TM. Stroke-related aphasias mistaken for psychotic speech: two case reports. J Geriatr Psychiatry Neurol 1994;7:144–7.
99. Knopman DS, Selnes OA, Niccum N, et al. A longitudinal study of speech fluency in aphasia: CT correlates of recovery and persistent nonfluency. Neurology 1983;33:1170–8.
100. Dickey L, Kagan A, Lindsay MP, et al. Incidence and profile of inpatient stroke-induced aphasia in Ontario, Canada. Arch Phys Med Rehabil 2010;91:196–202.
101. Maas MB, Lev MH, Ay H, et al. The prognosis for aphasia in stroke. J Stroke Cerebrovasc Dis 2012;21:350–7.
102. Tompkins CA. Rehabilitation for cognitive-communication disorders in right hemisphere brain damage [review]. Arch Phys Med Rehabil 2012;93:S61–9.
103. Beyn ES. Peculiarities of thought in patients with sensory aphasia. Lang Speech 1958;1:233–49.
104. Otsuki M, Soma Y, Yoshimura N, et al. How to improve repetition ability in patients with Wernicke's aphasia: the effect of a disguised task. J Neurol Neurosurg Psychiatry 2005;76:733–5.
105. Pedersen PM, Vinter K, Olsen TS. Aphasia after stroke: type, severity and prognosis. The Copenhagen Aphasia Study. Cerebrovasc Dis 2004;17: 35–43.

106. Weylman ST, Brownell HH, Gardner H. "It's what you mean, not what you say": pragmatic language use in brain-damaged patients. Res Publ Assoc Res Nerv Ment Dis 1988;66:229–43.
107. Barrett AM, Crucian GP, Raymer AM, et al. Spared comprehension of emotional prosody in a patient with global aphasia. Neuropsychiatry Neuropsychol Behav Neurol 1999;12:117–20.
108. van der Meulen I, van de Sandt-Koenderman ME, Ribbers GM. Melodic Intonation Therapy: present controversies and future opportunities [review]. Arch Phys Med Rehabil 2012;93:S46–52.
109. Allen L, Mehta S, McClure JA, et al. Therapeutic interventions for aphasia initiated more than six months post stroke: a review of the evidence. Top Stroke Rehabil 2012;19:523–35.
110. Elsner B, Kugler J, Pohl M, et al. Transcranial direct current stimulation (tDCS) for improving aphasia in patients with aphasia after stroke [review]. Cochrane Database Syst Rev 2015;(5):CD009760.
111. Meinzer M, Rodriguez AD, Gonzalez Rothi LJ. First decade of research on constrained-induced treatment approaches for aphasia rehabilitation [review]. Arch Phys Med Rehabil 2012;93:S35–45.
112. Johnson ML, Taub E, Harper LH, et al. An enhanced protocol for CI Aphasia Therapy: CIAT II—a case series. Am J Speech Lang Pathol 2014;23: 60–72.
113. Gorelick PB, Ross ED. The aprosodias: further functional-anatomical evidence for the organisation of affective language in the right hemisphere. J Neurol Neurosurg Psychiatry 1987;50:553–60.
114. Bryan KL. Language prosody and the right hemisphere. Aphasiology 1989;3: 285–99.
115. Van Lancker D, Sidtis JJ. The identification of affective-prosodic stimuli by left- and right-hemisphere-damaged subjects: all errors are not created equal. J Speech Hear Res 1992;35:963–70.
116. Alvarez G, Araya F, Verdugo R, et al. Prosody, socioeconomic level, and the right hemisphere [letter]. Arch Neurol 1989;46:480.
117. Knollman-Porter K. Acquired apraxia of speech: a review. Top Stroke Rehabil 2008;15:484–93.
118. Goodwin J, Kansu T. Vulpian's sign: conjugate eye deviation in acute cerebral hemisphere lesions. Neurology 1986;36:711–2.
119. Ostrow LW, Llinás RH. Eastchester clapping sign: a novel test of parietal neglect. Ann Neurol 2009;66:114–7.
120. Butter CM, Kirsch NL, Reeves G. The effect of lateralized dynamic stimuli on unilateral spatial neglect following right hemisphere lesions. Restor Neurol Neurosci 1990;2:39–46.
121. Starkstein SE, Fedoroff JP, Price TR, et al. Anosognosia in patients with cerebrovascular lesions. A study of causative factors. Stroke 1992;23:1446–53.
122. Bisiach E, Luzzatti C. Unilateral neglect of representational space. Cortex 1978; 14:129–33.
123. Lindell AB, Jalas JM, Tenovuo O, et al. Clinical assessment of hemispatial neglect: evaluation of different measures and dimensions. Clin Neuropsychol 2007;21:479–97.
124. Kinsella G, Ford B. Hemi-inattention and the recovery patterns of stroke patients. Int Rehabil Med 1985;7:102–6.
125. Punt TD, Riddoch MJ. Motor neglect: implications for movement and rehabilitation following stroke. Disabil Rehabil 2006;28:857–64.

126. Stone SP, Halligan PW, Greenwood RJ. The incidence of neglect phenomena and related disorders in patients with an acute right or left hemisphere stroke. Age Ageing 1993;22:46–52.
127. Aimola L, Schindler I, Simone AM. Near and far space neglect: task sensitivity and anatomical substrates. Neuropsychologia 2012;50:1115–23.
128. Shelton PA, Bowers D, Heilman KM. Peripersonal and vertical neglect. Brain 1990;113:191–205.
129. Mark VW, Heilman KM. Diagonal spatial neglect. J Neurol Neurosurg Psychiatry 1998;65:348–52.
130. Gottesman RF, Kleinman JT, Davis C, et al. Unilateral neglect is more severe and common in older patients with right hemispheric stroke. Neurology 2008;71:1439–44.
131. Cassidy TP, Lewis S, Gray CS. Recovery from visuospatial neglect in stroke patients. J Neurol Neurosurg Psychiatry 1998;64:555–7.
132. Luukkainen-Markkula R, Tarkka IM, Pitkänen K, et al. Comparison of the behavioural inattention test and the Catherine Bergego Scale in assessment of hemispatial neglect. Neuropsychol Rehabil 2011;21:103–16.
133. Hayes A, Chen CS, Clarke G, et al. Functional improvements following the use of the NVT Vision Rehabilitation program for patients with hemianopia following stroke. Neurorehabilitation 2012;31:19–30.
134. Vangkilde S, Habekost T. Finding Wally: prism adaptation improves visual search in chronic neglect. Neuropsychologia 2010;48:1994–2004.
135. Cantagallo A, Della Sala S. Preserved insight in an artist with extrapersonal spatial neglect. Cortex 1998;34:163–89.
136. Robertson IH. Do we need the "lateral" in unilateral neglect? Spatially nonselective attention deficits in unilateral neglect and their implications for rehabilitation. Neuroimage 2001;14:S85–90.
137. Campbell DC, Oxbury JM. Recovery from unilateral visuo-spatial neglect? Cortex 1976;12:303–12.
138. Hoffmann M. Higher cortical functions after stroke: an analysis of 1000 patients from a dedicated cognitive stroke registry. Neurorehabil Neural Repair 2001;15:113–27.
139. Rebok GW, Ball K, Guey LT, et al. Ten-year effects of the advanced cognitive training for independent and vital elderly cognitive training trial on cognition and everyday functioning in older adults. J Am Geriatr Soc 2014;62:16–24.
140. Bogousslavsky J. William Feinberg Lecture 2002: emotions, mood, and behavior after stroke [review]. Stroke 2003;34:1046–50.
141. Carota A, Rossetti A, Karapanayiotides T, et al. Catastrophic reaction in acute stroke: a reflex behavior in aphasic patients. Neurology 2001;57:1902–5.
142. Ross ED. Acute agitation and other behaviors associated with Wernicke aphasia and their possible neurological bases. Neuropsychiatry Neuropsychol Behav Neurol 1993;6:9–18.
143. Ross ED, Homan RW, Buck R. Differential hemispheric lateralization of primary and social emotions: implications for developing a comprehensive neurology for emotions, repression, and the subconscious. Neuropsychiatry Neuropsychol Behav Neurol 1994;7:1–19.
144. Robinson RG, Szetela B. Mood change following left hemisphere brain injury. Ann Neurol 1981;9:447–53.
145. Schwartz JA, Speed NM, Brunberg JA, et al. Depression in stroke rehabilitation. Biol Psychiatry 1993;33:694–9.

146. Eriksson M, Glader EL, Norrving B, et al. Poststroke suicide attempts and completed suicides: a socioeconomic and nationwide perspective. Neurology 2015;84:1732–8.

147. Pustokhanova L, Morozova E. Cognitive impairment and hypothymia in post stroke patients. J Neurol Sci 2013;325:43–5.

148. Robinson RG, Bolla-Wilson K, Kaplan E, et al. Depression influences intellectual impairment in stroke patients. Br J Psychiatry 1986;148:541–7.

149. Chemerinski E, Robinson RG, Kosier JT. Improved recovery in activities of daily living associated with remission of poststroke depression. Stroke 2001;32: 113–7.

150. Dennis M, O'Rourke S, Lewis S, et al. Emotional outcomes after stroke: factors associated with poor outcome. J Neurol Neurosurg Psychiatry 2000;68: 47–52.

151. Robinson RG, Benson DF. Depression in aphasic patients: frequency, severity, and clinical-pathological correlations. Brain Lang 1981;14:282–91.

152. Sinyor D, Jacques P, Kaloupek DG, et al. Poststroke depression and lesion location. An attempted replication. Brain 1986;109:537–46.

153. Turner-Stokes L, Hassan N. Depression after stroke: a review of the evidence base to inform the development of an integrated care pathway. Part 1: diagnosis, frequency and impact. Clin Rehabil 2002;16:231–47.

154. Watkins C, Daniels L, Jack C, et al. Accuracy of a single question in screening for depression in a cohort of patients after stroke: comparative study. BMJ 2001; 323:1159.

155. Starkstein SE, Mizrahi R, Power BD. Antidepressant therapy in post-stroke depression [review]. Expert Opin Pharmacother 2008;9:1291–8.

156. Choi-Kwon S, Kim JS. Poststroke fatigue: an emerging, critical issue in stroke medicine. Int J Stroke 2011;6:328–36.

157. Brooks BR, Crumpacker D, Fellus J, et al. PRISM: a novel research tool to assess the prevalence of pseudobulbar affect symptoms across neurological conditions. PLoS One 2013;8:e72232.

158. Schoedel KA, Morrow SA, Sellers EM. Evaluating the safety and efficacy of dextromethorphan/quinidine in the treatment of pseudobulbar affect [review]. Neuropsychiatr Dis Treat 2014;10:1161–74.

159. Fisher CM. Neurologic fragments. I. Clinical observations in demented patients. Neurology 1988;38:1868–73.

160. Pearce JMS. Misoplegia [review]. Eur Neurol 2007;57:62–4.

161. Jorge RE, Starkstein SE, Robinson RG. Apathy following stroke [review]. Can J Psychiatry 2010;55:350–4.

162. Starkstein SE, Fedoroff JP, Price TR, et al. Apathy following cerebrovascular lesions. Stroke 1993;24:1625–30.

163. Tang WK, Caeiro L, Lau CG, et al. Apathy and suicide-related ideation 3 months after stroke: a cross-sectional study. BMC Neurol 2015;15:60.

164. Skidmore ER, Whyte EM, Butters MA, et al. Strategy training during inpatient rehabilitation may prevent apathy symptoms after acute stroke. PM R 2015;7: 562–70.

165. Hillis AE. Inability to empathize: brain lesions that disrupt sharing and understanding another's emotions [review]. Brain 2014;137:981–97.

166. Eslinger PJ, Parkinson K, Shamay SG. Empathy and social-emotional factors in recovery from stroke [review]. Curr Opin Neurol 2002;15:91–7.

167. Taub E, Uswatte G, Mark VW, et al. The learned nonuse phenomenon: implications for rehabilitation [review]. Eura Medicophys 2006;42:241–55.

168. Uswatte G, Taub E, Morris D, et al. The motor activity log-28: assessing daily use of the hemiparetic arm after stroke. Neurology 2006;67:1189–94.
169. Taub E, Miller NE, Novack TA, et al. Technique to improve chronic motor deficit after stroke. Arch Phys Med Rehabil 1993;74:347–54.
170. Langhorne P, Coupar F, Pollock A. Motor recovery after stroke: a systematic review. Lancet Neurol 2009;8:741–54.
171. Jackson JH. Notes on the physiology and pathology of language. Med Times Gaz 1866;i:659.
172. Jackson JH. Remarks on non-protrusion of the tongue in some cases of aphasia. Lancet 1878;i:716.
173. Foix C, Chavany JA, Marie J. Diplégie facio-linguomasticatrice d'origine cortico sous-corticale sans paralysie des membres (contribution à l'étude de la localisation des centres de la face du membre supérieur), par MM. Rev Neurol (Paris) 1926;33:214–9.
174. Mao CC, Coull BM, Golper LA, et al. Anterior opercular syndrome. Neurology 1989;39:1169–72.
175. Bakar M, Kirshner HS, Niaz F. The opercular-subopercular syndrome: four cases with review of the literature. Behav Neurol 1998;11:97–103.
176. Mark VW, Heilman KM, Watson RT. Motor neglect: what do we mean? [letter]. Neurology 1996;46:1492–3.
177. Gold M, Adair JC, Jacobs DH, et al. Anosognosia for hemiplegia: an electrophysiologic investigation of the feed-forward hypothesis. Neurology 1994;44:1804–8.
178. Stone J, LaFrance WC, Brown R, et al. Conversion disorder: current problems and potential solutions for DSM-5. J Psychosom Res 2011;71:369–76.
179. Chou HY, Weng MC, Huang MH, et al. Conversion disorder in stroke: a case report. Kaohsiung J Med Sci 2006;22:586–9.
180. Nielsen G, Stone J, Matthews A, et al. Physiotherapy for functional motor disorders: a consensus recommendation. J Neurol Neurosurg Psychiatry 2015;86:1113–9.
181. Ambrosoni E, Sala SD, Motto C, et al. Gesture imitation with lower limbs following left hemisphere stroke. Arch Clin Neuropsychol 2006;21:349–58.
182. Pedersen PM, Jørgensen HS, Kammersgaard LP, et al. Manual and oral apraxia in acute stroke, frequency and influence on functional outcome. The Copenhagen Stroke Study. Am J Phys Med Rehabil 2001;80:685–92.
183. Dovern A, Fink GR, Weiss PH. Diagnosis and treatment of upper limb apraxia [review]. J Neurol 2012;259:1269–83.
184. Cantagallo A, Maini M, Rumiati RI. The cognitive rehabilitation of limb apraxia in patients with stroke [review]. Neuropsychol Rehabil 2012;22:473–88.
185. Rapcsak SZ, Ochipa C, Beeson PM, et al. Praxis and the right hemisphere. Brain Cogn 1993;23:181–202.
186. De Renzi E, Motti F, Nichelli P. Imitating gestures. A quantitative approach to ideomotor apraxia. Arch Neurol 1980;37:6–10.
187. Leiguarda R. Apraxias as traditionally defined. In: Freund HJ, Jeannerod M, Hallet M, et al, editors. Higher-order motor disorders. New York: Oxford University Press; 2005. p. 303–38.
188. Hayakawa Y, Yamadori A, Fujii T, et al. Apraxia of single tool use. Eur J Neurol 2000;43:76–81.
189. Della Sala S, Marchetti C, Spinnler H. Right-sided anarchic (alien) hand: a longitudinal study. Neuropsychologia 1991;29:1113–27.
190. Shereef H, Cavanna AE. The "brother's arm:" alien hand syndrome after right posterior parietal lesion [letter]. J Neuropsychiatry Clin Neurosci 2013;25(4):E02.

191. Feinberg TE, Schindler RJ, Flanagan NG, et al. Two alien hand syndromes. Neurology 1992;42:19–24.
192. Yuan JL, Wang SK, Guo XJ, et al. Acute infarct of the corpus callosum presenting as alien hand syndrome: evidence of diffusion weighted imaging and magnetic resonance angiography. BMC Neurol 2011;11:142.
193. Nishikawa T, Okuda J, Mizuta I, et al. Conflict of intentions due to callosal disconnection. J Neurol Neurosurg Psychiatry 2001;71:462–71.
194. Hoffmann M, Schmitt F, Bromley E. Comprehensive cognitive neurological assessment in stroke. Acta Neurol Scand 2009;119:162–71.
195. Kerkhoff G, Münßinger U, Meier EK. Neurovisual rehabilitation in cerebral blindness. Arch Neurol 1994;51:474–81.
196. De Renzi E, Faglioni P, Scotti G, et al. Impairment in associating colour to form, concomitant with aphasia. Brain 1972;95:293–304.
197. Cleland PG, Saunders M, Rosser R. An unusual case of visual perseveration. J Neurol Neurosurg Psychiatry 1981;44:262–3.
198. Pallis CA. Impaired identification of faces and places with agnosia for colours. J Neurol Neurosurg Psychiatry 1955;18:218–24.
199. Starrfelt R, Ólafsdóttir RR, Arendt IM. Rehabilitation of pure alexia: a review. Neuropsychol Rehabil 2013;23:755–79.
200. Cousins R. Prosopagnosia after stroke: potentials for impairment and treatment. Top Stroke Rehabil 2013;20:471–7 [review].
201. Van Lancker DR, Cummings JL, Kreiman J, et al. Phonagnosia: a dissociation between familiar and unfamiliar voices. Cortex 1988;24:195–209.

Cognitive and Psychiatric Disturbances in Parkinsonian Syndromes

Richard M. Zweig, MD*, Elizabeth A. Disbrow, PhD,
Vijayakumar Javalkar, PhD

KEYWORDS

- Parkinson • Dementia with Lewy Bodies (DLB) • Parkinsonian
- Progressive Supranuclear Palsy (PSP) • Multiple System Atrophy (MSA)
- Corticobasal degeneration (CBD)

KEY POINTS

- Executive dysfunction is often measurable in newly diagnosed Parkinson's disease.
- Treatment with dopaminergic medications, particularly dopamine agonists, has been associated with hallucinations and impulse control disorder.
- While sharing many pathological features with Alzheimer's disease, distinguishing clinical features of Dementia with Lewy bodies include episodic fluctuations of cognition, early hallucinations, and REM behavior disorder symptoms.
- Quetiapine appears to be effective for hallucinating patients, without worsening parkinsonism at lower dosages. Clozapine is also effective. The promising 5-HT2A inverse agonist pimavanserin is awaiting FDA approval.
- The neuropsychiatric profile of progressive supranuclear palsy may closely resemble that of the frontotemporal lobar degenerations.

INTRODUCTION

As is the case with all of the neurodegenerative disorders, the subset comprising the parkinsonian syndromes of Parkinson disease, dementia with Lewy bodies, progressive supranuclear palsy (PSP), corticobasal degeneration (CBD), and multiple system atrophy (MSA) are considered proteinopathies. In these disorders, disease-associated proteins accumulate in the wrong cellular or extracellular compartments, and are often

The authors have nothing to disclose.
Department of Neurology, Louisiana State University Health Sciences Center - Shreveport, 1501 King's Highway, Shreveport, LA 71103, USA
* Corresponding author.
E-mail address: rzweig@lsuhsc.edu

Neurol Clin 34 (2016) 235–246
http://dx.doi.org/10.1016/j.ncl.2015.08.010 **neurologic.theclinics.com**
0733-8619/16/$ – see front matter © 2016 Elsevier Inc. All rights reserved.

glycosylated, phosphorylated, ubiquinated, and misfolded, initiating or otherwise contributing to neuronal dysfunction and death. Moreover, misfolded proteins likely spread to other neuronal populations that are neighboring or networked, acting as prion-like templates corrupting native proteins, resulting in specific patterns of neuronal cell loss, with gliosis and atrophy.[1]

Patients with these syndromes also share certain clinical signs including akinesia/bradykinesia and rigidity, which are the hallmark clinical consequences of pathologic involvement of dopaminergic neurons of the substantia nigra pars compacta. These cells normally fire regularly, in pacemaker-like fashion, releasing dopamine in the striatum. Released dopamine is quickly taken back up by the presynaptic terminal through the dopamine transporter and stored in presynaptic vesicles, thus allowing for tight regulation of extracellular, synaptic dopamine. Based on the well-established direct/indirect pathway model of basal ganglia function,[2] this dopaminergic tone is necessary for the proper gain setting of this system, facilitating desired movement, without excessive inhibition of movement or excessive, unwanted movements.

During movement, neurons in normal basal ganglia modulate activity to specific parameters including velocity, direction selectivity, force, amplitude, and active versus passive movement,[3] and are organized somatotopically.[4] These patterns of specific movement-related modulation of activity have been described at multiple subcortical levels (for review, see Ref.[5]). In Parkinson disease, this level of specificity is lost, and inhibitory output from basal ganglia to thalamocortical circuitry seems to be increased. Thus, electrophysiologic recording data from humans and MPTP nonhuman primate animal models indicate that the relative number of pallidal cells showing movement-related activity is increased,[6] and the ratio of inhibited to activated cells in this basal ganglia outflow nucleus drops from 0.22 to 0.03.[7] Furthermore, somatotopy breaks down with an increase in kinesthetic cells responding to multiple joints or body parts and ipsilateral (in addition to contralateral) limbs.[4,8] Moreover, direct recording from the motor cortex of Parkinson disease patients undergoing deep brain stimulation therapy has demonstrated neuronal population spiking that is excessively synchronized to oscillations of subcortical basal ganglionic networks, which is reversed with successful deep brain stimulation.[9]

In 1923, the pathologist Fredrick Lewy described the characteristic target-shaped cytoplasmic inclusions found in dopaminergic and other neuronal populations affected in Parkinson disease. Following the identification of mutations in the gene encoding the protein α-synuclein in a small number of families with this disease[10] it was soon discovered that this protein is a component of Lewy bodies.[11] Thus, the distribution of these inclusions (and α-synuclein-containing Lewy neurites) could be determined using antibodies raised against this protein. Although the direct contribution of Lewy body inclusions is unclear, these inclusions occur preferentially in brain regions with neuronal dysfunction/death and atrophy. In 2004, using α-synuclein immunocytochemistry in an autopsy series of brains from individuals with Parkinson disease and clinically normal control subjects, Braak and colleagues[12] described six stages of Lewy inclusions. The first three stages were considered presymptomatic, with pathology confined to olfactory bulb/nucleus and lower brainstem, and (in stage 3) inadequate nigral pathology to result in motor symptoms. At the other end of the spectrum, Lewy inclusions were found in the amygdala as early as stage 4, and then in neocortex in the higher Braak stages of disease. However, the course of disease varies widely among patients.

This article discusses aspects of cognitive and psychiatric disturbances in patients with mild/early Parkinson disease without dementia. This is followed by a discussion of dementia in Parkinson disease: its anatomic/pathologic basis, relationship to dementia with Lewy bodies and to Alzheimer disease, and available treatments of resultant symptomatology. Finally, cognitive and psychiatric disturbances in the other parkinsonian syndromes are discussed.

COGNITIVE AND PSYCHIATRIC DISTURBANCES IN PATIENTS WITH MILD/EARLY PARKINSON DISEASE WITHOUT DEMENTIA

In recent years, there has been considerable study of nonmotor symptoms in patients with mild Parkinson disease, including retrospective review of these symptoms before onset of motor symptoms, presumably reflecting stages 1 to 3, and other early pathology.[13] Thus, many patients report difficulty with sense of smell and/or rapid eye movement (REM) behavior disorder symptoms while sleeping, starting years before onset of motor symptoms, presumably reflecting olfactory bulb and lower brainstem Lewy-related pathology. Likewise, early constipation presumably reflects Lewy-related pathology in the intestines.[14] A recent study[15] has suggested that the well-known negative relationship between cigarette smoking and risk of Parkinson disease may reflect a greater ease of quitting smoking than normal in presymptomatic patients, rather than a neuroprotective effect of nicotine or other ingredients in tobacco smoke. Whether this behavioral consequence, if verified, reflects early dopaminergic pathology or pathology elsewhere is unclear.

Although estimates vary, the prevalence of cognitive impairment in newly diagnosed Parkinson disease approximates 55%.[16] Affected domains include executive functions, such as memory, cognitive flexibility, and planning, and processing speed, verbal fluency, and visuospatial processing (for review see Ref.[17]). For example, task switching, or the ability to modify a plan because of evolving environmental conditions, has been shown to be impaired in Parkinson disease.[18–20] Patients with this disease show deficits on standard neuropsychological tests with a large task switching component, such as the Wisconsin Card Sort Test.[21,22] Nondeclarative, or procedural memory has also been associated with basal ganglia function, which is in contrast to declarative memory that is subserved by the hippocampus. There seems to be a relationship between cognitive and motor deficits in Parkinson disease. Producing a movement is a complex interplay between cognitive factors, such as flexibility and planning, and motor execution, and both are impaired in Parkinson disease. Cognitive (bradyphrenia) and motor (bradykinesia) slowing, and cognitive and motor inflexibility and perseveration are noted.[17]

The pathophysiology underlying parkinsonian executive dysfunction is not fully understood. However, basal ganglia dysfunction has a far reaching impact because of dense connectivity with the thalamus and cortex. In fact, anatomically segregated basal ganglia–thalamocortical circuits have been described in nonhuman primates that subserve specific functions based on cortical targets.[2,23] Thus, disruption of the motor circuit underlies motor deficits. In contrast, disruption of the executive control network with cortical targets in prefrontal cortex results in executive dysfunction, and parkinsonian cognitive deficits have been described as frontoexecutive.[17] Like motor dysfunction, executive dysfunction is reportedly dopamine responsive in Parkinson disease.[22] These include spatial working memory, planning, processing speed, and switching, which have been demonstrated to improve with dopamine replacement therapy.[22,24]

Dopaminergic nigral neurons projecting to the putamen are preferentially lost in Parkinson disease, with relative sparing of neurons projecting to the caudate. This is readily demonstrated using dopamine transporter radioimaging.[25] Yet in Parkinson disease and in the other parkinsonian syndromes, caudate projecting neurons are involved with disease progression. Other dopaminergic neuronal populations, such as the neighboring ventral tegmental area, are less consistently affected by the disease processes. Involvement of these "extra" putamenal projections may contribute to some of these cognitive disturbances, and to psychiatric comorbidities discussed later.

Parkinson disease has classically been staged clinically on the one-dimensional, five-level, Hoehn and Yahr scale,[26] where the higher scores mostly reflect increasing immobility, irrespective of presence or severity of cognitive impairment. A more comprehensive way of staging Parkinson disease might include two axes, one reflecting severity, with the other axis reflecting how widely distributed is the disease process (**Fig. 1**).

Thus, a typical patient with onset in the late 40s or 50s, presenting with levodopa-responsive asymmetrical resting tremor and perhaps micrographia, but few additional symptoms, would have mild, focal disease. Over the years, if this patient developed increasing levodopa-responsive motor symptoms, but also "wearing off" of levodopa benefit between dosages (sometimes with unpredictable response or rapid wearing off) and levodopa-induced dyskinesias, but without significant cognitive disturbances, he or she would have severe, focal disease. Pathology would likely be severe Braak Stage 4 disease.

Although by this scenario the patient would not have dementia, he or she might have one or more psychiatric/behavioral disturbances related either to the underlying disease state or side effects of medications used. These include depression, with or without anxiety, and possibly resulting from or worsened by a disturbance of sleep and/or daytime sleepiness. Psychiatric comorbidities, such as depression, anxiety, and apathy, are difficult to identify in Parkinson disease because of symptomatic overlap with the associated movement disorder (for review, see Ref.[27]), thus it is not surprising that estimates of prevalence vary wildly. A large study by Aarsland and colleagues[28] evaluated neuropsychiatric symptoms in 537 Parkinson disease patients. They reported depression in 58%, apathy in 54%, anxiety (sometimes with associated internal tremor) in 49%, and hallucinations in 44% of participants. A community-based prospective study noted that of 137 individuals with Parkinson disease, 60% developed hallucinations or delusions by the end of the 12-year study (many also with dementia).[29]

Treatment with dopaminergic medicates, and in particular dopamine agonists, has been associated with hallucinations.[30] Although more common in patients with frank dementia, visual hallucinations can occur as a complication of dopamine agonist use in otherwise cognitively intact patients, particularly at higher dosages. These may be fleeting, and are sometimes described as "off the corner of the eye," just out of view. Other patients may have recurrent, vivid, visual hallucinations, which may or may not

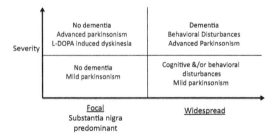

Fig. 1. The spectra of Parkinson disease and dementia with Lewy bodies. L-DOPA, levodopa.

be troublesome to the patient or family. These typically subside with reduction of dopamine agonist dosage. In addition, treatment with dopamine agonists can result in the development of impulse control disorders (ie, compulsive behaviors) that can be problematic.[31] This has also been described with the drug amantadine.[32] These can occur at any dosage of medication, sometimes improving with dosage reduction, but not always. Common compulsive behaviors include compulsive gambling, shopping, and compulsive interest in sex. It is imperative that these complications be screened for regularly during office visits, and their absence be corroborated if possible by the patient's spouse or others accompanying the patient.

DEMENTIA IN PARKINSON DISEASE AND DEMENTIA WITH LEWY BODIES

When clear cognitive impairment begins within 1 year after the onset of parkinsonian motor symptoms, or precedes the onset of motor symptoms, the diagnosis of dementia with Lewy bodies is used rather than Parkinson disease.[33] This distinction between Parkinson disease (with later-onset dementia) and dementia with Lewy bodies is arbitrary, but useful clinically (eg, dopamine agonists should be used with great caution, or not at all, in patients with dementia with Lewy bodies). Nevertheless, with few exceptions, autopsy series have failed to distinguish pathologically patients with dementia with Lewy bodies from Parkinson disease patients with dementia early in the course of disease.[34]

A major determinant of early widespread Lewy body deposition, and early dementia, seems to be presence of Alzheimer disease–related pathology: amyloid plaques and tau-containing neurofibrillary tangles. For example, of 87 patents coming to autopsy from the prospective Sydney Multicenter Study of Parkinson disease,[35] 83% of those meeting clinical criteria for dementia with Lewy bodies and 80% of patients with Parkinson disease with dementia dying within 10 years of disease onset had significant amyloid plaque formation. Patients with dementia living longer than 10 years had an increasingly lower percentage with amyloid plaques. By contrast, none of the patients with Parkinson disease dying within 15 years of disease onset and without dementia had amyloid plaque formation. In another study of 56 pathologically confirmed Parkinson disease cases,[36] including 29 who had developed dementia, a combination of cortical Lewy body score, amyloid plaque burden, and Braak Alzheimer tau stage[37] was better than any of the individual measures in predicting presence of dementia. However, of the three measures, higher Braak tau stages correlated best with severity of dementia within the last year of life (as is also seen with Alzheimer disease). Of note, amyloid scores and age at death were tightly correlated, and both predicted a faster progression to dementia, whereas carriers of the Alzheimer disease genetic risk factor APOE-4 also had higher amyloid scores. Thus, it seems that older age, presence of APOE-4 gene, and/or other factors result in amyloid plaque deposition that, in turn, accelerates cortical Lewy body and tau pathology, linking dementia with Lewy bodies and Parkinson disease dementia (particularly early in the course) with Alzheimer disease.

Despite the pathologic link between dementia with Lewy bodies and Parkinson disease with dementia (especially early in the course) on the one hand, and Alzheimer disease on the other hand, there are clinical distinctions between these conditions. A "core" clinical feature of Dementia with Lewy Bodies is episodic fluctuations of cognition or clouding of consciousness, sometimes resembling delirium. Though this sign can be quite alarming to family and physicians, it has been difficult to define formally or measure. Another core feature, visual (and less often, other) hallucinations, tends to occur early in the course of dementia with Lewy bodies, often before the start of dopaminergic medications, which can worsen this symptom. In an autopsy series of patients with dementia with Lewy bodies and Parkinson disease with and without dementia,[38] dementia with Lewy body cases had highest Lewy body densities in the parahippocampal gyrus, amygdala, and particularly in the inferior temporal cortex, which was also associated with the presence of well-formed visual hallucinations early in the course of disease. Of note, no pathologic correlates of fluctuating cognition were found. In another study of Parkinson disease patients that included a large autopsy series, hallucinations typically occurring late in the course of disease were also associated with temporal lobe Lewy body deposition, and Lewy bodies in the middle frontal and anterior cingulate gyri.[39] However, in a more recent MRI study controlling for dementia, hallucinations were associated with cortical atrophy in visual perceptual pathways rather than mesial temporal lobe.[40] Clinical correlates of presence of hallucinations, in addition to cognitive impairment, included sleep disorders (including REM behavior disorder and excessive daytime sleepiness), depression, higher age at disease onset, and duration of disease (for review, see Ref.[41]).

Although not originally considered a core feature of dementia with Lewy bodies, REM behavior disorder is a common, distinguishing feature of the α-synucleinopathies, including MSA, and in Parkinson disease, is a marker for earlier onset of dementia.[42] Other nighttime sleep disturbances occur commonly in Parkinson disease including restless leg syndrome, obstructive sleep apnea, and insomnia. Other patients have motor "wearing off" during the night, associated with difficulty turning and sometimes with pain, including from dystonic posturing (often in the more symptomatic foot). Patients often have low back pain and urinary frequency at night, aggravating the sleep disturbance. Daytime sleepiness is also very common, sometimes caused by or aggravated by medications (dopamine agonists in particular, but also levodopa in some patients). Sudden, narcolepsy-like sleepiness may occur, and may be particularly problematic in patients still driving.[43]

As in Alzheimer disease, there is a profound cholinergic deficit in dementia with Lewy bodies and in Parkinson disease with dementia, even in patients with minimal Alzheimer-related pathology.[44] Treatment with cholinesterase inhibitors has been shown to be efficacious in these patients, with best evidence for rivastigmine.[45] However, the effect seems to be modest and some of the potential side effects are particularly problematic in this group of patients. These include gastrointestinal (diarrhea, weight loss); sleep disturbances including daytime sleepiness; increased drooling; and worsening of parkinsonian motor symptoms, including tremor. There is also some evidence for benefit from the N-methyl-D-aspartate receptor antagonist memantine[45]; however, the potential side effect of confusional episodes may mimic the episodic fluctuations of cognition from the disease state.

Treatment of hallucinations in Parkinson disease with dementia and in dementia with Lewy bodies can be challenging, particularly because most neuroleptics, including so-called "atypical" neuroleptics, greatly worsen parkinsonism in these patients. Although sometimes relatively benign (with insight and/or where the patient can be easily redirected), hallucinations are often problematic, particularly if the patient becomes delusional and agitated. Psychotic symptoms in Parkinson patients often contribute to nursing home placement.[46] The first steps in management include screening for underlying stressors, such as medical illness (including dehydration and infection), worsening depression or anxiety, worse sleep, or others. Parkinson and other medications must be reviewed: the dosage of dopamine agonist should be reduced or the medication should be stopped, with increase in levodopa dosage as needed for control of parkinsonian symptoms. Elimination of amantadine and probably monoamine oxidase-B inhibitors should be considered. Anticholinergics, including quaternary formulations, which are less likely to cross the blood-brain barrier, can cause or worsen hallucinations, and should be eliminated if possible. Although often helping sleep, benzodiazepines can also trigger hallucinations in some vulnerable patients.

The usual first-line atypical neuroleptic used in this group of patients is quetiapine, which seems to be effective in many patients, even at a low dosage (although there is no class 1 or 2 evidence of efficacy available). In an open label series of Parkinson patients with hallucinations, the average dosage used was 54 mg nightly,[47] with a typical range from 12.5 nightly to, in some patients, well over 100 mg daily in divided dosages. This medication typically worsens parkinsonism only to a small degree, and only at higher dosages. Clozapine is also effective in many patients, and does not worsen parkinsonism.[48] However, the requirement for frequent white blood count assessments (including weekly for the first 6 months), has undoubtedly dampened use of this medication. In addition, both of these medications (and other neuroleptics) can be oversedating. The 5-HT2A receptor inverse agonist pimavanserin is currently awaiting Food and Drug Administration approval for Parkinson disease psychosis, and should be a welcome addition when it is available. In clinical trials, this medication effectively reduced psychotic symptoms, and improved nighttime sleep, without daytime sedation.[49]

Various selective serotonin reuptake inhibitor or serotonin-norepinephrine reuptake inhibitor antidepressants have also been shown to be beneficial for depression, which occurs commonly in Parkinson disease, with class 1 evidence for patients without dementia.[50] Benefit for depression and other nonmotor symptoms may be enhanced when treatment also includes the monoamine oxidase-B inhibitor rasagiline.[51] There is also evidence that aerobic exercise may improve not only motor function, but additionally mood and executive control in Parkinson disease,[52] reflecting the neuroplasticity of basal ganglia circuitry.[53]

NEUROPSYCHIATRIC MANIFESTATIONS IN MULTIPLE SYSTEM ATROPHY, PROGRESSIVE SUPRANUCLEAR PALSY, AND CORTICOBASAL DEGENERATION

Cognitive impairment, and in particular executive dysfunction, occurs in patients with the other α-synucleinopathy, MSA. These patients can also have some impairment of memory and spatial skills.[54] This may occur early in the course of disease. In one study, about 22% of patients with early stages of MSA had cognitive impairment.[55] The type of cognitive impairment may vary between the types of MSA. In one study,[56] patients with a parkinsonian presentation (ie, MSA-P) showed involvement of visuospatial, constructional, verbal fluency, and executive skills, whereas those with a cerebellar presentation (ie, MSA-C) demonstrated visuospatial and constructional dysfunction only. The same study also showed that patients with MSA-P have more severe and widespread problems with cognitive dysfunction than patients with MSA-C. The cognitive deficits in MSA may correlate with frontal atrophy and duration of the disease.[57] The pathologic basis of cognitive impairment in this disease is not clear. In one report there was no difference in the severity of MSA-related pathologic finds (eg, glial and neuronal cytoplasmic inclusions) in patients with, versus those without, cognitive impairment.[58] However, another study noted that in patients with MSA, cortical thickness was reduced in the same areas as observed in Alzheimer disease and in Parkinson disease with dementia.[59] Similarly, a PET study showed reduced glucose metabolism in frontal, temporal, and parietal cortices in patients with MSA.[60]

Patients with MSA can have anxiety and depression in addition to executive dysfunction. The severity of anxiety and depression may differ between the two subtypes of MSA. In one study, patients with MSA-P reported abnormally increased levels of depression and anxiety, whereas patients with MSA-C reported higher anxiety levels than healthy adults. The authors correlated this with reduced executive regulation, abstract reasoning, and episodic learning.[61] Other behavioral changes reported in patients with MSA include emotional incontinence, panic attacks, and suicidal ideation.[62]

PSP and CBD are two of a family of tauopathies that also includes tau variants of the frontotemporal lobar degenerations (FTD). In patients with PSP, cognitive slowing, executive impairments, and inefficient memory recall have been identified in most patients.[63,64] The neuropsychiatric profile may closely resemble that of FTD.[63,65] For example, the prevalence of antisocial behavior in PSP may be comparable with those with FTD.[65] The pattern of cortical atrophy may also be similar between PSP and the behavior variant of FTD (bvFTD), with decrease in gray matter volume in widespread frontal areas and in the temporal uncus in bvFTD, and decrease in the frontal and temporal lobes and in the thalamus (and brainstem) in PSP.[66] Other neuropsychiatric manifestations observed in PSP include apathy and disinhibition.[67] Apathy has been associated in PSP with executive dysfunction.[68] Depression also occurs commonly in patients with this disease.[69] Patients with PSP may have deficits in emotion recognition and this has been correlated with the severity of other cognitive disturbances rather than duration of disease.[70]

Patients with CBD also demonstrate impairments in executive functions and memory, but more distinguishing are deficits in language, visuospatial dysfunction, such as apraxias and "alien hand," and social cognition difficulties (for review, see Ref.[71]). Depression (73%) and irritability (20%) were noted to occur more commonly in patients with CBD than with PSP. Apathy and agitation was also common, with anxiety, disinhibition, delusional activity, or aberrant motor behaviors (eg, pacing) noted less commonly with CBD.[72]

REFERENCES

1. Luk KC, Lee VM. Modeling Lewy pathology propagation in Parkinson's disease. Parkinsonism Relat Disord 2014;20:S85–7.
2. Alexander GE, Crutcher MD. Functional architecture of basal ganglia circuits: neural substrates of parallel processing. Trends Neurosci 1990;13: 266–71.
3. Delong MR, Crutcher MD, Georgopoulos AP. Primate globus pallidus and subthalamic nucleus: functional organization. J Neuropysiol 1985;53:530–43.
4. Baker KB, Lee JY, Mavinkurve G, et al. Somatotopic organization in the internal segment of the globus pallidus in Parkinson's disease. Exp Neurol 2010;222: 219–25.
5. Bronfeld M, Bar-Gad I. Loss of specificity in basal ganglia related movement disorders. Front Syst Neurosci 2011;5:38.
6. Erez Y, Tischler H, Belelovsky K, et al. Dispersed activity during passive movement in the globus pallidus of the 1-methyl-4-phenyl-1,2,3,6-tetrahydropyridine (MPTP)-treated primate. PLoS One 2011;6:e16293.
7. Boraud T, Bezard E, Bioulac B, et al. Ratio of inhibited-to-activated pallidal neurons decreases dramatically during passive limb movement in the MPTP-treated monkey. J Neurophysiol 2000;83:1760–3.
8. Levy R, Dostrovsky JO, Lang AE, et al. Effects of apomorphine on subthalamic nucleus and globus pallidus internus neurons in patients with Parkinson's disease. J Neurophysiol 2001;86:249–60.

9. De Hemptinne C, Swann NC, Ostrem JL, et al. Therapeutic deep brain stimulation reduces cortical phase-amplitude coupling in Parkinson's disease. Nat Neurosci 2015;18:779–86.

10. Polymeropoulos MH, Lavedan C, Leroy E, et al. Mutation in the alpha-synuclein gene identified in families with Parkinson's disease. Science 1997;276:2045–7.

11. Spillantini MG, Schmidt ML, Lee VM, et al. Alpha-synuclein in Lewy bodies. Nature 1997;388:839–40.

12. Braak H, Ghebremedhin E, Rub U, et al. Stages in the development of Parkinson's disease-related pathology. Cell Tissue Res 2004;318:121–34.

13. Iranzo A. Parkinson disease and sleep: sleep-wake changes in the premotor stage of Parkinson disease; impaired olfaction and other prodromal features. Curr Neurol Neurosci Rep 2013;13:373.

14. Clairembault T, Leclair-Visonneau L, Neunlist M, et al. Enteric glial cells: new players in Parkinson's disease? Mov Disord 2015;30:494–8.

15. Ritz B, Lee PC, Lassen CF, et al. Parkinson disease and smoking revisited: ease of quitting is an early sign of the disease. Neurology 2014;83:1396–402.

16. Janvin C, Aarsland D, Larsen JP, et al. Neuropsychological profile of patients with Parkinson's disease without dementia. Dement Geriatr Cogn Disord 2003;15: 126–31.

17. Robins TW, Cools R. Cognitive deficits in Parkinson' disease: a cognitive neuroscience perspective. Mov Disord 2014;29:597–607.

18. Cools R, Barker RA, Sahakian BJ, et al. L-DOPA medication remediates cognitive inflexibility, but increases impulsivity in patients with Parkinson's disease. Neuropsychologia 2003;41:1431–41.

19. Disbrow EA, Sigvardt KA, Franz EA, et al. Movement activation and inhibition in Parkinson's disease: a functional imaging study. J Parkinsons Dis 2013;3: 181–92.

20. Kehagia AA, Cools R, Barker RA, et al. Switching between abstract rules reflects disease severity but not dopaminergic status in Parkinson's disease. Neuropsychologia 2009;47:1117–27.

21. Monchi O, Petrides M, Doyon J, et al. Neural basis of setshifting deficits in Parkinson's disease. J Neurosci 2004;24:702–10.

22. Shook SK, Franz EA, Higginson CL, et al. Dopamine dependency of intradimensional and extradimensional switching operations in Parkinson's patients. Neuropsychologia 2005;43:1990–9.

23. Alexander GE, Delong MR, Strick PL. Parallel organization of functionally segregated circuits linking basal ganglia and cortex. Annu Rev Neurosci 1986;9: 357–81.

24. Lange KW, Robbins TW, Marsden CD, et al. L-dopa withdrawal in Parkinson's disease selectively impairs cognitive performance in tests sensitive frontal lobe dysfunction. Psychopharmacology 1992;107:394–404.

25. Marek KL, Seibyl JP, Zoghbi SS, et al. [1231] beta-CIT/SPECT imaging demonstrates bilateral loss of dopamine transporters in hemi-Parkinson's disease. Neurology 1996;46:231–7.

26. Hoehn M, Yahr M. Parkinsonism: onset, progression and mortality. Neurology 1967;17:427–42.

27. Gallager DA, Schrag A. Psychosis, apathy, depression and anxiety in Parkinson's disease. Neurobiol Dis 2012;46:581–9.

28. Aarsland D, Bronnick K, Ehrt U, et al. Neuropsychiatric symptoms in patients with Parkinson's disease and dementia: frequency, profile and associated care giver stress. J Neurol Neurosurg Psychiatry 2007;78:36–42.

29. Forsaa EB, Larsen JP, Wentzel-Larsen T, et al. A 12-year population-based study of psychosis in Parkinson disease. Arch Neurol 2010;67:996–1001.

30. Fenelon G, Mahieux F, Huon R. Hallucinations in Parkinson's disease: prevalence, phenomenology and risk factors. Brain 2000;123:733–45.

31. Weintraub D, Koester J, Potenza MN, et al. Impulse control disorders in Parkinson disease: a cross-sectional study of 3090 patients. Arch Neurol 2010;67:589–95.

32. Weintraub D, Sohr M, Potenza MN, et al. Amantadine use associated with impulse control disorders in Parkinson disease in cross-sectional study. Ann Neurol 2010;68:963–8.

33. McKeith G, Galasko D, Kosaka K, et al. Consensus guidelines for the clinical and pathologic diagnosis of dementia with Lewy bodies (DLB): report of the consortium on DLB international workshops. Neurology 1996;47:1113–24.

34. Tsuiboi Y, Dickson DW. Dementia with Lewy bodies and Parkinson's disease with dementia: are they different? Parkinsonism Relat Disord 2005;11(Suppl 1): S47–51.

35. Halliday G, Hely M, Reid W, et al. The progression of pathology in longitudinally followed patients with Parkinson's disease. Acta Neuropathol 2008;115:409–15.

36. Compta Y, Parkkinen L, O'Sullivan SS, et al. Lewy-and Alzheimer-type pathologies in Parkinson's disease dementia: which is more important? Brain 2011; 134:1493–505.

37. Braak H, Braak E, Bohl J. Staging of Alzheimer-related cortical destruction. Eur Neurol 1993;33:403–8.

38. Harding AJ, Broe GA, Halliday GM. Visual hallucinations in Lewy body disease relate to Lewy bodies in the temporal lobe. Brain 2002;125:391–403.

39. Gallagher DA, Parkkinen L, O'Sullivan SS, et al. Testing an aetiological model of visual hallucinations in Parkinson's disease. Brain 2011;134:3299–309.

40. Goldman JG, Stebbins GT, Dinh V, et al. Visuoperceptive region atrophy independent of cognitive status in patients with Parkinson's disease with hallucinations. Brain 2014;137:849–59.

41. Aarsland D, Taylor JP, Weintraub D. Psychiatric issues in cognitive impairment. Mov Disord 2014;29:651–62.

42. Marion MH, Qurashi M, Marshall G, et al. Is REM sleep behavior disorders (RBD) a risk factor of dementia in idiopathic Parkinson's disease? J Neurol 2008;255:192–6.

43. Paus S, Brecht HM, Koster J, et al. Sleep attacks, daytime sleepiness, and dopamine agonists in Parkinson's disease. Mov Disord 2003;18:659–67.

44. Hall H, Reyes S, Landeck N, et al. Hippocampal Lewy pathology and cholinergic dysfunction are associated with dementia in Parkinson's disease. Brain 2014;137: 2493–508.

45. Wang HF, Yu JT, Tang SW, et al. Efficacy and safety of cholinesterase inhibitors and memantine in cognitive impairment in Parkinson's disease, Parkinson's disease dementia, and dementia with Lewy bodies: systematic review with metaanalysis and trail sequential analysis. J Neurol Neurosurg Psychiatry 2015;86: 135–43.

46. Factor SA, Feustel PJ, Friedman JH, et al. Longitudinal outcome of Parkinson's disease patients with psychosis. Neurology 2003;11:1756–61.

47. Reddy S, Factor SA, Molho ES, et al. The effect of quetiapine on psychosis and motor function in parkinsonian patients with and without dementia. Mov Disord 2002;17:676–81.

48. Pollak P, Tison F, Rascol O, et al. Clozapine in drug induced psychosis in Parkinson's disease: a randomized, placebo controlled study with open follow up. J Neurol Neurosurg Psychiatry 2004;75:689–95.

49. Hacksell U, Burstein ES, Mcfarland K, et al. On the discovery and development of pimavanserin: a novel drug candidate for Parkinson's psychosis. Neurochem Res 2014;39:2008–17.

50. Richard IH, McDermott MP, Kurlan R, et al. A randomized, double-blind, placebo-controlled trail of antidepressants in Parkinson disease. Neurology 2012;78: 1229–36.

51. Smith KM, Eyal E, Weintraub D, et al. Combined rasagiline and antidepressant use in Parkinson disease in the ADAGIO study: effects on nonmotor symptoms and tolerability. JAMA Neurol 2015;72:88–95.

52. Uc EY, Doerschug KC, Magnotta V, et al. Phase I/II randomized trial of aerobic exercise in Parkinson disease in a community setting. Neurology 2014;83: 413–25.

53. Petzinger GM, Fisher BE, McEwen S, et al. Exercise-enhanced Neuroplasticity targeting motor and cognitive circuitry in Parkinson's disease. Lancet Neurol 2013;12:716–26.

54. Stankovic I, Krismer F, Aleksandar J. Cognitive impairment in multiple system atrophy: a position statement by the Neuropsychology Task Force of the MDS Multiple System Atrophy (MODIMSA) study group. Mov Disord 2014;29:857–67.

55. Brown RG, Lacomblez L, Landwehrmeyer BG. Cognitive impairment in patients with multiple system atrophy and progressive supranuclear palsy. Brain 2010; 133:2382–93.

56. Kawai Y, Suenaga M, Takeda A. Cognitive impairments in multiple system atrophy: MSA-C vs MSA-P. Neurology 2008;70:1390–6.

57. Chang CC, Chang YY, Chang WN. Cognitive deficits in multiple system atrophy correlate with frontal atrophy and disease duration. Eur J Neurol 2009;16: 1144–50.

58. Asi YT, Ling H, Ahmed Z. Neuropathological features of multiple system atrophy with cognitive impairment. Mov Disord 2014;29:884–8.

59. Kim HJ, Jeon BS, Kim YE. Clinical and imaging characteristics of dementia in multiple system atrophy. Parkinsonism Relat Disord 2013;19:617–21.

60. Otsuka M, Ichiya Y, Kuwabara Y. Glucose metabolism in the cortical and subcortical brain structures in multiple system atrophy and Parkinson's disease: a positron emission tomographic study. J Neurol Sci 1996;144:77–83.

61. Balas M, Balash Y, Giladi N. Cognition in multiple system atrophy: neuropsychological profile and interaction with mood. J Neural Transm 2010;117:369–75.

62. Fanciulli A, Wenning GK. Multiple-system atrophy. N Engl J Med 2015;372: 249–63.

63. Kobylecki C, Jones M, Thompson JC. Cognitive-behavioural features of progressive supranuclear palsy syndrome overlap with frontotemporal dementia. J Neurol 2015;262:916–22.

64. Gerstenecker A, Mast B, Duff K. Executive dysfunction is the primary cognitive impairment in progressive supranuclear palsy. Arch Clin Neuropsychol 2013; 28:104–13.

65. Yatabe Y, Hashimoto M, Kaneda K. Neuropsychiatric symptoms of progressive supranuclear palsy in a dementia clinic. Psychogeriatrics 2011;11:54–9.

66. Lagarde J, Valabregue R, Corvol JC. Are frontal cognitive and atrophy patterns different in PSP and bvFTD? A comparative neuropsychological and VBM study. PLoS One 2013;8:e80353.

67. Aarsland D, Litvan I, Larsen JP. Neuropsychiatric symptoms of patients with progressive supranuclear palsy and Parkinson's disease. J Neuropsychiatry Clin Neurosci 2001;13:42–9.

68. Litvan I, Mega MS, Cummings JL. Neuropsychiatric aspects of progressive supranuclear palsy. Neurology 1996;47:1184–9.
69. Bloise MC, Berardelli I, Roselli V. Psychiatric disturbances in patients with progressive supranuclear palsy: a case-control study. Parkinsonism Relat Disord 2014;20:965–8.
70. Ghosh BCP, Rowe JB, Calder AJ. Emotion recognition in progressive supranuclear palsy. J Neurol Neurosurg Psychiatry 2009;80:1143–5.
71. Burrell JR, Hodges JR, Rowe JB. Cognition in corticobasal syndrome and progressive supranuclear palsy: a review. Mov Disord 2014;29:684–93.
72. Litvan I, Cummings JL, Mega M. Neuropsychiatric features of corticobasal degeneration. J Neurol Neurosurg Psychiatry 1998;65:717–21.

Neuropsychiatric Features in Primary Mitochondrial Disease

Samantha E. Marin, MD[a], Russell P. Saneto, DO, PhD[b,c],*

KEYWORDS

- Mitochondrial • Neuropsychiatric • Behavioral • Autism • Depression • Anxiety
- Bipolar disorder • Schizophrenia

KEY POINTS

- There is some evidence to suggest that mitochondrial dysfunction plays a role in neuropsychiatric illness; however, the data are inconclusive.
- Onset of psychiatric illness often proceeds onset of mitochondrial disease symptoms.
- Many classic mitochondrial syndromes are associated with psychiatric illness.
- Children and adults have co-morbid mitochondrial disease and psychiairic illness.

INTRODUCTION

Mitochondrial diseases are a clinically heterogeneous group of disorders that ultimately result from dysfunction of the mitochondrial respiratory chain. The respiratory chain (also known as the electron transport chain) is a series of 5 protean complexes

Disclosure Statement: S.E. Marin has received funding as part of a mitochondrial fellowship from the National Institutes of Health (NIH 2U54NS078059-04). She is involved in the North American Mitochondrial Disease Consortium (NAMDC). She has been a nonpaid member of pharmaceutical company sponsored clinical studies, including those sponsored by Edison Pharmaceuticals, Raptor Pharmaceuticals, and Stealth Peptides. R.P. Saneto has received grant funding to perform clinical studies on mitochondrial diseases from National Institutes of Health (NIH 2U54NS078059-04) and Edison Pharmaceuticals. He is a nonpaid member of the DSMB board for REATA Pharmaceuticals 408-C-1402 and 408-C-1403.

[a] Department of Neurosciences, University of California, San Diego (UCSD), 9500 Gilman Drive #0935, La Jolla, CA 92093-0935, USA; [b] Department of Neurology, Seattle Children's Hospital, University of Washington, 4800 Sand Point Way Northeast, Seattle, WA 98105, USA; [c] Department of Pediatrics, Seattle Children's Hospital, University of Washington, 4800 Sand Point Way Northeast, Seattle, WA 98105, USA
* Corresponding author. Department of Pediatric Neurology, 4800 Sand Point Way Northeast, Box MB 7.420, Seattle, WA 98105.
E-mail address: russ.saneto@seattlechildrens.org

that are linked together to reduce molecular oxygen to water (oxidation) and phosphorylate adenosine diphophosphate to adenosine triphosphate (ATP).[1] The active shuttling of electrons begins when complex I (nicotinamide adenine dinucleotide with hydrogen [NADH] dehydrogenase or NADH:ubiquinone oxidoreductase) accepts electrons from NADH produced in the Krebs cycle and passes them to coenzyme Q10 (ubiquinone). Ubiquinone also receives electrons from reduced flavin adenine dinucleotide ($FADH_2$) via complex II (succinate dehydrogenase: SDH). Electrons are then shuttled from ubiquinone to complex III (cytochrome bc_1 complex) and then to complex IV (cytochrome c oxidase: COX), which reduces molecular oxygen to water. An electrochemical gradient is produced as protons are pumped to the intermembrane space between the inner and outer mitochondrial membrane as electrons shuttle between complexes I to IV. Using this proton gradient, complex V (ATP synthase) acts as an ion channel allowing for proton flux back into the mitochondrial matrix, resulting in the release of free energy, which drives ATP synthesis (**Fig. 1**).

The mitochondria are considered the "power plants" of the cell; the majority of cellular energy is in the form of ATP. The proteins required for mitochondrial structure and function are derived from both nuclear DNA (nDNA) and mitochondrial DNA (mtDNA) encoded genes.[2] Unlike nDNA, which exists as a single copy within the nucleus of each cell, the mtDNA exists as multiple copies within the mitochondria of each cell. Human mtDNA is a circular, double-stranded molecule containing approximately 16,569 base pairs and encodes for 37 genes: 22 transfer ribonucleic acids (tRNAs), 2 ribosomal RNAs (rRNAs), and 13 polypeptides that are incorporated into the electron transport chain subunits I, III, IV, and V (see **Fig. 1**).[3,4] These 13 polypeptides are important for efficient generation of ATP, but represent a small fraction of the total number of respiratory chain subunits, the remainder of which are encoded by nDNA.

The dependence on both nuclear and mitochondrial gene products, combined with the unique physiology of mitochondrial function, can create a wide range of disease expression. Mitochondrial disorders owing to mtDNA-encoded mutations differ from those secondary to nDNA mutations in various ways. Inheritance of mtDNA is through the maternal lineage rather than following classic Mendelian genetics. However, because mitochondrial disease may be secondary to nuclear-encoded mutations, absence of maternal inheritance does not rule out the possibility of an underlying mitochondrial disease. Second, unique mitochondrial physiology can alter disease expression. Every cell contains hundreds to thousands of mtDNA molecules. When mutations arise, a mixture of wild-type and mutant mtDNA (heteroplasmy) can exist that are then randomly distributed to daughter cells through mitotic segregation. This random segregation of normal and mutant mtDNA results in different mutation loads in various tissues (see **Fig. 1**).[5,6] When the mutation load reaches a certain "threshold," features of mitochondrial dysfunction in that tissue become apparent.[7] The percentage level of mutant mtDNA may vary among individuals within the same family, and also among organs and tissues within the same individual.[8] The energetic requirement between organs varies and, therefore, expression of organ dysfunction can vary within the individual. Additionally, the mtDNA is susceptible to a higher mutation and base pair substitution rate compared with nDNA owing to the lack of histones and DNA repair mechanisms and has been considered by some as the "weak point" of the human genome.[9] A high level of polymorphisms in mtDNA have been reported, some of which have been linked to susceptibility to certain diseases.[10]

The understanding of mitochondrial disorders is in its youth, with the first pathogenic mutation identified fewer than 30 years ago.[11] Mitochondrial disorders were previously

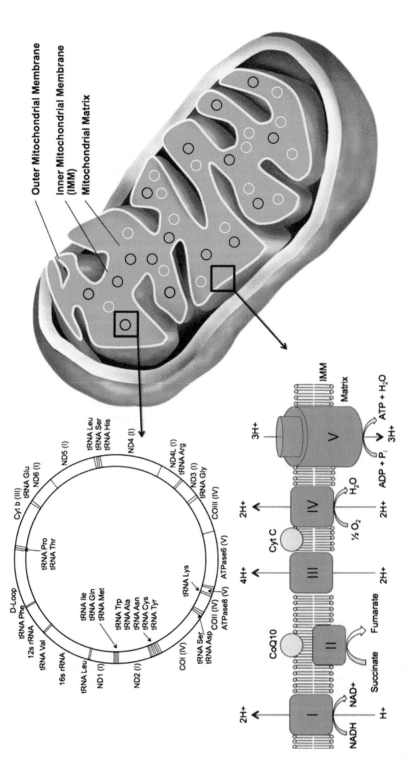

Fig. 1. Structure of the mitochondrion (*right*), including the layout of the outer mitochondrial membrane (OMM), mitochondrial matrix, and inner mitochondrial membrane (IMM). Within the mitochondrial matrix, the circular mitochondrial DNA (mtDNA) is shown. There is often a combination of wild-type (*white circles*) and mutant (*black circles*) mtDNA in each mitochondrion, a feature known as heteroplasmy. In the upper left hand corner, the mtDNA with the 37 mtDNA genes is depicted. In the bottom left corner, the electron transport chain (complex I–V) is shown. ADP, adenosine diphosphate; ATP, adenosine triphosphate; ATPase, adenosine triphosphatase; COI, complex I; COII, complex II; CoQ10, coenzyme Q10; Cyt b, cytochrome b; COIII; Cyt C, cytochrome C; COIV; COV NAD, nicotinamide adenine dinucleotide; NADH, nicotinamide adenine dinucleotide plus hydrogen; rRNA, ribosomal RNA; tRNA, transfer RNA.

thought to be rare, but are now regarded as among the most common inborn errors of metabolism, with a birth incidence of approximately 1 in 2000 in the population.[12,13] More recent studies suggest that the incidence of pathological mtDNA mutations may be even greater; a study from the United Kingdom looking at the frequency of 10 common pathogenic mtDNA mutations in 3148 neonatal cord samples determined an incidence of 1 in 200.[14] However, the presence of these mutations is not necessarily congruent with disease. Ultimately, disease depends on heteroplasmy, organ threshold, and environmental factors.

Mitochondrial disorders are typically suspected based on their clinical presentations; however, disease confirmation is often difficult, requiring extensive clinical and laboratory evaluation.[15,16] Diagnostic criteria based on biochemical, immunohistochemical, and enzymatic analyses; neuroimaging findings; and clinical symptoms have been proposed to assist in the identification of mitochondrial disease.[17,18] However, these criteria are imperfect and do not take into account the recent advances in genetic testing. Diagnosis is further complicated by the use of different methods and lack of standardization among different laboratories worldwide with respect to enzymatic analysis.[16,19] The pediatric population adds further complexity to the diagnosis of mitochondrial disorders because age-related tissue changes have not yet occurred and, to date, most diseases are secondary to nDNA mutations rather than mtDNA mutations.[20] To assist in simplifying the diagnosis in patients meriting workup for a mitochondrial disease, a diagnostic algorithm has been proposed.[16]

Mitochondrial disorders have been divided classically into particular syndromes based on common clinical features, biochemical alterations, pathologic findings, and more recently genetic underpinnings. Mitochondrial syndromes described in the literature include, but are not restricted to, mitochondrial encephalopathy, myopathy with lactic acidosis and strokelike episodes (MELAS); Leber hereditary optic neuropathy (LHON); myoclonic epilepsy with ragged red fibers (MERRF); mitochondrial neurogastrointestinal encephalomyopathy (NMGIE); sensory ataxia, neuropathy, dysarthria, and ophthalmoplegia (SANDO); neuropathy, ataxia, and retinitis pigmentosa (NARP); chronic progressive external ophthalmoplegia (CPEO); Kearns–Sayre syndrome (KSS); and Leigh syndrome.[21–25] Although some patients do fall into these particular phenotypes, it is now recognized that patients with particular gene mutations present with a large spectrum of clinical features that may not fit into a particular phenotype and that a particular phenotype may be associated with several different gene mutations.

In disorders of oxidative phosphorylation, organs with the greatest requirements for energy are often the most vulnerable, including the brain, heart, and skeletal muscle.[26] The brain depends on mitochondrial energy production for various functions, including the maintenance of the transmembrane potential across neurons and glia, signal transduction, synaptic plasticity, and calcium homeostasis.[27–30] Therefore, it is not unexpected that disorders resulting from mitochondrial dysfunction manifest with neuropsychiatric symptomatology. Central nervous system (CNS) manifestations that are common to mitochondrial disorders include epilepsy, movement disorders, visual impairment, episodic encephalopathy, behavioral abnormalities, and cognitive impairment.[31] The association of psychiatric symptoms in mitochondrial disorders, however, has received little systematic evaluation. As such, the prevalence of psychiatric illness in patients with mitochondrial disorders is not known. This article summarizes the available literature published in the area of neuropsychiatric manifestations in both children and adults with primary mitochondrial disease, with a focus on autism spectrum disorder (ASD) in children and mood disorders and schizophrenia in adults.

NEUROPSYCHIATRIC FEATURES IN PRIMARY MITOCHONDRIAL DISEASE IN CHILDREN
Autism

ASD are a group of developmental disorders characterized by 2 core clinical characteristics: (1) persistent deficits in social communication and social interaction across various contexts and (2) restricted and repetitive patterns of behavior, interests, and/or activities that impair everyday functioning.[32,33] ASD typically manifest early in childhood and are persistent across the lifespan. The *Diagnostic and Statistical Manual of Mental Disorders*, 5th edition (DSM V) merged formerly separate diagnostic entities (autistic disorder, Asperger's disorder, and pervasive developmental disorder not otherwise specified) into a single dimension.[33] Rigorous epidemiologic studies have demonstrated that the prevalence of autism has increased in recent years.[34–36] The Centers for Disease Control and Prevention now estimate that 14.7 per 1000 (1 in 68) children in the United States fulfill the diagnostic criteria for ASD.[37] The etiology of ASD is considered to be multifactorial, resulting from the complex interplay of biological mechanisms, genetic vulnerabilities, and environmental factors.[38,39] Although a majority of cases of ASD are diagnosed in otherwise healthy-appearing children, there is a growing body of evidence suggesting that a proportion of patients presenting with ASD have an underlying genetic or metabolic etiology.[40,41]

As knowledge about mitochondrial diseases has expanded in recent years, substantial attention has been focused on a potential link between ASD and mitochondrial disease. Current evidence suggests that the prevalence of mitochondrial disorders in patients with ASD is much greater than that of the general population (5%–7%).[42,43] Multiple lines of evidence exist to support the role of mitochondrial dysfunction in ASD, including (1) similar biochemical changes seen in patients with autism and mitochondrial disease, (2) the high prevalence of autism and autistic features in patients with definite primary mitochondrial disease, and (3) the identification of shared genetic loci in both mtDNA and nDNA implying an underlying dysfunction in oxidative phosphorylation.

Biochemical alterations in patients with autism

Within the published literature, evidence suggests that a subset of individuals with ASD exhibit biochemical alterations seen with dysfunction of mitochondrial oxidative phosphorylation.[42–54] Dysfunction of the respiratory chain in patients with mitochondrial disease results in a decrease in the level of ATP. In the presence of low ATP levels owing to inefficient respiratory chain activity, an upregulation of glycolysis occurs, resulting in an overproduction of pyruvate that is either transaminated to alanine or reduced to lactate.[55] As such, the common biochemical alterations noted in patients with ASD suggestive of mitochondrial dysfunction are an elevated plasma lactate, elevated pyruvate, and elevated alanine.

The first to suggest a possible link between mitochondrial disorders and autism on the basis of serologic evidence of disordered oxidative phosphorylation (respiratory chain dysfunction) was Coleman and Blass.[47] In a series of patients diagnosed with autism over an 8-year period, 4 of 80 (5%) demonstrated persistent elevations in lactate and pyruvate.[47] They hypothesized that this subgroup of patients had an "abnormality in the utilization of sugar" and postulated that "the autistic syndrome" can be associated with a family of disorders of carbohydrate metabolism."[47] They urged that studies of lactate and pyruvate be part of the routine evaluation of autistic children. Similar rates of lactic acidemia (4%) were subsequently found in another cohort of autistic children.[56] Other authors have reported rates of hyperlacticacidemia and hyperpyruvatemia in other groups of children with ASD have been as high as 43% and 30%, respectively.[48] However, it is unclear what percentages of these children were later diagnosed with a definite mitochondrial disease, or even if the diagnosis of a primary mitochondrial disorder was pursued. Two studies found that a diagnosis of a mitochondrial disease was given to 19%[57] and 43%[42] patients with only the combination of ASD and elevated lactate; however, only a percentage of these children underwent a subsequent workup for mitochondrial disease.

The finding of an elevated lactate in patients who meet diagnostic criteria for ASD and are diagnosed with a definite mitochondrial disease is a common occurrence.[42,45] In their population-based study, Oliveira and colleagues[42] found an elevated lactate (defined as >2.5 mmol/L) in 20.3% of their mitochondrial disease cohort who also had ASD. Weissman and colleagues[45] suggested a higher rate of lactic acidosis in patients with a dual diagnosis and reported at least 1 elevated lactate level in 76%. Of their cases with an elevated lactate, 52% had persistently elevated lactate levels and 56% had lactate level of greater than 3 mmol/L.[45]

Lactic acidosis is the most recognized biochemical abnormality seen in patients with primary mitochondrial disorders. Jackson and colleagues[58] reported a rate of lactic acidosis in 50% of pediatric and adult cases with mitochondrial disorders. However, lactic acidosis is found more frequently in patients with mtDNA mutations rather than nDNA mutations impacting mitochondrial function.[59] In the pediatric population, mtDNA mutations account for less than 10% of all mitochondrial disorders[60]; therefore, the incidence of lactic acidosis found in this study is likely an overestimate of the true incidence of lactic acidosis in affected pediatric patients. In the absence of other, better biochemical markers, it is still recommended that lactate be considered as a biochemical test in the workup of suspected mitochondrial disorders; however, the following caveats should be considered: (1) frequently in mitochondrial disorders, lactate may be normal outside of a metabolic crisis or after exercise,[61] (2) patients with genetically or biochemically proven mitochondrial disorders may have consistently normal or only minimally elevated lactate levels (owing to insensitivity), and (3) elevated lactate has been shown not specific to primary mitochondrial disease.[16] Furthermore, a frequent cause for a spuriously elevated plasma lactate is from poor collection conditions or techniques, such as a struggling child.[16] In children with ASD, thrashing and writhing during a blood collection may not be infrequent and may contribute to a falsely elevated lactate. We suggest caution with findings of isolated elevated lactate levels, but further clinical investigation is warranted.

Pyruvate is another screening test frequently completed in patients with suspected mitochondrial disease. Pyruvate is elevated in pyruvate metabolism defects such as pyruvate dehydrogenase deficiency or pyruvate carboxylase deficiency, but can also be elevated in various other primary mitochondrial disorders. Lactate/pyruvate ratios indirectly reflect the NADH/nicotinamide adenine dinucleotide (NAD) plus cytoplasmic redox state,[61] and may be helpful in identifying patients with defective oxidative phosphorylation. Unfortunately, pyruvate is unstable and blood specimens must be taken and handled carefully for accurate measurement.[16] In the series by Weissman and colleagues,[45] an elevated pyruvate was identified in 53% of their patient cohort who had both ASD and primary mitochondrial disease. Oliveira and colleagues[42] found that 82% of their cohort had an elevated lactate:pyruvate ratio; however, this number was much higher than the lactate:pyruvate ratio identified by Weissman and colleagues[45] in patient fibroblasts (20%).

Other measures frequently used to indicate the possible presence of a mitochondrial disorder are specific changes plasma amino acids (PAA) and urinary organic acids. Elevated plasma alanine is a useful indicator of longstanding pyruvate accumulation and therefore redox state.[16] Hence, an absolute elevation in alanine (>450 μmol/L) is part of the Nijmegen diagnostic criteria to assist in the diagnosis of mitochondrial diseases.[18] According to 1 series, 36% of patients with both mitochon-drial disorders and ASD had an elevated alanine on PAA.[45] However, similar to elevated lactate levels and other biochemical markers of mitochondrial dysfunction, the sensitivity of an elevated alanine is low and it may only be increased during times of physiologic stress. Urinary organic acid analysis may also suggest a mitochondrial disorder. Organic acids are byproducts of the catabolism of proteins, carbohydrates, and fats. Frequently seen metabolites in mitochondrial disorders include tricarboxylic acid cycle intermediates, ethylmalonate, 3-methyl-glutaconate, and dicarboxylic acids.[16] Unlike plasma lactic acid, lactic acid elevation on urine organic acid analysis is not a good discriminator (low sensitivity) for mitochondrial cytopathies.[62]

In one of the most comprehensive reviews of biochemical alterations in patients with ASD, Filipek and colleagues[44] completed a retrospective chart review of 100 cases that had available metabolic tests documented in their charts (including total and free carnitine, lactate, pyruvate, ammonia, and PAA). In their cohort, several metabo-lites differed between children with ASD and control subjects. They found evidence of anaerobic conversion of pyruvate to lactate (with 88% of pyruvate below the mean and 52% of lactate above the mean) and a finding of an elevated alanine (in 80%) on PAA. In addition, within their autistic cohort, there was a significant decrease in both total and free carnitine levels. Carnitine plays an essential role in the transportation of long chain fatty acids across the outer and inner mitochondrial membrane to partici-pate in beta-oxidation in the mitochondrial matrix.[63] Frequently, total plasma carnitine is decreased in patients with mitochondrial disease. Similarly, a study by Rossignol and Frye[43] identified that patients with autism showed the following biochemical alter-ations: elevated lactate (31.1%), elevated pyruvate (13.6%), elevated lactate/pyruvate ratio (27.6%), elevated alanine (8.3%), low total carnitine (90%), elevated creatine phosphokinase (47%), and abnormal liver function tests in approximately 45%. Taken as a whole, these data provide evidence supporting the presence of mitochondrial induced biochemical abnormalities in a subgroup of ASD children.

Further support for a role of mitochondrial dysfunction in autism comes from abnormal findings on muscle biopsy, particularly when investigating the enzyme activ-ity of the respiratory chain complexes. Compromised respiratory chain enzymatic ac-tivity is considered one of the major criteria for the diagnosis of frank mitochondrial disease.[17] Oliveira and colleagues[42] completed a muscle biopsy in 11 patients in their cohort with ASD and an elevated lactate identified on biochemical screening. Seven were identified to have a deficiency of 1 or more respiratory chain complexes, most frequently involving complex V (3/7; 43%), complex IV (2/7; 29%), and complex I (2/7; 29%). Five of the 6 patients in their cohort had enzyme complex activity of less than 20% of the normal mean (a major laboratory criteria) and one of the patients had enzyme complex activity between 20% and 30% (a minor laboratory criteria).[17] Similarly, decreased enzyme activity was identified in 7 of 8 patients in another cohort, with complex III deficiency being the most common (6/7; 86%), followed by complex IV (1/7; 14%). More recent studies completed using more sophisticated enzyme ana-lyses revealed that complex I deficiency is the most commonly found enzymatic defect in patients with ASD, identified in 50% to 64%, followed by complex III defi-ciency (20%–36%), complex II deficiency (8%), and complex IV deficiency (4%).[45,51,64] The differences in electron transport chain enzymatic deficiencies be-tween studies may be secondary to the use of different laboratories that have differ-ential methodologies and techniques of assessing components of the electron transport chain. In 1 study analyzing 5 diagnostic test centers in the United States, inconstant diagnostic interpretations resulted from different laboratories, suggesting the need for comparative testing in multiple laboratories.[65]

Despite the findings of biochemical and enzymatic abnormalities in a cohort of patients with ASD, extensive diagnostic investigations may be unnecessary and unwarranted.[66] Current practice guidelines suggest that metabolic testing should be considered only in patients who have an atypical presentation or if uncharacteristic features develop in someone who has already received a diagnosis of an ASD.[66] This suggestion is supported by studies attempting to further characterize the clinical features in patients with "mitochondrial autism" (see The Clinical Phenotype in Patients with "Mitochondrial Autism").[45,64,67] These studies suggest that the presence of the following characteristics in patients with ASD may warrant further investigation for a mitochondrial disorder: (1) presence of multiorgan system disease (particularly those with severe gastrointestinal [GI] dysfunction) and (2) presence of autistic regression.[67] However, 7.2% of patients with ASD identified as having definite mitochondrial disorders in 1 cohort, displayed "typical autism" without other organ involvement, autistic regression, seizures, or neurologic examination abnormalities that would have otherwise prompted a workup for an underlying metabolic or genetic etiology.[42] Additionally, Rossignol and Frye[43] identified that, in a metaanalysis looking at patients with both ASD and mitochondrial disease, 92% of patients were diagnosed with ASD before the diagnosis of mitochondrial disorders. Therefore, clinicians should have a low threshold to initiate further testing of possible underlying mitochondrial dysfunction in children with autism, even in the absence of "atypical" autistic features.

The clinical phenotype in patients with "mitochondrial autism"

"Mitochondrial autism" is a term Weissman and colleagues[45] coined to describe patients with probable or definite mitochondrial disease, as defined by the Modified Walker Criteria[17] and/or the Nijmegan Criteria,[18] who also meet DSM-IV-TR[32] diagnostic criteria for either Autistic Disorder or Pervasive Developmental Disorder, Not Otherwise Specified (PDD-NOS). To attempt to define the phenotype of patients with mitochondrial autism to assist in the selection of patients with ASD, these authors explored features seen in a 25 patients with the dual diagnosis. Type I error is very likely in this study owing to small numbers, but may be helpful in the initial assessment of this disorder. In their cohort, 96% of patients displayed at least 1 major clinical finding uncommon in ASD. They found that 84% of patients had involvement of at least 1 non-CNS organ system, 32% of had at least 2 non-CNS organ systems, and 60% of patients presented with at least 1 neurologic finding uncommon to ASD. Biochemical evidence of mitochondrial dysfunction was seen in a large proportion of patients, including elevated lactate (76%), pyruvate (53%), alanine (36%), and abnormal nonspecific urine organic acids (42%). The most common neurologic manifestations included fatigability/exercise intolerance (68%), marked gross motor delay (32%), seizures (20%), oculomotor abnormalities (16%), dysarthria (12%), sensorineural hearing loss (12%), ptosis (8%), and movement disorders (8%). Nonneurologic features included GI dysfunction (reflux, constipation) (64%), cardiovascular anomalies (28%), growth restriction (20%), hematologic abnormalities (8%), renal dysfunction (8%), and endocrine dysfunction (8%). Although it is certainly helpful that other manifestations are common in patients with mitochondrial disorders and ASD, none of these features are specific to or sensitive for mitochondrial disorders. Epilepsy, for example, has been reported in 16% to 44% of all patients with ASD without an associated mitochondrial disorder.[68–70] However, these clinical and biochemical findings suggest a starting place for further investigation.

Similarly, in an attempt to define the phenotype of patients with mitochondrial autism, Shoffner and colleagues[64] identified 28 pediatric cases (1.5–19.3 years) with a dual diagnosis of ASD and mitochondrial disease. Clinically, 46.4% exhibited motor developmental delay and hypotonia, 42.9% exhibited exercise-induced fatigue, 39.3% and had a diagnosis of epilepsy, and 11% had growth delay or failure to thrive. A family history was exhibited in 36% (affected siblings). Biochemical findings included elevated lactate, pyruvate, and alanine in 46% of patients. MRI of the brain was normal in all patients for whom neuroimaging was available. Muscle biopsy was completed in all patients. Routine pathology was normal or nonspecific in all patients, including absence of ragged red fibers or cytochrome c oxidase-deficient fibers. The following distribution of oxidative phosphorylation enzyme defects was observed: isolated complex I defect in 50%, combined complexes I and III defects in 17.9%, combined complexes I, III, and IV defects in 17.9%, and an isolated complex V defect in 14.3%. Western blot of electron transport chain protein subunits was abnormal in 71% of patients. Muscle mtDNA depletion was identified in 5%. Muscle coenzyme Q10 deficiency was isolated in 7.1%.

Rossignol and Frye[43] also looked at features present in patients with autism and mitochondrial disorders. Similarly to Weissman and colleagues and Shoffner and colleagues, there was a high prevalence of motor delay (51%), regression (52%), fatigue/lethargy (54%), ataxia (58%), and GI abnormalities (74%).[43,45,64] Interestingly, there was not a significant difference in the prevalence of hypotonia between patients with ASD and a primary mitochondrial disorder compared with ASD in isolation, which was a feature commonly seen in cohort described by Shoffner and colleagues.[64] Compared with patients with mitochondrial disorders without ASD, patients with the dual diagnosis had significantly higher levels of lethargy, ataxia, GI abnormalities, and elevated lactate but not rates of male gender, developmental regression, seizures, hypotonia, cardiomyopathy, or myopathy. There was no difference in the prevalence of respiratory chain (complex I-V) deficiencies between the 2 groups. The most common deficiency noted in patients with the dual diagnosis was complex I (53%). Muscle pathologic studies suggested that the presence of abnormal histology was more frequent with an isolated mitochondrial disease over those with a dual diagnosis, supporting the findings by Shoffner and colleagues[64] in their cohort.

In patients with autism spectrum disorder, special attention has been paid to patients with an autistic regression. The occurrence of developmental regression in patients with autism has been discussed in the literature since its early reports in 1964.[71] The significance of this regression is not fully understood. In a recent metaanalysis of 85 articles representing 29,035 individuals with ASD, the prevalence rate of autistic regression was estimated to be 32.1%.[72] An "autistic regression" typically involves the loss of previously acquired language and social skills, in keeping with the archetypal features of the autism diagnosis. Similarly, in patients with primary mitochondrial disorders, metabolic decompensation associated with neurodegeneration is a frequent manifestation.[67] Psychomotor regression often occurs after encountering stressors, such as fever or infection. In a prior cohort of patients with mitochondrial disorders, intercurrent infection was a precipitant of neurodegeneration in 33% of patients and 72% of all metabolic decompensations occurred in the setting of an infection.[73] The mechanism of infection-mediated metabolic decompensation in mitochondrial disease is also unknown. However, considering that regression is a common manifestation of mitochondrial disease, authors have sought to determine whether the regression found in a subset of patients with ASD could be secondary to an underlying mitochondrial disorder.

Studies looking at the patterns of regression in patients with "mitochondrial autism" compared with those with an isolated ASD diagnosis have suggested that regression is more common and often atypical in the former. Regression of previously acquired skills has been identified in more than one-half of patients ($\leq$61%) with a dual diagnosis of a mitochondrial disorder and ASD,[45,64] which is nearly double the figures described in the general ASD populace. Of the patients who exhibit regression, Weissman and colleagues[45] found that atypical features of the regression included (1) a late-onset regression (>3 years) in 43% (6/14), (2) simultaneous motor regression in addition to language and/or social regression in 43% (6/14), and (3) multiple regressions in 64% (9/14). Considering the commonality of regression in patients with a dual diagnosis, its presence should alert the clinician to the possibility of a mitochondrial underpinning to the patient's autism diagnosis.[67]

Illness-induced reduced electron transport chain enzyme activity or oxidative phosphorylation (OXPHOS) activity with increased temperature, particularly in cell lines extracted from patients with identified mitochondrial disease who have established dysfunctional OXPHOS at baseline.[74–77] Similarly, in some patients with ASD who have an autistic regression, the deterioration in social and/or language skills seems to follow an infection-induced fever. In a small percentage of these patients, a definite diagnosis of mitochondrial disease is later established. Shoffner and colleagues completed a retrospective chart review and identified 28 patients that met diagnostic criteria for both ASD (DSM-IV-TR[32]) and definite mitochondrial disease.[17,18,64] In the patients who exhibited an autistic regression, fever secondary to a presumed infection was temporally associated to the deterioration in 70.6%.[64] Similarly, Weissman and colleagues[45] determined that 50% of patients who exhibited regression did so in the face of an infection or another metabolic stressor. Physicians managing patients with mitochondrial disease are routinely aggressive with fever control and hydration; therefore, it is important to find those patients with autism who may have an underlying mitochondrial disease.

Although fever often develops in the presence of an immunization, the association of immunizations and regression, particularly in patients with a dual diagnosis of ASD and mitochondrial disease, is an area of controversy. At this time, there is no evidence that the immunization itself is associated with the development of either ASD or mitochondrial disease.

Genetics in mitochondrial autism

With the expansion of our capacity to perform sophisticated genetic testing, the genetic underpinning of autism has become a leading research question. It has long been identified that autism has a strong genetic component.[78–84] Twin studies suggest a 70% to 90% concordance rate in monozygotic twins and 10% for dizygotic twins, a 25-fold risk in other siblings, and a high incidence of autistic behavioral traits.[85] Within the last decade, enhanced genetic testing has elucidated the genetic changes of a subset of patients with ASD.[40,41] However, no single genomic change seems to account for more than 1% to 2% of ASD cases. All genetic defects considered together may explain 10% to 20% of ASD cases.[85,86] Recently, interest has been given to the role of both mitochondrial genes and nuclear genes involved in mitochondrial function in the etiology of autism.

The role of mtDNA encoded mutations in patients with ASD has been suggested by multiple case reports.[50,53,54] The most frequently associated mutation in the literature associated with neuropsychiatric disorders is the m.3243A>G mutation. The m.3243A>G mutation is within the coding region of mtDNA for the gene *MT-TL1*, the specific tRNA for leucine (tRNA$^{Leu(UUR)}$). Although considered the "common MELAS mutation," depending on the heteroplasmy of the mtDNA-encoded mutation, it can also give rise to other phenotypically distinct syndromes, such as maternally inherited diabetes and deafness (MIDD).[87–92] In addition, the m.3243 A>G mutation can give rise to other clinical findings in patients who do not meet the criteria for one of the specific syndromes.[87–92] Pons and colleagues[54] screened for the m.3243A>G mutation in 5 patients with ASD and a family history suggestive of maternal inheritance or with a known family history of a mitochondrial disorder. The m.3243A>G mutation was identified in 2 of 5 patients (in hair follicles in 1 patient and in muscle, blood, urinary sediment, oral mucosa, and hair follicles in another). Two other patients were negative for the m.3243A>G mutation in any tissue sampled, but the mutation was identified in samples from their mothers. Considering the association of the m.3243A>G mutation and other psychiatric diagnoses and the suggestion that psychiatric features often precede the development of more typical features of MELAS or the other phenotypes associated with this mutation, the authors proposed that the ASD may be an early clinical presentation in children harboring the m.3243A>G mutation. The genetic background is likely important, because many patients with this mutation do not have ASD. In a study of 810 individuals with ASD, only 0.2% of individuals had a mutation in m.3243A>G.[93] Similarly, in another study of 129 individuals with Asperger syndrome and 138 mothers of patients with Asperger syndrome, no m.3243A>G mutation was identified.[94]

Another mtDNA mutation that has been implicated in ASD is the m.8363G>A mutation, which is in the coding region of the gene, *MT-TK*, which encodes for the tRNA (tRNA^{Lys}). Graf and colleagues[53] found the m.8363G>A mutation in a family that presented with variable neuropsychiatric features, including a child with autism. The affected child presented with language delay, with the inability to speak more than 10 to 20 single words or 2-word phrases. He developed a regression in his second year of life, with the loss of speech and play skills, and was subsequently diagnosed as autistic. At the time he was evaluated at the age of 3.5 years, he still had absence of all functional and expressive language, demonstrated hyperactive and injurious behavior, and had developed focal seizures. One of the authors (R.P.S.) had followed this patient until he was 18 years of age and his phenotype had not changed. All biochemical studies were within normal limits and his muscle biopsy showed nonspecific changes. Heteroplasmy analysis revealed the presence of the m.8363G>A mutation at 60% in blood and 61% in muscle. In the literature, the m.8363G>A mutation has been associated with cardiomyopathy, hearing loss, myopathy, ataxia, MERRF, and Leigh syndrome.[95–100] This case was the first, and currently the only, association of autism with this mutation.

Deletions and duplications of small chromosomal segment(s) result in an abnormal variation in the number of copies of one or more sections of DNA, known as copy number variations (CNVs). These variations are the most prevalent type of structural variations in the human genome, accounting for approximately 13% of human genomic nDNA, and range from 1 kilobase to several megabases in size.[101–103] CNVs are emerging as important etiologic factors in various neuropsychiatric disorders, including autism.[50,54,104–112] Research on CNVs altering mtDNA functioning is only beginning to be investigated. Fillano and colleagues[50] analyzed a group of 12 children presenting with hypotonia, epilepsy, autism, and developmental delay (HEADD) and identified multiple mtDNA deletions or a large 7.4-kb mtDNA deletion in 42% of a small sample of patients. Similarly, Smith and colleagues[110] found mtDNA deletions of varying length (9.7–13.7kb) in 67% of children (8/12) with ASD. Recently, increased copy numbers of 3 mtDNA-encoded genes (*ND1* and *ND4* encoding for complex I subunits and *CytB* encoding for a complex III subunit) were identified in lymphocytes in 50% of subjects with autism in on cohort secondary to mtDNA overreplication.[111] To identify if mtDNA CNVs existed in pathologic brain samples, Gu and colleagues[105] investigated post mortem frontal lobe cortical samples from 14 autistic subjects and identified increased copy numbers of *ND1, ND4,* and *CytB* mtDNA segments in 44%. Small deletions were identified in *ND4* and *CytB* in 44% and 33%, respectively. It is hypothesized that increased mtDNA copy number variants in autism may represent a mechanism to compensate for decreased complex I or III activity, which has been reported by multiple studies, that may result in chronic oxidative stress.[45,51,64,105] Alternatively, the higher mtDNA copy number may result from a compensatory mechanism to increase wild-type mtDNA templates so that normal levels of mitochondrial transcripts can be maintained.[113] CNV occurs not only in the mtDNA segments, but also in nDNA segments of children with autism.[104,106–109,114] Sebat and colleagues[108] reported a strong association of de novo CNVs in in nDNA and autism. CNVs involving duplications at 1q21.1, 7q11.23, 15q11-13, and 22q11.21 and deletions at 16p11.2 have been suggested as risk factors.[106,115–118] The role of CNVs (both mtDNA and nDNA) in autism is a blooming area of research and more studies are anticipated.

The role of nDNA mutations that impact mitochondrial function has been less systematically reviewed in the ASD population. Three candidate genes have also been further explored in autism: *IMMP2L, SLC25A12,* and *MARK1.* Two studies have examined the inner mitochondrial peptidase 2-like gene (*IMMP2L*).[119,120] Eleven studies have investigated the role of expression or single nucleotide polymorphisms (SNPs) in the gene for calcium-dependent mitochondrial aspartate/glutamate carrier isoform 1 (*SLC25A12*).[57,121–130] The evidence for the role of either of these genes was mixed and inconclusive. It is suggested that this may be secondary to small sample size and the clinical/genetic heterogeneity of the populations involved.[43] The other nDNA gene involved in mitochondrial function that has been linked to autism is the gene for the microtubule affinity regulating kinase 1 gene (*MARK1*), which is associated with mitochondrial trafficking. Several SNPs have been associated with ASD. Additionally, overexpression of *MARK1* was demonstrated in post mortem samples from the frontal cortex of individuals with ASD.[131] mtDNA depletion, which is typically secondary to nDNA mutations, has been found in a single patient with autism and mitochondrial dysfunction. A 72% mtDNA depletion was found in skeletal of this patient, but the mechanism was not noted.[52] At this time, no critical association between ASD and an nDNA gene associated with mitochondrial function has been found.

Overall, in a recent metaanalysis, only 21% of children with a confirmed ASD and primary mitochondrial disorder diagnosis had an identifiable mtDNA, nDNA, or chromosomal abnormality.[43] Therefore, although there have been advances in the understanding of the genetics in both primary mitochondrial disease and ASD, there remain many patients who are left without a known genetic underpinning.

NEUROPSYCHIATRIC FEATURES IN PRIMARY MITOCHONDRIAL DISEASE IN ADULTS

Many adult patients with primary mitochondrial disorders exhibit psychiatric comorbidities. Two large cohorts of patients with disorders of oxidative phosphorylation have been investigated for psychiatric comorbidities. Fattal and colleagues[132] found that the lifetime prevalence of neuropsychiatric diagnoses in their cohort of 36 patients with mitochondrial cytopathy far exceeded the rates seen in the general population, including major depressive disorder (MDD; 54%), bipolar disorder (17%), and panic disorder (11%). Psychiatric symptoms preceded the diagnosis of a mitochondrial disorder by an average of 7.5 years.[132] Similarly, an overall lifetime prevalence of psychiatric diagnoses in patients with mitochondrial disease was 47% in a separate cohort of 19 patients.[133] Most recently, Anglin and colleagues[134] completed a thorough review of the literature investigating the presentation of different psychiatric illnesses in patients with mitochondrial disorders. From their case series of 12 patients and the 50 cases identified in the literature, the most common neuropsychiatric manifestations were those of MDD (44%), psychotic disorders (34%), and anxiety disorders (12%). In a majority of patients, psychiatric symptoms preceded the development of physical symptoms associated with, and the diagnosis of, their underlying mitochondrial disorder, providing support for the notion that psychiatric features were secondary to the mitochondrial disease diagnosis.

In adult patients with psychiatric diagnoses, several features should prompt consideration of an underlying mitochondrial disorder.[134] These features include a past history of multiple medical problems affecting several organs; a significant family medical history of mitochondrial symptoms, multiple medical problems, or unusual neurologic symptoms (not limited to maternal inheritance); and treatment resistance or worsening clinical status with psychotropic medications. The presence of comorbid psychiatric disorders in patients with mitochondrial diseases is associated with a worse overall prognosis, with significantly more hospital admissions, more medical conditions, and a lesser quality of life compared with patients with mitochondrial disease without coexistent psychiatric diagnoses.[132] This confluence suggests that the identification of psychiatric comorbidities in patients with mitochondrial disease or the identification of an underlying mitochondrial disorder in patients presenting with psychiatric features is paramount so that effective treatment for both the psychiatric condition and the primary mitochondrial disorder can be instituted.

MOOD DISORDERS
Depression

MDD is characterized by 1 or more episodes of depressed mood, anhedonia, poor concentration, changes in appetite, sleep, and/or energy, feelings of worthlessness or guilt, and suicidality.[33] The DSM-IV-TR previously recognized dysthymia as an entity to describe a milder, albeit more chronic low mood; however, this has recently been replaced in the DSM-V with persistent depressive disorder.[32,33] Both MDD and persistent depressive disorder have a major impact on quality of life. The lifetime prevalence of MDD is 16.2%, with a majority of patients (72.1%) also meeting criteria for a comorbid DSM diagnosis.[135] The etiology of depression, much like many other psychiatric diagnoses, is believed to be a combination of an underlying genetic predisposition with the contribution of environmental factors. Depression is known to be a comorbid symptom of various somatic diseases, including hypothyroidism, Parkinson disease, Huntington disease, migraine, and dementia.[136–138] Additionally, illness in general and chronic disease in particular increases the risk for depression in vulnerable individuals.[139,140] The role of mitochondrial dysfunction in the pathophysiology of depression has garnered significant interest in recent years, with particular attention paid to the area of genetics.

Mitochondrial genetics in patients with depression
Evidence suggests that patients with primary mitochondrial disease secondary to either nDNA-encoded or mtDNA-encoded mutations can have affective symptoms.[141–149] Patients with proven mitochondrial disorders demonstrate a 3.9 times increased risk for the comorbidity of major depression, with a lifetime prevalence in these patients of 54%.[132,150] Although it may be difficult at times to distinguish between a mental reaction to a physical disorder and a primary mental disorder diagnosis, the high comorbidity data suggest that psychiatric conditions in patients with mitochondrial disease may be directly related to primary nuclear or mtDNA alteration.[132,150]

Multiple case reports in the literature suggest that pathogenic mtDNA-encoded point mutations are associated with the development of depressive symptoms.[148,149,151,152] Koene and colleagues[153] evaluated 35 patients for a history of depression in patients in whom a genetically confirmed mtDNA- or nDNA-encoded mitochondrial disease had been established. Of the 35 patients, a diagnosis of MDD was confirmed in 14.3%. Two patients had point mutations in mtDNA, m.3460G>A in the gene encoding for NADH dehydrogenase subunit 1 (*ND1*), commonly seen in Leber hereditary optic neuropathy, and m.8344A>G in the gene encoding for tRNA^Lys (*MT-TK*), commonly associated with MERRF.[154] Subsequently, a second case of depressed mood in associated with the m.8344A>G mutation was described.[151] Molnar and colleagues[151] presented a case series of a mother and her twin sons with the m.8344A>G mutation who all suffered from depression and anxiety before the development of neurologic features (proximal muscle weakness, sensorineural hearing loss, peripheral neuropathy, and ataxia). The heteroplasmy of the m.8344A>G mutation was correlated with the degree of severity of the psychiatric symptoms, with the mother showing the largest heteroplasmy (82% in muscle, 46% in blood) and the most severe psychiatric symptoms (recurrent episodes of psychotic depression). None of the patients developed typical features associated with the MERRF phenotype.

Patients with the m.3243A>G in *MT-TL1*, encoding for a specific tRNA (tRNA^Leu(UUR))[148,149,155] seem to be overrepresented in the literature describing neuropsychiatric manifestations of mitochondrial disease, including depression. Anglin and colleagues[134] completed a thorough review of the literature on patients with mitochondrial disorders presenting with prominent psychiatric symptoms. In their review, they determined that the m.3243A>G mutation was the most common mitochondrial syndrome associated with a mental disorder presentation (52%). Onishi and colleagues[149] described a 22-year-old man with a family history of maternal diabetes and a personal history of sensorineural hearing loss and Wolff–Parkinson–White syndrome, who presented with depressed mood, anxiety, and generalized fatigue. After initially responding to antidepressant therapy, he developed a major depressive episode 1 year later. He was found to have m.3243A>G at 37% heteroplasmy in blood. His depressive symptoms and cerebral blood flow as measured by single photon emission computed tomography gradually improved on a combination of coenzyme Q10 and idebenone. Subsequently, Miyaoka and colleagues[148] assessed patients presenting with diabetes for comorbid mood or anxiety disorders and the m.3243A>G mutation. Of 205 patients with diabetes mellitus, 9 (4.4%) were found to be positive for the m.3243A>G mutation. Of these, 44.4% had comorbid mental disorders, including a patient presenting with recurrent major depressive episodes beginning at age 47 years. However, depressive disorders have been described in 8.5% to 18% of patients with diabetes[156,157]; therefore, it is difficult to discern whether the patient's symptoms in this particular case were secondary to mitochondrial dysfunction rather than the diabetes itself. It has been proposed that white matter abnormalities, which are seen in up to 90% of patients with mitochondrial disorders[158] and are common in patients with the m. 3243A>G mutation, may play an important role in psychiatric presentations of mitochondrial disease. Disruption of pathways connecting different parts of the brain involved in emotion, thought, and behavior may be paramount to the pathophysiology.[134]

Another mtDNA-encoded mutation that can give rise to the MELAS syndrome, m.3271T>C in the *MT-TL1* gene encoding for tRNA (tRNA^Leu(UUR)), has also been seen in association with depressive features. Anglin and colleagues[155] presented a case of a woman presenting with recurrent and treatment-resistant MDD with psychotic features and borderline personality disorder beginning in adolescence. She had persistent fatigue and developed diabetes, progressive cognitive decline, ptosis, dystonia, muscle weakness, and ataxia as an adult. Her family history revealed mental illness in her mother and 3 siblings and dementia of unknown etiology in maternal relatives. An MRI revealed significant white matter pathology, prompting an evaluation for an underlying cause of her neuropsychiatric features. Genetic testing revealed the m.3271T>C mutation in the *MT-TL1* gene in fibroblasts, which was not found in the patient's blood on 2 separate occasions. This case calls attention to the fact that tissue and urine samples are often more sensitive in demonstrating mtDNA mutations that may be missed if only blood is tested.

In addition to the role of single mtDNA mutations, there is some suggestion that accumulation of mtDNA deletions can also predispose to affective disorders. Suomalainen and colleagues[144] presented the case of a patient with severe, recurrent episodes of major depression who later developed ptosis and ophthalmoplegia. She had multiple family members (including her mother, 4 siblings, and 3 nieces and nephews) with similar symptoms, including a "tendency to depressive mood." Autopsy demonstrated multiple mtDNA deletions on Southern blot from various tissues, including the frontal cortex and basal ganglia, which were analyzed specifically owing to her predominant symptom of altered mood. These findings suggest that the development of depressive disorder may be associated with the accumulation of multiple mtDNA deletions in areas of the brain that play a predominant role in mood and affect. A subsequent study by the Suomalainen and colleagues[159] reported 2 patients fulfilling criteria for MDD in an 11-subject cohort with autosomal dominant CPEO and multiple mtDNA deletions. Ciafaloni and colleagues[143] similarly reported a mother and daughter pair with CPEO and affective disorder who demonstrated multiple DNA deletions in muscle tissue. However, pathologic samples from the brain were not assessed. Gardner and colleagues[150] identified a higher load of mtDNA deletions in the muscle of patients with depressive disorder compared with controls. However, 2 studies looking at pathologic samples from the frontal cortices of patients with MDD failed to find a higher deletion load.[160,161] Therefore, at this point, the evidence for the role of mtDNA deletions in MDD is controversial and requires further investigation.

The role of single nucleotide variants (SNVs) in the mtDNA genome in major depression has been investigated. An SNV is a variation at a single nucleotide base within a DNA sequence, either mtDNA or nDNA. When seen at a frequency of greater than 1% in the population, an SNV is considered a polymorphism (SNP). Two studies of mtDNA sequence variants in post mortem brain tissue in patients with major depression have been undertaken.[162,163] Neither study found any association between sequence variants or mutations in the mtDNA and MDD. A single study sequenced the mitochondrial genome in a single case with depression and epilepsy with a maternal psychiatric history and identified 34 base substitutions.[164] However, no mitochondrial impairment could be identified in transmitochondrial cybrids; therefore, the relevance of this finding is unclear. At the current time, the role of SNVs in the mtDNA genome in depression is uncertain.

Mood disorders have also been reported in patients with nDNA genes that are involved in mtDNA replication and integrity, such as *POLG1*. *POLG1* encodes the only known mtDNA polymerase. Transgenic mice expressing a mutant *POLG1* gene and resulting mtDNA deletions show characteristic behavioral patterns associated with depression, including reduced appetite, reduced wheel running, a distorted circadian rhythm, and a robust periodic activity pattern associated with the estrous cycle.[165] In a series of patients with *POLG1* and a mitochondrial recessive ataxia syndrome (MIRAS) phenotype, Hakonen and colleagues[166] noted that more than one-half of the cases in their series had evidence of psychiatric symptoms, including depression. Koene and colleagues[153] also reported on a single patient who had a mutation in *POLG1* who developed depressive symptoms. She presented with muscle cramps, epilepsy, and migraine, and subsequently developed dysphoria and apathy. She died of fulminant hepatic failure when valproic acid (VPA) was initiated for the combination of seizures and hallucinations.

Differential expression of mitochondria-related genes may also be involved in the pathogenesis of depression. Shao and colleagues[161] found a significantly decreased expression of mitochondrial-related transcripts in the dorsolateral prefrontal cortex. Their findings continued to be statistically significant after adjustment for age, gender, and pH. Vawter and colleagues[167] initially found a lesser expression of mitochondrial-related transcripts in patients with depression; however, they were no longer be significant after adjustment for pH. Three additional studies failed to demonstrate altered mitochondria-related gene expression in the frontal cortex or the hippocampus.[162,168,169] Despite these results, there is some suggestion that alteration of complex I subunit expression may be important. Complex I subunit mRNA expression was increased in the parietooccipital cortex, unchanged in the striatum, and decreased in the cerebellum.[170,171]

Depression in children differs from depression in adults in multiple ways. Depression in children is much less common, with a prevalence of 1% to 4%.[172] In pediatric patients with mitochondrial disease, it seems that the risk for depressive mood or depressive behaviors exceeds that which would be expected in chronic diseases or other inborn errors of metabolism. Morava and colleagues[152] investigated the psychological characteristics of 18 pediatric patients diagnosed with a primary mitochondrial disorder using a Child Behavior Checklist. These authors found that children with a mitochondrial disease diagnosis exhibited a significantly higher rate of withdrawn, depressive behavior compared with both a control group of children with a nonprogressive, chronic neurologic condition (Sotos syndrome) and children with inborn errors of metabolism (fatty acid oxidation disorders, galactosemia, organic acidemias, glycogen storage disorders, and phenylketonuria). The occurrence of depressive behavior showed no correlation with the clinical severity or degree of mitochondrial dysfunction assessed by biochemical analysis of skeletal muscle. However, the authors rightfully questioned whether the overlap of certain features of oxidative phosphorylation disorders and those of depression (such as decreased activity, fatigue, poor sleep) could contribute to a bias in the data.

Bipolar Disorder

Bipolar disorder is a psychiatric condition in which there are extreme shifts in mood, resulting in periods of emotional highs (mania) and lows (depression), producing marked impairment in daily functioning.[33] Bipolar disorder is believed to affect approximately 1% of the population. Although the etiology of bipolar disorder is unknown, it is believed to result from a combination of genetic and environmental factors.[173,174] Several candidate loci have been linked with bipolar disorder[175]; however, no single gene has been identified as causative. Recently, there has been significant interest in the role of mitochondrial dysfunction in the pathophysiology of bipolar disorder.

Studies suggested that an abnormality in mitochondrial function existed in a subset of patients with bipolar owing to (1) structural abnormalities in mitochondria identified in patients with bipolar disorder, (2) abnormal brain phosphorus metabolism detected by ^{31}P magnetic resonance spectroscopy (MRS), (3) altered markers of oxidative stress in bipolar disorder, (4) possible contribution of parent-of-origin effect in the transmission of bipolar disorders in families, (5) increased levels of mitochondrial polymorphisms, point mutations, and deletions in serum or post mortem brain samples from patients with bipolar disorder, (6) phenotypes of animal models with mitochondrial dysfunction, and (7) comorbidity of affective disorders in patients with established primary mitochondrial disease diagnoses.

Mitochondrial structural and functional abnormalities in bipolar disorder

One of the first lines of evidence suggesting a link between mitochondrial dysfunction and bipolar disorder is the demonstration of structural abnormalities of the mitochondria in bipolar disorder affected patients.[176–178] Uranova and colleagues[176,177] investigated the ultrastructural appearance of pathologic samples from patients with bipolar disorder and schizophrenia. They found decreased numbers and size of mitochondria within oligodendrocytes in the caudate nucleus and prefrontal cortex.[177] However, it is unclear whether these changes were related directly to their underlying diagnosis or if they were secondary to medication effect. Subsequently, Cataldo and colleagues[178] investigated the appearance of mitochondria in post mortem brain and peripheral samples from patients with bipolar disorder. They found changes in mitochondrial size and distribution: intracranial mitochondria were significantly smaller in area compared with controls and extracranial mitochondria were concentrated within the perinuclear region. These changes seemed to be independent of lithium exposure and independent of changes of surrounding neuropil structure. Further studies are required to delineate the structural changes of mitochondria found in larger populations of patients with bipolar disorder.

Additional support for abnormal oxidative phosphorylation in patients with bipolar disorder comes from neuroimaging studies. Studies using ^{31}P MRS in patients with bipolar disorder have demonstrated decreased intracellular pH in the euthymic state and decreased phosphocreatine in the depressed state within the frontal lobes, which is hypothesized to be secondary to mitochondrial dysfunction.[179–181] Dager and colleagues[182] demonstrated that patients with bipolar disorder exhibited significantly increased gray matter lactate levels compared with healthy controls, suggesting a shift from oxidative phosphorylation toward glycolysis. However, these findings are inconsistent; other studies using proton MRS have failed to find similar changes in patients with bipolar disorder compared with controls.[183] One of the most convincing lines of neuroradiologic evidence suggesting that mitochondrial dysfunction in specific brain regions can give psychiatric symptoms is from Anglin and associates.[184] These authors demonstrated that there were altered metabolite signals in the hippocampus and cingulate cortex on proton MRS in patients with mitochondrial disease and concurrent psychiatric diagnoses. Overall impairment of functioning owing to the psychiatric symptoms correlated with metabolic markers in the cingulate cortex.

Altered markers of oxidative stress in bipolar disorder

There is some evidence that oxidative stress is thought to mediate neuropathologic processes of a number of neuropsychiatric disorders, including bipolar disorder. The mitochondria play a role in producing reactive oxygen species (ROS). Under normal conditions, the mitochondria are a major source of ROS, produced in the complexes of the respiratory chain. However, if sufficient ROS are generated to overwhelm the innate antioxidant systems, oxidative stress results in inhibition of the respiratory chain, resulting in a decreased production of ATP and cellular dysfunction. The brain is particularly vulnerable to ROS production because it metabolizes 20% of total body oxygen and has a limited amount of antioxidant capacity.[185] Multiple studies have reported increased products of lipid peroxidation and alterations of the major antioxidant enzymes in patients with bipolar disorder.[186–194] Wang and colleagues[190] demonstrated a significant increase of 4-hydroxynonenal (a product of lipid peroxidation) in post mortem samples from the anterior cingulate in patients with bipolar disorder, suggesting a role for oxidative dysfunction. Decreased levels of mitochondrial complex I subunits and increased protein oxidation and nitration in post mortem samples from the prefrontal cortex in patients with bipolar disorder was subsequently found by other groups.[192,195] Although oxidative stress markers as a means to determine bipolar disorder vulnerability have generated interest,[196] further studies are required before implementation in clinical practice.

Parent-of-origin effects in bipolar disorder

Multiple studies investigating the heritability of bipolar disorder in families have suggested a gender-specific mode of transmission. In early studies of bipolar disorder, male-to-male transmission was deemed rare.[197] Therefore, an X-linked inheritance was presumed. In the 1960s, it was believed that X-linkage alone could not explain the pattern of inheritance of bipolar disorder and a mitochondrial inheritance was considered a possibility after the discovery of mtDNA.[198] Then in the mid 1990s linkage studies suggested a maternal "parent-of-origin" effect, with affected mothers being more common than affected fathers.[199–201] The parent-of-origin effect is the phenomenon in which gender of the transmitting patent affects the expression of illness in their offspring without following Mendelian laws. Further studies supported the idea of a parent-of-origin effect by showing that more maternal relatives are affected by bipolar disorder than paternal relatives.[199,202] Although this finding is not universal in all studies investigating the genetic contribution to bipolar disease, there is some suggestion that maternal inheritance is present at least in some patients afflicted with the disorder.

Single nucleotide polymorphisms and haplotypes in bipolar disorder

Various mtDNA SNPs are believed to play a role in the pathophysiology of bipolar disorder.[203–208] Many of those identified as playing a role in bipolar disorder involve mtDNA SNPs in complex I subunits. McMahon and associates[207] investigated mtDNA SNPs in pedigrees from patients with bipolar disorder in whom maternal inheritance was evident. They identified 4 SNPs that were more common in probands. Although not significant in this study, other subsequent studies have demonstrated their significance. Studies by Kato and colleagues[203,204] demonstrated that the m.10398A>G SNP was associated significantly with the bipolar disorder compared with controls. This SNP alters an evolutionarily conserved threonine into an alanine in the mitochondrial-encoded NADH dehydrogenase (complex I) subunit-3 (MT-ND3) gene. This SNP is reported at polymorphism frequencies in various ethnicities (30%–64%)[209,210] and is not likely to be of etiologic importance in mitochondrial disease, although its effects on NADH dehydrogenase have not been examined.[211] There is also some evidence that it plays a role in intracellular calcium dynamics[212] and glucose utilization.[213] There is also a suggestion that patients with this polymorphism may have better response to lithium.[214]

A second SNP, m.5178C>A, has also been identified as being more frequently seen in patients with bipolar disorder compared with control subjects.[203] The nucleotide change results in the substitution of a methionine instead of leucine in the NADH-dehydrogenase (complex I) subunit-2 gene (ND2). This SNP was significantly more common in leukocytes in patients with bipolar disorder compared with controls.[203]

The presence of both the m.10398A>G and m.5178C>A polymorphisms, known as the C/A haplotype, may increase the susceptibility to bipolar disorder than each polymorphism alone.[204] Kato and colleagues[204] found that the coexpression of both polymorphisms was significantly more common in those with bipolar disorder. The C/A haplotype was found in 33.6% of subjects, compared with 16.8% of control patients (a relative risk of 2.4). However, more studies are required to determine the significance of the synergistic effect of these polymorphisms in the etiology of bipolar disease.

One other polymorphism that warrants mention is the m.3644T>C in the gene for a complex I NADH dehydrogenase subunit 1 subunit (*ND1*). This polymorphism was identified as being significantly associated with bipolar disorder. Munakata and colleagues[208] identified several homoplasmic, nonsynonymous SNPs in 6 patients with bipolar disorder and symptoms suggestive of mitochondrial disorder. Multiple other mtDNA SNPs have been reported in bipolar disorder patients at a lower frequency including those in complex I subunits (m.3316G>A and m.3394T>C in the ND1 subunit; m.10084T>C and m.10398A>G in the ND3 subunit; complex V subunits (m.8537A>G, m.8563A>G in ATPase6); tRNA genes (m.1662C>T, m.5539A>G, m.5592A>G, m.5773G>A, m.5821G>A, m.10410T>C, and m.10427G>A); rRNA genes (m.63A>G, m.709G>A, m.769G>A, m.794T>C, m.3206C>T); a variant in the L-strand replication site (m.5747A>G); and several silent polymorphisms.[204] Three of these variants (m.5539A>G in tRNA^{Trp}, m.5747A>G in the L-strand replication site, and m.8537A>G in ATPase6) may be of more significance because they cause amino acid substitutions at evolutionarily conserved sites and merit further investigation.[204] However, it is difficult to interpret the significance of these variants without larger samples of bipolar patients.

Not all studies have identified mtDNA SNPs in their bipolar disorder patient cohorts.[206] Kirk and colleagues[206] sequenced the entire mitochondrial genome in 25 probands of maternally inherited pedigrees with bipolar disorder, but found no associated polymorphisms or variants attaining significance. It should also be noted, that although associations of SNPs and bipolar disorder have been explored, it is unclear how these mtDNA polymorphisms affect the vulnerability to bipolar disorder. If and how these variants lead to changes to protein structure and function needs to be elucidated to establish any pathophysiologic significance.

In addition to polymorphisms reported in the mtDNA in patients with bipolar disorder, there is some evidence to suggest that polymorphic variants in nDNA-encoded mitochondrial genes may also have a role in bipolar genetic susceptibility.[170,214–217] Several prior studies have provided evidence for the linkage of chromosome 18 with bipolar disorder.[201,218–225] *NDUFV2*, encoding the 24-kDa subunit of complex I in the respiratory chain (NADH dehydrogenase flavoprotein 2) is located at chromosome 18p11,[226,227] close to the loci identified in prior linkage studies. Therefore, it has been hypothesized that polymorphisms in *NDUFV2* may be associated with psychiatric illness. Washizuka and colleagues[214,216,228] identified 5 polymorphisms in *NDUFV2* (c.602A>G, c.3542G>A, c.3245T>G, c.3041T>C and c.2694A>G) associated with bipolar disorder in different ethnicities. The CTAT haplotype for 4 polymorphisms in *NDUFV2* that are strongly linked (c.796C>G, c.795T>G, c.602G>A, and c.233T>C) is significantly less common in those with bipolar disorder compared with control subjects.[216] Although the effect of these polymorphisms on complex I activity has not been thoroughly explored, many of these polymorphisms exist around the promoter region of *NDUFV2*. The c.602A>G polymorphism, also associated with a higher likelihood of being diagnosed with bipolar disorder, has been shown to promote activity through a loss of binding capacity to a transcription factor.[216] Doyle and colleagues[215] also concluded that promoter haplotypes seem to be associated with bipolar disorder in the Caucasian population. However, the exact mechanism by which this alters complex I activity and leads to a higher susceptibility to bipolar disorder is inconclusive.

The role of mtDNA haplogroups has been investigated in patients with bipolar disorder without consensus for disease association. A particular combination of SNPs in an individual's mtDNA (haplotype) is used to identify ancestral heritage and divide people into groups that share a common maternal ancestor. Three studies have investigated the role of haplogroups in bipolar disorder; however, no consistent findings have emerged. Kazuno and colleagues[205] identified an overrepresentation of haplogroup N9a in patients with bipolar disorder compared with controls. Alternatively, Rollins and colleagues[163] found a possible association between the pre-HV haplogroup and bipolar disorder. However, another study did not find any differences in haplogroup frequencies in patients with bipolar disorder.[207]

Mitochondrial DNA deletions and copy number variations in bipolar disorder

Deletions in the mitochondrial genome have been implicated in the pathogenesis of bipolar disorder.[147,162–164,207,208,214,229–233] Kato and Takahashi[147] reported that 2 of 35 patients (5.7%) with bipolar disorder harbored the common 4997 base-pair deletion in mtDNA isolated from leukocytes, suggesting that deletions of mtDNA in the brain may result in affective symptoms. Kato and colleagues[234] later reported that there was a significant increase in the 4997 base-pair deletion in mtDNA in autopsied brains of patients with bipolar disorder compared with normal controls. Although the ratio of partially deleted mtDNA was small (<0.6%), this seemed to be a reflection of increased free radical generation, resulting in an increased accumulation of mtDNA deletion in these patients. These findings were replicated by Shao and colleagues,[161] who identified a greater proportion of the common deletion in the dorsolateral prefrontal cortex of patients with bipolar disorder. Three subsequent studies have been unable to replicate these findings.[160,233,235]

Mitochondrial mtDNA CNVs have also been investigated in patients with various neuropsychiatric disorders. Each human cell contains hundreds to thousands of mitochondria, each of which contains multiple copies of mtDNA. Studies have suggested that maintaining an adequate mtDNA copy number may be important for cell viability.[236] Two studies have investigated the role of mitochondrial mtDNA copy numbers in patients with major depression, bipolar disorder, and schizophrenia.[167,233] Vawter and colleagues[167] looked at mtDNA copy number in the dorsolateral prefrontal cortex and identified a nonsignificant trend toward a lower copy number in patients with bipolar disorder compared with controls, which was not seen in patients with depression. Similarly, Kakiuchi and colleagues[233] found a nonsignificant trend toward decreased mtDNA copy number in patients with bipolar disorder but not schizophrenia. Overall, the current evidence for a role of mitochondrial mtDNA copy numbers in psychiatric illness is not persuasive.

Mitochondrial DNA mutations in bipolar disorder

Similar to depression, there seems to be an association between pathogenic mutations in mtDNA genes encoding for mitochondrial tRNAs and bipolar disorder. Munakata and colleagues[162] reexamined the DNA microarray data from post mortem prefrontal cortices from patients with various psychiatric diagnoses, including bipolar disorder, and the mtDNA m.3243A>G mutation.[237] In their series, they identified an increased expression of LARS2 (human leucyl-tRNA synthetase 2), which is responsible for the aminoacylation of tRNA^{Leu}. It is possible that LARS2 expression was a compensatory upregulation owing to accumulation of the mutation, m.3243A>G, which has been shown to decrease the efficiency of processing and aminoacylation of tRNA^{Leu}.[238–240] Interestingly, the detection of the m.3243A>G mutation may be related to the sensitivity of the testing used. This mutation was not identified in the prefrontal cortex or liver using conventional restriction fragment length polymorphism polymerase chain reaction (RFLP-PCR), but was identified using peptide nucleic acid–clamped RFLP-PCR, which has a much lower detection limit of 0.1%.[162] Further studies using the more sensitive detection methodology are necessary to investigate mtRNA and bipolar disorder.

Nuclear DNA mutations in bipolar disorder

Bipolar disorder has been reported in a subset of patients diagnosed with mtDNA depletion secondary to various pathogenic nDNA mutations involved in mitochondrial integrity and maintenance.[241–243] Siciliano and colleagues[241] reported on a 44-year-old woman who had a history of bipolar affective disorder with an onset in her teens. Lithium therapy was ineffective and she had frequent episodes of psychotic mania. At the age of 40 years, she developed ptosis and migraine headaches. She had an exaggerated lactate elevation during moderate exercise and a muscle biopsy demonstrating increased ragged red fibers and multiple cytochrome oxidase–negative fibers (>15%). Southern blot demonstrated multiple mtDNA deletions (accounting for 28% of mtDNA). Her older sister was similarly affected. Multiple family members demonstrated different combinations of ptosis, memory difficulties, and migraine headaches. Bipolar disorder was also diagnosed in 3 additional family members. The proband and her affected family members were subsequently found to harbor a pathologic mutation in ANT1 (p. L98P), which has been seen in patients with autosomal-dominant progressive external ophthalmoplegia. Psychiatric disturbances were also reported in a large Finnish family harboring a mutation in C10orf2 (encoding for Twinkle)[242] and a large Belgian family carrying a mutation in POLG1 (encoding for mitochondrial polymerase gamma).[243]

Differential expression of mitochondria-related nDNA genes has also been investigated in bipolar disorder. Studies have suggested that there is differential mitochondria-related gene expression in bipolar disorder compared with controls in post mortem samples from the prefrontal cortex[229,244]; however, these findings have not been replicated by other investigators.[161,162] Other authors have demonstrated inconsistent findings with respect to the expression of nuclear genes encoding subunits of the respiratory chain.[169,245,246] Authors have also investigated mRNA content as a maker of gene expression and have found significantly lower mRNA content for complex I subunits.[171] However, Karry and colleagues[170] reported the presence of a higher protein content of complex I subunits in the ventral parietooccipital cortex that was not associated with a higher mRNA expression.

Summary of mitochondrial dysfunction and affective disorders

Overall, multiple lines of evidence have suggested a role for mitochondrial dysfunction in some patients with depression and bipolar disorder. However, the mechanism by which mitochondrial dysfunction leads to a presentation of affective disorders is unclear. Genetic studies, particularly those investigating the genetic underpinnings of bipolar and depression, have been completed with small numbers of patients, different methodologies, and different endpoints giving inconsistent results. Considering the impact that affective disorders have on quality of life, particularly in those with a concurrent chronic illness (mitochondrial disease), it is important that large-scale, highly powered, and methodologically strong studies be completed to try to identify the link between affective disorders and mitochondrial dysfunction.

SCHIZOPHRENIA

Schizophrenia, one of the most devastating psychiatric disorders, has a lifetime prevalence of approximately 1% worldwide. Schizophrenia is believed to result from a combination of genetic vulnerability and environmental factors.[173,247,248] Genetic factors have long been proposed to be causal to the development of schizophrenia. First-degree relatives of schizophrenia are at higher risk for developing the illness (odds ratio [OR], 9.8) and the heritability of susceptibility of schizophrenia has been proposed to be 70% to 80%.[249-253] Recent studies attempting to identify the underlying genetic cause of schizophrenia have identified several possible involved polymorphisms and mutations.[254,255] However, delineation of the exact genetic cause of schizophrenia remains elusive, but is likely multifactorial in nature.

There are multiple pieces of evidence to suggest that mitochondrial dysfunction could be involved in the pathophysiology of schizophrenia[256,257]: (1) alterations in mitochondrial morphology, brain energy metabolism, and enzymatic activity of the respiratory chain in patients with schizophrenia, suggestive of mitochondrial dysfunction,[258,259] (2) the rates of schizophrenia are higher among relatives of female patients compared with relatives of male patients, implying possible maternal inheritance and a role of mtDNA,[257,260-270] (3) lower marriage rates and offspring production in probands with schizophrenia, suggesting its persistence could be explained only if genetic susceptibility variants are transmitted by mtDNA in female siblings,[271-280] (4) major psychiatric disorders in adult patients with mitochondrial disease,[256,281,282] and (5) sequence variants in the mitochondrial genome found in patients with schizophrenia.[147,162,163,228,229,233,283-285]

Mitochondrial Structural and Functional Abnormalities in Schizophrenia

Studies of mitochondrial structure and function in patients with schizophrenia have provided evidence for mitochondrial dysfunction in the etiology of the disorder. Several studies have demonstrated ultrastructural abnormalities in patients with schizophrenia.[176,177,286-291] These studies have demonstrated mitochondrial swelling and hyperplasia[286,287,289] as well as decreased mitochondrial density[176,177,288,290,291] in patients with schizophrenia compared with controls. Additionally, altered mitochondrial oxidative phosphorylation has been suggested in some patients with schizophrenia.[192,292-295] Several studies investigating patients with schizophrenia have suggested that altered complex I activity is associated with disease-symptoms.[292-294] Complex I and III activity has been shown to be significantly lower in post mortem temporal cortex and basal ganglia in patients with schizophrenia.[296] However, other studies of complex I activity in post mortem prefrontal cortices and the basal ganglia have not shown convincing findings of altered complex I activity.[192,295] Studies looking at cytochrome c oxidase (complex IV) activity have been similarly inconclusive. Some investigators have found lower complex IV activity in post mortem caudate, frontal, and temporal cortices and greater complex IV activity in the putamen and the nucleus accumbens in patients with schizophrenia.[295-297] However, another study found no demonstrable alterations in enzyme activity of any of the electron transport chain complexes in the dorsolateral prefrontal cortex in patients with schizophrenia.[298] Some authors have suggested that the dissimilar findings in post mortem studies may result from changes in complex activity with delay post mortem or may be the effects of different patterns in antipsychotic use in patients with schizophrenia.[299,300] Further studies are warranted to determine if any consistent patterns can be identified.

Parent-of-Origin Effects in Schizophrenia

Similar to bipolar disorder, there has been suggestion of a maternal parent-of-origin inheritance pattern in patients with schizophrenia. Reed and colleagues[265] first reported that mothers with psychosis produced approximately twice as many offspring with psychosis compared with fathers with psychosis. Shimizu and colleagues[260] reviewed the medical records or completed personal interviews with 1691 parents and siblings of inpatients meeting DSM-III criteria for schizophrenia. They found that 16.4% of the schizophrenic probands had at least 1 first-degree relative with schizophrenia, the risk of which was significantly greater in female compared with male probands. Multiple additional studies subsequently confirmed a greater risk of schizophrenia in relatives of female probands compared with male probands.[266–268]

Further studies have been published on the transmission patterns of schizophrenia using more strict diagnostic criteria, adjusted for gender-dependent age-of-onset differences, and adjusted for the effects of schizophrenia on fertility. Similar to prior studies, an increased risk to relatives of female probands was noted.[261,264,269,270] Goldstein and colleagues[301] reported that the rate of schizophrenia, schizophreniform, and schizoaffective disorders was significantly higher in relatives of affected schizoaffective females compared with affected males. However, when schizotypal personality disorder was included in the analysis, the sex differences in risk were less evident, suggesting relatives of female probands were only at risk for the psychotic forms of the illness spectrum.

Recently, Verge and colleagues[257] interviewed 100 patients with a DSM-IV diagnosis of schizophrenia and 147 of their relatives. Of the patients interviewed, 37% had familial schizophrenia ($\geq$1 first- or second-degree relative). Of the familial cases, 46% displayed strong evidence of a matrilineal pattern of inheritance (ie, only maternal relatives had a schizophrenia diagnosis) and an additional 32% had an affected maternal relative. In terms of familial risk, there was a significantly higher risk of presenting with schizophrenia if family members shared mtDNA with the proband compared with those that did not share mtDNA (OR = 3.05). Female relatives of the proband who shared mtDNA were also significantly at risk for other psychiatric disorders, including unipolar depression (OR, 10.19), panic attacks (OR = 15.52), and other anxiety disorders (OR = 4.14) compared with female relatives of the proband who did not share mtDNA. Risk of bipolar disorder and intellectual disability was not significantly greater in females who shared mtDNA compared with those that do not. Interestingly, male relatives of the proband who shared mtDNA were not at risk for any of these psychiatric conditions. This may be reflective of the fact that females are more susceptible to these disorders in general.

Mitochondrial DNA Single Nucleotide Polymorphisms, Synonymous Base Pair Substitutions, Haplogroups, and Mitochondrial DNA Gene-related Expression in Schizophrenia

Several groups have investigated sequence variations in the mitochondrial genome and schizophrenia. There seems to be a role for SNPs in the susceptibility for schizophrenia. Five studies have evaluated the entire mtDNA genome sequence in patients with schizophrenia.[283,284,302–304] Lindholm and colleagues[302] sequenced 2 patients with schizophrenia and low complex IV activity identified in post mortem brain pathologic samples and 2 related patients demonstrating possible mitochondrial inheritance. They identified 5 previously unreported substitutions in coding regions; however, these regions were not associated with schizophrenia in a larger sample.[302] They did identify 2 mutations in the mtDNA cytochrome b gene (*CytB*) at positions m.14793 and m.15218 that appeared at an increased frequency among patients with schizophrenia in 3 of 4 European cohorts, but this was not significant. Ueno and colleagues[303] identified 3 rare, nonsynonymous, homoplasmic variants (m.8843T>C, m.8902G>A, and m.8945T>C) in the subunit 6 of the ATP synthase (*MT-ATP6*) gene in patients with schizophrenia that were not present in controls. The amino acid substitutions identified were in highly conserved (>90%) areas of the gene and their physicochemical differences between the original and altered amino acid residues were relatively high, suggesting they were likely deleterious. In addition, 3 novel heteroplasmic variants were identified: m.1227G>A in *MT-RNR1* (encoding for 12S rRNA), m.5578T>C in the tRNA *MT-TW* gene, and the m.13418G>A in the NADH-dehydrogenase (complex I) *MT-ND5* gene.[303] Although the functional role of the 1227G>A mutation remains unclear, there is a role for the 5578T>C change in affecting tRNA end processing[305] and dysfunction of complex I in the 13418G>A SNP.[303] Martorell and colleagues[284] sequenced the mtDNA of 6 patients with an apparent maternal inheritance of schizophrenia and identified a large number (50) of sequence variants, including 6 novel variants and 3 missense variants, which were also present in the mtDNA of the schizophrenic mothers. In their cohort, the m.12096T>A variant in the NADH-dehydrogenase (complex I) *MT-ND4* gene was found in 5 mother–offspring pairs. Bamne and colleagues[283] did not find any mtDNA sequence differences between patients with schizophrenia and controls. Another study investigated 7 patients with acute confusion, emotional instability, and psychomotor changes ("atypical psychosis") and found no associated pathogenic mtDNA mutations.[304] Additionally, when investigating 3 polymorphisms (m.5460G>A and m.5460G>T in the *ND2* gene and polymorphisms in 12S rRNA) previously reported by other groups in a large sample of both Caucasian and African American cases, no association was found.[306] Together, these studies suggest that there is insufficient evidence at this time to support the involvement of a particular mtDNA polymorphism in schizophrenia.

Recently, the prevalence of synonymous base pair substitutions in schizophrenia has been investigated. Although these types of substitutions are often considered silent, in some cases, they may alter transcription, splicing, mRNA transport, or translation leading to disease. Rollins and colleagues[163] assessed mtDNA sequence variants in the dorsolateral prefrontal cortex from 77 patients with psychiatric conditions (schizophrenia, bipolar disorder, and major depression). The rate of synonymous base pair substitutions in the coding regions of the mtDNA genome was significantly higher (22%) in patients with schizophrenia compared with controls. A majority of the base pair substitutions were in complex I subunits, with a synonymous substitution in the NADH-dehydrogenase (complex I) *ND2* gene (m.4769G>A) showing a strong association with schizophrenia,[163] a finding concordant with those of previous studies.[283–285] Decreased complex I mitochondrial transcripts have been seen in the DLPFC in patients with schizophrenia, a finding that would support the possibility that these mutations may not be entirely silent.[161] However, it should be noted that this is potentially secondary to medication effect.

Other studies using post mortem samples also suggest evidence for mitochondrial involvement in schizophrenia. Six studies have found altered mitochondrial-related gene expression in the prefrontal or frontal cortex in schizophrenia.[161,168,170,229,307–309] Ben-Shachar and Kerry[171] found that there was significantly lesser expression of mRNA encoding for complex I subunits in the striatum but not cerebellum, which contrasts with their findings in patients with bipolar disorder. Distinct brain region expression of mitochondrial-encoded genes has been found between psychiatric disorders. Konradi and colleagues[245] also found no altered expression of mitochondria-related genes in the hippocampus, which is also different from patients with bipolar disorder. Another study found that there was overexpression of mtDNA genes in the frontal cortex of patients with schizophrenia: cytochrome-c oxidase subunit 2, 12S rRNA, and 16S rRNA.[307] Subsequent studies have also suggested altered expression of cytochrome-c oxidase subunit 2 in patients with schizophrenia[168,297]; however, Cavelier and colleagues[297] identified decreased cytochrome c oxidase activity rather than an increased expression. It was questioned whether or not the decreased expression of cytochrome c oxidase subunit 2 identified by this group could be secondary to poorly matched controls.[168]

The role of mtDNA haplogroups has been investigated in patients with schizophrenia without consensus for causality. Among Israeli-Arab patients, Amar and colleagues[310] reported an association between the HV haplogroup and schizophrenia (OR = 1.8). Conversely, Magri and colleagues[311] did not find any differences in haplogroup frequency but did identify that patients with the J-T haplogroup showed an earlier age of onset of their psychosis compared with other haplogroups. As mentioned, Rollins and colleagues[163] reported a higher rate of the pre-HV haplogroup in patients with bipolar disorder and schizophrenia; however, only 1 patient in that cohort had schizophrenia. Therefore, it is likely that the association was driven by the 3 patients with bipolar who had the pre-HV haplogroup in their cohort. Finally, Ueno and colleagues[303] found no association between mtDNA haplogroup and schizophrenia in their cohort.

Mitochondrial DNA deletions in schizophrenia
Similar to the affective disorders, the role of mtDNA deletions in the pathogenesis of schizophrenia has been explored.[160,161,233,235,297] None of the studies found convincing evidence for an overabundance of mtDNA deletions as playing a role in schizophrenia. However, Kakiuchi and colleagues[233] did find the absence of normal, age-related accumulation of mtDNA deletions in patients with schizophrenia. However, the relevance of this finding in schizophrenia is unclear.

Mitochondrial DNA mutations in psychosis and schizophrenia
Throughout the literature, various case reports have described patients with definite primary mitochondrial disease that present with symptoms of psychosis. Several case reports exist of patients harboring the m.3243A>G mutation that present with psychotic features.[281,312] Suzuki and colleagues[312] reported one of the first cases of a patient presenting with recurrent agitation, auditory hallucinations, delusions of persecution, and disorganized behavior preceding the development of more typical features of MELAS. Later, Inagaki and colleagues[281] described a case of a 37-year-old man with a history of short stature, mediocre school performance, sensorineural hearing loss (onset at 29 years), Wolff–Parkinson–White syndrome (onset at 31 years), and diabetes mellitus. His family history was significant for diabetes and sensorineural hearing loss in multiple maternal relatives. He presented at the age of 31 years with his first episode of psychosis, during which time he developed auditory hallucinations and delusions of persecution that resolved with haloperidol treatment and blood glucose control. Subsequent episodes occurred at the age of 35 and 37 years. With each subsequent episode of psychosis, his intelligence quotient progressively declined and he became completely dependent on others for his activities of daily living. It was identified that he carried the m.3243A>G mutation and was diagnosed with MIDD. Treatment with idebenone led to improvement of his neuropsychiatric symptoms. Although case reports exist linking the known pathologic mtDNA mutations to patients with psychosis, studies assessing cohorts of patients with schizophrenia in attempts

to identify a mtDNA mutation at nucleotide position 3243 have not been successful in the Japanese population.[313]

ANXIETY DISORDERS

In a small case series, 44.4% of patients with the common m.3243A>G mutation and diabetes had mental disorders, and 33.3% of these patients presented with various anxiety disorder diagnoses.[148] In this series, 1 woman presented with panic disorder with agoraphobia at age 37 years, another woman presented with a social phobia with an onset at age 25 years, and the final patient developed simple phobia (related to dental treatment) at age 35 years. In all patients, the anxiety disorder predated the onset of diabetes.[148]

OBSESSIVE–COMPULSIVE DISORDER

Obsessive–compulsive disorder (OCD) involves obsessions and compulsions that require a considerable amount of time and get in the way of social activities and personal values.[33] In the DSM-IV-TR, OCD was classified as an anxiety disorder.[32] In the current DSM-V,[33] OCD has been granted its own section owing to increasing understanding of the disorder and the features associated with it.

Very little research has looked at the connection of OCD and mitochondrial disease. Lacey and Salzberg[314] reported 2 patients with the m.3243A>G mutation who were subsequently diagnosed with OCD. The first patient was a 30-year-old man who came to medical attention because of a combination of short stature, migraine, epilepsy, left homonymous hemianopia, sensorineural hearing loss, elevation of cerebrospinal fluid lactate, and an MRI showing T2-weighted signal abnormalities in his temporal and occipital lobes. Genetic testing in serum demonstrated the m.3243A>G mutation at a 27% heteroplasmic load. Although he was previously described as having a "perfectionistic and obsessional" personality at the time of diagnosis, over the following 6 years he developed obsessions of perfectionism and contamination with compulsions with associated compulsions of grooming and hand washing, respectively. He was subsequently unable to work primarily owing to his OCD-associated features, in conjunction with recurrent strokelike episodes and progressive hearing loss as part of his MELAS syndrome. The features associated with his OCD did not respond to conventional therapies, including cognitive–behavioral therapy, 3 different selective serotonin reuptake inhibitors, and 2 antipsychotics (quetiapine, olanzapine).[314]

The second patient in their series was a 51-year-old man who presented with short stature, sensorineural deafness, right hemiplegia, dysphagia, diabetes mellitus, and seizures. Blood and hair specimens identified a heteroplasmy load of 25% for the common m.3243A>G mutation. Two years before his diagnosis, it was noted that he had obsessions but was never seen in consultation by a psychiatrist. He subsequently exhibited progressive neurocognitive decline. He began to exhibit episodic agitation owing to interruption of ritualistic and repetitive behaviors associated with hoarding, eating, and dressing. Similar to their other case, he did not respond to therapy with selective serotonin reuptake inhibitors or antipsychotics.

Considering that OCD is an uncommon association with mitochondrial disease, the fact that both of these patients had MELAS with associated stroke-like episodes deserves merit. The onset of or reactivation of OCD has been reported after a variety of brain insults[315,316] and with assorted brain lesions affecting the orbitofrontal area, anterior cingulate, dorsolateral prefrontal cortex, caudate, thalamus, and subthalamic nucleus.[317–320] Therefore, it could be hypothesized that patients with stroke-like episodes in associated eloquent brain areas associated with OCD may be sufficient to allow for clinical expression in a subgroup of patients. However, considering that the prevalence of OCD in the adult population is 1%, it cannot be excluded that the appearance of OCD in this small group of patients is unrelated to their MELAS diagnosis.[135]

PERSONALITY DISORDERS

Very few studies have investigated the frequency of personality disorders in patients with mitochondrial disease. One of the early reports was from Suomalainen and colleagues described 64% of their 11-patient cohort with autosomal-dominant CPEO and multiple mtDNA deletions had avoidant personality disorder, avoidant personality traits, explosive behavior, or histrionic personality disorder (as per DSM-III-R diagnostic criteria).[144] Later, Inczedy-Farkas and colleagues[133] demonstrated a significantly greater proportion of patients with a known mtDNA mutation meeting diagnostic criteria for a personality disorder compared with a control group with hereditary sensorimotor neuropathy. In their cohort, 42% of patients met the diagnostic criteria for a personality disorder. The types of personality disorders were variable: 3 patients had avoidant personality disorder, 2 patients had obsessive-compulsive personality disorder, and 3 patients having personality disorders not otherwise specified (NOS).

TREATMENT IMPLICATIONS OF COMORBID NEUROPSYCHIATRIC ILLNESS IN PATIENTS WITH MITOCHONDRIAL DISEASE

Although there is no standardized treatment for patients with primary mitochondrial diseases, patients are often placed on a 'mitochondrial cocktail' consisting of vitamins that are cofactors for various components of oxidative phosphorylation. These vitamins include free radical scavengers, such as alpha-lipoic acid, vitamin E, and vitamin C; riboflavin, which is added because complex I, complex II, fatty acyl-coenzyme A dehydrogenase, and electron transfer factor dehydrogenase are flavoproteins; coenzyme Q10, which is integral to the shuttling of electrons from complex I and II to complex III in the electron transport chain; and creatine monohydrate, an alternative energy sources to assist in ATP generation.[321–328] Other agents that have been used in select groups of patients with mitochondrial disease include dichloroacetate,[329–331] dimethylglycine,[332] and EPI-743.[333–336] Two large, systematic reviews have been completed to investigate the use of different therapies for primary mitochondrial diseases that have been subjected to controlled trials.[321,322] Despite the conclusion that there was "no clear evidence supporting the use of any intervention in mitochondrial disorders," this is likely secondary to the difficulty of completing randomized trials in patients with heterogeneous genotypes and phenotypes rather than a true lack of efficacy.[322] Therefore, when a diagnosis of a mitochondrial disorder is suspected or confirmed, the initiation of vitamins and cofactors is recommended. Moreover, there are multiple promising clinical trails that would be available to patients with a definite mitochondrial disease diagnosis.

The diagnosis of a mitochondrial disorder has particularly important treatment implications for patients with psychiatric illness. There is some evidence that psychiatric symptoms in patients with mitochondrial disorders are more resistant to, and may actually worsen when exposed to, traditional therapies[134,155,299,300]; many medications used to treat these disorders may inhibit mitochondrial function.[337] Additionally, the side effect profile of many of these medications complicates the symptoms of the underlying mitochondrial disorder (eg, the metabolic syndrome in patients with diabetes or anticholinergic side effects in patients with dysautonomia and cognitive dysfunction). Therefore, in patients with psychiatric illness and mitochondrial disorders, some of these agents should be used with caution. If a patient presents with comorbid symptoms suggestive of underlying mitochondrial dysfunction or matrilineal inheritance is suggested by medical history, a diagnosis of a mitochondrial disorder should be explored to guide treatment decisions. Certain agents warrant particular mention, because they have been associated with mitochondrial toxicity in the literature.

Amitriptyline and Selective Serotonin Reuptake Inhibitors

Amitriptyline is a tricyclic antidepressant that is used frequently in patients with depression. Recent studies suggest that it may induce oxidative stress and mitochondrial dysfunction both in vitro and in vivo.[338,339] It is hypothesized that amitriptyline induces an acquired coenzyme Q10 deficiency and acquired mitochondrial dysfunction seen with amitriptyline can be reversed with a combination of coenzyme Q10 and alpha-tocopherol administration.[338,339] Selective serotonin reuptake inhibitors, alternatively, inhibit mitochondrial function in animal models and may produce dysfunction of the respiratory chain at high doses.[340,341]

Lithium

Lithium is effective in the prevention of depressive and manic episodes in patients with bipolar disorder and, as such, it remains the drug of choice in patients with this diagnosis. The exact mechanism of action of lithium, an alkaline metal ion, is not fully elucidated. Unfortunately, more than 50% of patients diagnosed with bipolar disorder do not show full response to lithium therapy.[214] Kato and colleagues[342] found that decreased intracellular pH, as measured by ^{31}P MRS, was associated with lithium response in patients with bipolar disorder, suggesting that mitochondrial dysfunction may alter medication response. Subsequently, Washizuka and colleagues[214] identified a possible relationship between mtDNA polymorphisms and lithium efficacy. They demonstrated patients carrying the m.10398A>G polymorphism, encoding for the ND3 subunit of complex I, showed a significantly better response to lithium. It is proposed that mitochondrial dysfunction results in calcium-dependent superoxides that modulate nuclear cyclic adenosine monophosphate–responsive element-binding protein (CREB) phosphorylation and alter signaling of hippocampal neurons.[343] This pathway has shown to be important in modulation of mood.[344] It is hypothesized that patients with this SNP may have altered intracellular calcium signaling leading to a higher lithium efficacy.

Valproic Acid

VPA is occasionally used as a pharmacologic agent for the treatment of mood disorders, particularly bipolar disorder. Recent evidence suggests it may be as efficacious as lithium, but associated with fewer patients discontinuing therapy.[345] There should be extreme caution used with using VPA as a pharmacologic agent in patients with mitochondrial diseases.[346] Studies have shown that VPA has pleotropic antimitochondrial effects, decreases beta-oxidation in the liver, and induces a secondary carnitine deficiency.[347–349] Detrimental effects have been reported in patients with MELAS exposed to VPA, including an increased frequency of seizures.[350] Patients with Alpers–Huttenlocher syndrome secondary to POLG1 mutations are at extremely high risk of fatal hepatotoxicity with valproate exposure. Therefore, in this subset of patients, VPA should be avoided altogether.[346]

Antipsychotics

Studies suggest that the typical or classical antipsychotics may inhibit mitochondrial complex I activity and alter production of ROS.[351–353] Haloperidol, and to a lesser degree chlorpromazine, fluphenazine, and risperidone, have been found to inhibit complex I in a mouse model.[351] The atypical antipsychotic, clozapine, did not seem to have the same effect complex I activity.[351] Similarly, in brain tissue samples from patients with a diagnosis of schizophrenia, neuroleptics (including haloperidol and flupenthixol) were found to reduce complex I activity.[352] Therefore, it may be that the atypical antipsychotics should be used preferentially over more typical agents in patients with documented complex I–associated mitochondrial disease, if at all possible.

SUMMARY AND FUTURE DIRECTIONS

The increasing understanding of the human genome, the availability of more advanced genetic testing within the last few decades, and research investigating the genetic underpinning of psychiatric disorders is rapidly advancing. However, despite these efforts, the exact genetic cause of these disorders remains elusive. More recently, the focus has turned to the mitochondrial genome and nuclear genes that play a role in mitochondrial function. Various clinical, genetic, ultrastructural, and biochemical studies have investigated the role of mitochondrial dysfunction in various neuropsychiatric illness, including autism in the pediatric population and mood disorders and psychotic disorders in the adult population.

There is currently a large body of evidence investigating mitochondrial involvement in psychiatric illness. Multiple clinical studies and case reports have suggested a high rate of comorbidity between mitochondrial disorders and psychiatric illness. Additionally, subsets of patients with psychiatric illness have been found to have biochemical and ultrastructural changes (such as abnormalities in mitochondrial morphology and density), suggestive of mitochondrial dysfunction. Genetic studies have shown a maternal inheritance pattern in some neuropsychiatric disorders, particularly mood disorders in adults. However, there is currently insufficient evidence to implicate any particular mtDNA mutation or polymorphism with any particular neuropsychiatric illness. Perhaps the most promising genetic studies have been in the area of particular mitochondrial haplotypes implicated in psychiatric illness (such as the pre-HV, HV, or N9a haplotypes); however, initial findings require validation with larger samples and more rigorous studies.

Unfortunately, many of the studies that have been completed to try and isolate the precise role of mitochondrial dysfunction in psychiatric illness have had methodologic flaws. Owing to the large range in genotypes and phenotypes in patients with mitochondrial disorders, it is difficult to generate sufficient populations of patients with a single genotype/phenotype disorder that may allow for more robust comparisons between cases. Additionally, in genome-wide association studies, selection of patients with specific phenotypes at greater risk for mitochondrial mutations (such as patients with multisystemic symptoms in addition to psychiatric illness) is required. Studies of oxidative phosphorylation in cohorts with psychiatric illness have been completed in different laboratories using varied methodologies to determine enzymatic defects. It has been shown that there is poor consistency between different laboratory interpretations, necessitating the need to confirm findings in multiple laboratories. Additionally, some studies have suggested complex V to be the most commonly affected in psychiatric illness; however, it is very difficult to confirm complex V deficiency in a laboratory setting. Furthermore, many patients with psychiatric illness who have been found to have ultrastructural abnormalities suggestive of mitochondrial dysfunction have been on psychotropic medications that result in mitochondrial toxicity. It is, therefore, not surprising that the current studies have yielded inconclusive results.

One of the greatest obstacles facing research in this area is producing studies with sufficient sample sizes to yield adequate results. Several studies have found potentially pathogenic mtDNA variants associated with psychiatric disorders; however, the sample sizes have been insufficient to make concrete conclusions and these findings have not been replicated in larger populations. To achieve adequate power, much larger sample sizes (in the range of thousands to tens of thousands of individuals) than those seen in the largest studies to date (a few hundred individuals) are needed. Current research suggests that the prevalence of mitochondrial disorders is 1 in 2000 in the population; therefore, studies with large samples are feasible but require collaboration between multiple centers. The creation of mitochondrial disorder consortia, networks, and national databases has made studies of this nature possible.

The available literature suggests that mitochondrial dysfunction is a possible etiologic factor in psychiatric illness. The current consensus is that psychiatric illness is multifactorial without clear strict Mendelian inheritance. Mitochondrial dysfunction may only play a partial role in the etiology of some of these disorders. Larger and more rigorous studies are also needed to determine what role mtDNA mutations, polymorphisms or haplotypes; mitochondria-related nDNA expression; ultrastructural abnormalities; and impaired oxidative phosphorylation might play in the etiology of psychiatric illness. Identification of the role of mitochondrial dysfunction in psychiatric illness could result in the development of preventative and therapeutic strategies that are desperately needed in this population.

REFERENCES

1. Berg JM, Tymoczko JL, Stryer L. Oxidative phosphorylation. Biochemistry. 5th edition. New York: W.H. Freeman; 2002.
2. DiMauro S, Schon EA. Mitochondrial respiratory-chain diseases. N Engl J Med 2003;348:2656–68.
3. Anderson S, Bankier AT, Barrell BG, et al. Sequence and organization of the human mitochondrial genome. Nature 1981;290:457–65.
4. Larsson NG, Clayton DA. Molecular genetic aspects of human mitochondrial disorders. Annu Rev Genet 1995;29:151–78.
5. Holt IJ, Harding AE, Morgan-Hughes JA. Deletions of muscle mitochondrial DNA in patients with mitochondrial myopathies. Nature 1988;331:717–9.
6. Holt IJ, Harding AE, Petty RK, et al. A new mitochondrial disease associated with mitochondrial DNA heteroplasmy. Am J Hum Genet 1990;46:428–33.
7. Schon EA, Bonilla E, DiMauro S. Mitochondrial DNA mutations and pathogenesis. J Bioenerg Biomembr 1997;29:131–49.
8. Macmillan C, Lach B, Shoubridge EA. Variable distribution of mutant mitochondrial DNAs (tRNA(Leu[3243])) in tissues of symptomatic relatives with MELAS: the role of mitotic segregation. Neurology 1993;43:1586–90.
9. Kato T. The other, forgotten genome: mitochondrial DNA and mental disorders. Mol Psychiatry 2001;6:625–33.
10. Chinnery PF, Schon EA. Mitochondria. J Neurol Neurosurg Psychiatry 2003;74:1188–99.
11. Wallace DC, Singh G, Lott MT, et al. Mitochondrial DNA mutation associated with Leber's hereditary optic neuropathy. Science 1988;242:1427–30.

12. Schaefer AM, Taylor RW, Turnbull DM, et al. The epidemiology of mitochondrial disorders–past, present and future. Biochim Biophys Acta 2004;1659:115–20.
13. Schaefer AM, McFarland R, Blakely EL, et al. Prevalence of mitochondrial DNA disease in adults. Ann Neurol 2008;63:35–9.
14. Elliott HR, Samuels DC, Eden JA, et al. Pathogenic mitochondrial DNA mutations are common in the general population. Am J Hum Genet 2008;83:254–60.
15. Haas RH, Parikh S, Falk MJ, et al. Mitochondrial disease: a practical approach for primary care physicians. Pediatrics 2007;120:1326–33.
16. Mitochondrial Medicine Society's Committee on Diagnosis, Haas RH, Parikh S, et al. The in-depth evaluation of suspected mitochondrial disease. Mol Genet Metab 2008;94:16–37.
17. Bernier FP, Boneh A, Dennett X, et al. Diagnostic criteria for respiratory chain disorders in adults and children. Neurology 2002;59:1406–11.
18. Wolf NI, Smeitink JA. Mitochondrial disorders: a proposal for consensus diagnostic criteria in infants and children. Neurology 2002;59:1402–5.
19. Gellerich FN, Mayr JA, Reuter S, et al. The problem of interlab variation in methods for mitochondrial disease diagnosis: enzymatic measurement of respiratory chain complexes. Mitochondrion 2004;4:427–39.
20. DiMauro S, Hirano M. Mitochondrial encephalomyopathies: an update. Neuromuscul Disord 2005;15:276–86.
21. Wallace DC. Mitochondrial diseases in man and mouse. Science 1999;283: 1482–8.
22. Moraes CT, DiMauro S, Zeviani M, et al. Mitochondrial DNA deletions in progressive external ophthalmoplegia and Kearns-Sayre syndrome. N Engl J Med 1989; 320:1293–9.
23. Zeviani M, Moraes CT, DiMauro S, et al. Deletions of mitochondrial DNA in Kearns-Sayre syndrome. Neurology 1988;38:1339–46.
24. Montagna P, Gallassi R, Medori R, et al. MELAS syndrome: characteristic migrainous and epileptic features and maternal transmission. Neurology 1988; 38:751–4.
25. Chinnery PF. Mitochondrial disorders overview. In: Pagon RA, Adam MP, Ardinger HH, et al, editors. GeneReviews(R). Seattle (WA): University of Washington; 1993.
26. Smeitink JA, Zeviani M, Turnbull DM, et al. Mitochondrial medicine: a metabolic perspective on the pathology of oxidative phosphorylation disorders. Cell Metab 2006;3:9–13.
27. Kuroda Y, Sako W, Goto S, et al. Parkin interacts with Klokin1 for mitochondrial import and maintenance of membrane potential. Hum Mol Genet 2012;21: 991–1003.
28. Cali T, Ottolini D, Brini M. Mitochondria, calcium, and endoplasmic reticulum stress in Parkinson's disease. BioFactors 2011;37:228–40.
29. Parihar MS, Brewer GJ. Mitoenergetic failure in Alzheimer disease. Am J Physiol Cell Physiol 2007;292:C8–23.
30. Smaili SS, Ureshino RP, Rodrigues L, et al. The role of mitochondrial function in glutamate-dependent metabolism in neuronal cells. Curr Pharm Des 2011;17: 3865–77.
31. Finsterer J. Central nervous system manifestations of mitochondrial disorders. Acta Neurol Scand 2006;114:217–38.
32. American Psychiatric Association. Diagnostic and statistical manual of mental disorders: DSM-IV-TR. 4th edition. Washington, DC: American Psychiatric Association; 2000.

33. American Psychiatric Association. DSM-5 Task Force. Diagnostic and statistical manual of mental disorders DSM-5. Available at: http://myaccess.library. utoronto.ca/login?url=http://dsm.psychiatryonline.org/doi/book/10.1176/appi. books.97808904255962013. Accessed September 11, 2015.

34. Bertrand J, Mars A, Boyle C, et al. Prevalence of autism in a United States population: the Brick Township, New Jersey, investigation. Pediatrics 2001;108: 1155–61.

35. Chakrabarti S, Fombonne E. Pervasive developmental disorders in preschool children. JAMA 2001;285:3093–9.

36. Baird G, Charman T, Baron-Cohen S, et al. A screening instrument for autism at 18 months of age: a 6-year follow-up study. J Am Acad Child Adolesc Psychiatry 2000;39:694–702.

37. Developmental Disabilities Monitoring Network Surveillance Year Principal Investigators, Centers for Disease Control and Prevention. Prevalence of autism spectrum disorder among children aged 8 years - autism and developmental disabilities monitoring network, 11 sites, United States, 2010. Morbidity Mortality Weekly Rep Surveill Summ 2014;63:1–21.

38. Volkmar FR, Pauls D. Autism. Lancet 2003;362:1133–41.

39. Dhillon S, Hellings JA, Butler MG. Genetics and mitochondrial abnormalities in autism spectrum disorders: a review. Curr Genomics 2011;12:322–32.

40. O'Roak BJ, Vives L, Fu W, et al. Multiplex targeted sequencing identifies recurrently mutated genes in autism spectrum disorders. Science 2012;338:1619–22.

41. Lee BH, Smith T, Paciorkowski AR. Autism spectrum disorder and epilepsy: disorders with a shared biology. Epilepsy Behav 2015;47:191–201.

42. Oliveira G, Diogo L, Grazina M, et al. Mitochondrial dysfunction in autism spectrum disorders: a population-based study. Dev Med Child Neurol 2005;47: 185–9.

43. Rossignol DA, Frye RE. Mitochondrial dysfunction in autism spectrum disorders: a systematic review and meta-analysis. Mol Psychiatry 2012;17:290–314.

44. Filipek PA, Juranek J, Nguyen MT, et al. Relative carnitine deficiency in autism. J Autism Dev Disord 2004;34:615–23.

45. Weissman JR, Kelley RI, Bauman ML, et al. Mitochondrial disease in autism spectrum disorder patients: a cohort analysis. PLoS One 2008;3:e3815.

46. Guevara-Campos J, Gonzalez-Guevara L, Puig-Alcaraz C, et al. Autism spectrum disorders associated to a deficiency of the enzymes of the mitochondrial respiratory chain. Metab Brain Dis 2013;28:605–12.

47. Coleman M, Blass JP. Autism and lactic acidosis. J Autism Dev Disord 1985;15: 1–8.

48. Laszlo A, Horvath E, Eck E, et al. Serum serotonin, lactate and pyruvate levels in infantile autistic children. Clin Chim Acta 1994;229:205–7.

49. Nissenkorn A, Zeharia A, Lev D, et al. Neurologic presentations of mitochondrial disorders. J child Neurol 2000;15:44–8.

50. Fillano JJ, Goldenthal MJ, Rhodes CH, et al. Mitochondrial dysfunction in patients with hypotonia, epilepsy, autism, and developmental delay: HEADD syndrome. J child Neurol 2002;17:435–9.

51. Filipek PA, Juranek J, Smith M, et al. Mitochondrial dysfunction in autistic patients with 15q inverted duplication. Ann Neurol 2003;53:801–4.

52. Poling JS, Frye RE, Shoffner J, et al. Developmental regression and mitochondrial dysfunction in a child with autism. J child Neurol 2006;21:170–2.

53. Graf WD, Marin-Garcia J, Gao HG, et al. Autism associated with the mitochondrial DNA G8363A transfer RNA(Lys) mutation. J child Neurol 2000;15:357–61.

54. Pons R, Andreu AL, Checcarelli N, et al. Mitochondrial DNA abnormalities and autistic spectrum disorders. J Pediatr 2004;144:81–5.
55. Koenig MK. Presentation and diagnosis of mitochondrial disorders in children. Pediatr Neurol 2008;38:305–13.
56. Fattal-Valevski A, Kramer U, Leitner Y, et al. Characterization and comparison of autistic subgroups: 10 years' experience with autistic children. Dev Med Child Neurol 1999;41:21–5.
57. Correia C, Coutinho AM, Diogo L, et al. Brief report: high frequency of biochemical markers for mitochondrial dysfunction in autism: no association with the mitochondrial aspartate/glutamate carrier SLC25A12 gene. J Autism Dev Disord 2006;36:1137–40.
58. Jackson MJ, Schaefer JA, Johnson MA, et al. Presentation and clinical investigation of mitochondrial respiratory chain disease. A study of 51 patients. Brain 1995;118(Pt 2):339–57.
59. Munnich A, Rotig A, Chretien D, et al. Clinical presentation of mitochondrial disorders in childhood. J Inherit Metab Dis 1996;19:521–7.
60. Lamont PJ, Surtees R, Woodward CE, et al. Clinical and laboratory findings in referrals for mitochondrial DNA analysis. Arch Dis Child 1998;79:22–7.
61. Debray FG, Mitchell GA, Allard P, et al. Diagnostic accuracy of blood lactate-to-pyruvate molar ratio in the differential diagnosis of congenital lactic acidosis. Clin Chem 2007;53:916–21.
62. Thorburn DR, Smeitink J. Diagnosis of mitochondrial disorders: clinical and biochemical approach. J Inherit Metab Dis 2001;24:312–6.
63. Bremer J. Carnitine–metabolism and functions. Physiol Rev 1983;63:1420–80.
64. Shoffner J, Hyams L, Langley GN, et al. Fever plus mitochondrial disease could be risk factors for autistic regression. J child Neurol 2010;25:429–34.
65. Chen X, Thorburn DR, Wong LJ, et al. Quality improvement of mitochondrial respiratory chain complex enzyme assays using *Caenorhabditis elegans*. Genet Med 2011;13:794–9.
66. Filipek PA, Accardo PJ, Ashwal S, et al. Practice parameter: screening and diagnosis of autism: report of the Quality Standards Subcommittee of the American Academy of Neurology and the Child Neurology Society. Neurology 2000;55:468–79.
67. Haas RH. Autism and mitochondrial disease. Developmental Disabilities Res Rev 2010;16:144–53.
68. Jokiranta E, Sourander A, Suominen A, et al. Epilepsy among children and adolescents with autism spectrum disorders: a population-based study. J Autism Dev Disord 2014;44:2547–57.
69. Levy SE, Giarelli E, Lee LC, et al. Autism spectrum disorder and co-occurring developmental, psychiatric, and medical conditions among children in multiple populations of the United States. J Dev Behav Pediatr 2010;31:267–75.
70. Woolfenden S, Sarkozy V, Ridley G, et al. A systematic review of two outcomes in autism spectrum disorder - epilepsy and mortality. Dev Med Child Neurol 2012;54:306–12.
71. Wolff S, Chess S. A behavioural study of schizophrenic children. Acta Psychiatr Scand 1964;40:438–66.
72. Barger BD, Campbell JM, McDonough JD. Prevalence and onset of regression within autism spectrum disorders: a meta-analytic review. J Autism Dev Disord 2013;43:817–28.
73. Edmonds JL, Kirse DJ, Kearns D, et al. The otolaryngological manifestations of mitochondrial disease and the risk of neurodegeneration with infection. Arch Otolaryngol Head Neck Surg 2002;128:355–62.

74. Possekel S, Marsac C, Kadenbach B. Biochemical analysis of fibroblasts from patients with cytochrome c oxidase-associated Leigh syndrome. Biochim Biophys Acta 1996;1316:153–9.

75. Kadenbach B, Barth J, Akgun R, et al. Regulation of mitochondrial energy generation in health and disease. Biochim Biophys Acta 1995;1271:103–9.

76. Brasseur G, Coppee JY, Colson AM, et al. Structure-function relationships of the mitochondrial bc1 complex in temperature-sensitive mutants of the cytochrome b gene, impaired in the catalytic center N. J Biol Chem 1995;270:29356–64.

77. Vinogradov AD, Sled VD, Burbaev DS, et al. Energy-dependent complex I-associated ubisemiquinones in submitochondrial particles. FEBS Lett 1995;370: 83–7.

78. Blomquist HK, Bohman M, Edvinsson SO, et al. Frequency of the fragile X syndrome in infantile autism. A Swedish multicenter study. Clin Genet 1985;27: 113–7.

79. Remschmidt H, Oehler C. The significance of genetic factors in the etiology of early infantile autism. Z Kinder Jugendpsychiatr 1990;18:216–23 [in German].

80. Smalley SL. Genetic influences in autism. Psychiatr Clin North Am 1991;14: 125–39.

81. Folstein SE, Piven J. Etiology of autism: genetic influences. Pediatrics 1991;87: 767–73.

82. Perrot A, Lenoir P, Carmagnat F, et al. Genetic factors in autism. Soins Psychiatr 1992;27–33 [in French].

83. Herault J, Martineau J, Petit E, et al. Genetic markers in autism: association study on short arm of chromosome 11. J Autism Dev Disord 1994;24:233–6.

84. Bailey A, Le Couteur A, Gottesman I, et al. Autism as a strongly genetic disorder: evidence from a British twin study. Psychol Med 1995;25:63–77.

85. Abrahams BS, Geschwind DH. Advances in autism genetics: on the threshold of a new neurobiology. Nat Rev Genet 2008;9:341–55.

86. Kakinuma H, Sato H. Copy-number variations associated with autism spectrum disorder. Pharmacogenomics 2008;9:1143–54.

87. Pavlakis SG, Phillips PC, DiMauro S, et al. Mitochondrial myopathy, encephalopathy, lactic acidosis, and strokelike episodes: a distinctive clinical syndrome. Ann Neurol 1984;16:481–8.

88. Goto Y, Horai S, Matsuoka T, et al. Mitochondrial myopathy, encephalopathy, lactic acidosis, and stroke-like episodes (MELAS): a correlative study of the clinical features and mitochondrial DNA mutation. Neurology 1992;42:545–50.

89. Ballinger SW, Shoffner JM, Hedaya EV, et al. Maternally transmitted diabetes and deafness associated with a 10.4 kb mitochondrial DNA deletion. Nat Genet 1992;1:11–5.

90. Reardon W, Ross RJ, Sweeney MG, et al. Diabetes mellitus associated with a pathogenic point mutation in mitochondrial DNA. Lancet 1992;340:1376–9.

91. Guillausseau PJ, Massin P, Dubois-LaForgue D, et al. Maternally inherited diabetes and deafness: a multicenter study. Ann Intern Med 2001;134:721–8.

92. van den Ouweland JM, Lemkes HH, Ruitenbeek W, et al. Mutation in mitochondrial tRNA(Leu)(UUR) gene in a large pedigree with maternally transmitted type II diabetes mellitus and deafness. Nat Genet 1992;1:368–71.

93. Serajee FJ, Zhang H, Huq A. Prevalence of common mitochondrial point mutations in autism. Neuropediatrics 2006;37:S127.

94. Kent L, Lambert C, Pyle A, et al. The mitochondrial DNA A3243A>G mutation must be an infrequent cause of Asperger syndrome. J Pediatr 2006;149: 280–1.

95. Santorelli FM, Mak SC, El-Schahawi M, et al. Maternally inherited cardiomyopathy and hearing loss associated with a novel mutation in the mitochondrial tRNA(Lys) gene (G8363A). Am J Hum Genet 1996;58:933–9.
96. Ozawa M, Nishino I, Horai S, et al. Myoclonus epilepsy associated with ragged-red fibers: a G-to-A mutation at nucleotide pair 8363 in mitochondrial tRNA(Lys) in two families. Muscle Nerve 1997;20:271–8.
97. Arenas J, Campos Y, Bornstein B, et al. A double mutation (A8296G and G8363A) in the mitochondrial DNA tRNA (Lys) gene associated with myoclonus epilepsy with ragged-red fibers. Neurology 1999;52:377–82.
98. Shtilbans A, Shanske S, Goodman S, et al. G8363A mutation in the mitochondrial DNA transfer ribonucleic acidLys gene: another cause of Leigh syndrome. J child Neurol 2000;15:759–61.
99. Graf WD, Sumi SM, Copass MK, et al. Phenotypic heterogeneity in families with the myoclonic epilepsy and ragged-red fiber disease point mutation in mitochondrial DNA. Ann Neurol 1993;33:640–5.
100. Virgilio R, Ronchi D, Bordoni A, et al. Mitochondrial DNA G8363A mutation in the tRNA Lys gene: clinical, biochemical and pathological study. J Neurol Sci 2009; 281:85–92.
101. Stankiewicz P, Lupski JR. Structural variation in the human genome and its role in disease. Annu Rev Med 2010;61:437–55.
102. Iafrate AJ, Feuk L, Rivera MN, et al. Detection of large-scale variation in the human genome. Nat Genet 2004;36:949–51.
103. Redon R, Ishikawa S, Fitch KR, et al. Global variation in copy number in the human genome. Nature 2006;444:444–54.
104. Cho SC, Yim SH, Yoo HK, et al. Copy number variations associated with idiopathic autism identified by whole-genome microarray-based comparative genomic hybridization. Psychiatr Genet 2009;19:177–85.
105. Gu F, Chauhan V, Kaur K, et al. Alterations in mitochondrial DNA copy number and the activities of electron transport chain complexes and pyruvate dehydrogenase in the frontal cortex from subjects with autism. Translational Psychiatry 2013;3:e299.
106. Crespi BJ, Crofts HJ. Association testing of copy number variants in schizophrenia and autism spectrum disorders. J neurodevelopmental Disord 2012; 4:15.
107. Griswold AJ, Ma D, Cukier HN, et al. Evaluation of copy number variations reveals novel candidate genes in autism spectrum disorder-associated pathways. Hum Mol Genet 2012;21:3513–23.
108. Sebat J, Lakshmi B, Malhotra D, et al. Strong association of de novo copy number mutations with autism. Science 2007;316:445–9.
109. Smith M, Flodman PL, Gargus JJ, et al. Mitochondrial and ion channel gene alterations in autism. Biochim Biophys Acta 2012;1817:1796–802.
110. Smith M, Spence MA, Flodman P. Nuclear and mitochondrial genome defects in autisms. Ann N Y Acad Sci 2009;1151:102–32.
111. Giulivi C, Zhang YF, Omanska-Klusek A, et al. Mitochondrial dysfunction in autism. JAMA 2010;304:2389–96.
112. Roberts JL, Hovanes K, Dasouki M, et al. Chromosomal microarray analysis of consecutive individuals with autism spectrum disorders or learning disability presenting for genetic services. Gene 2014;535:70–8.
113. Williams RS. Mitochondrial gene expression in mammalian striated muscle. Evidence that variation in gene dosage is the major regulatory event. J Biol Chem 1986;261:12390–4.

114. Devlin B, Scherer SW. Genetic architecture in autism spectrum disorder. Curr Opin Genet Dev 2012;22:229–37.

115. Miller DT, Shen Y, Weiss LA, et al. Microdeletion/duplication at 15q13.2q13.3 among individuals with features of autism and other neuropsychiatric disorders. J Med Genet 2009;46:242–8.

116. Sanders SJ, Ercan-Sencicek AG, Hus V, et al. Multiple recurrent de novo CNVs, including duplications of the 7q11.23 Williams syndrome region, are strongly associated with autism. Neuron 2011;70:863–85.

117. Weiss LA, Shen Y, Korn JM, et al. Association between microdeletion and micro-duplication at 16p11.2 and autism. N Engl J Med 2008;358:667–75.

118. Glessner JT, Wang K, Cai G, et al. Autism genome-wide copy number variation reveals ubiquitin and neuronal genes. Nature 2009;459:569–73.

119. Maestrini E, Pagnamenta AT, Lamb JA, et al. High-density SNP association study and copy number variation analysis of the AUTS1 and AUTS5 loci implicate the IMMP2L-DOCK4 gene region in autism susceptibility. Mol Psychiatry 2010;15:954–68.

120. Petek E, Schwarzbraun T, Noor A, et al. Molecular and genomic studies of IMMP2L and mutation screening in autism and Tourette syndrome. Mol Genet genomics 2007;277:71–81.

121. Palmieri L, Papaleo V, Porcelli V, et al. Altered calcium homeostasis in autism-spectrum disorders: evidence from biochemical and genetic studies of the mito-chondrial aspartate/glutamate carrier AGC1. Mol Psychiatry 2010;15:38–52.

122. Ramoz N, Reichert JG, Smith CJ, et al. Linkage and association of the mitochon-drial aspartate/glutamate carrier SLC25A12 gene with autism. Am J Psychiatry 2004;161:662–9.

123. Segurado R, Conroy J, Meally E, et al. Confirmation of association between autism and the mitochondrial aspartate/glutamate carrier SLC25A12 gene on chromosome 2q31. Am J Psychiatry 2005;162:2182–4.

124. Blasi F, Bacchelli E, Carone S, et al. SLC25A12 and CMYA3 gene variants are not associated with autism in the IMGSAC multiplex family sample. Eur J Hum Genet 2006;14:123–6.

125. Rabionet R, McCauley JL, Jaworski JM, et al. Lack of association between autism and SLC25A12. Am J Psychiatry 2006;163:929–31.

126. Lepagnol-Bestel AM, Maussion G, Boda B, et al. SLC25A12 expression is asso-ciated with neurite outgrowth and is upregulated in the prefrontal cortex of autistic subjects. Mol Psychiatry 2008;13:385–97.

127. Ramoz N, Cai G, Reichert JG, et al. An analysis of candidate autism loci on chromosome 2q24-q33: evidence for association to the STK39 gene. Am J Med Genet Part B, Neuropsychiatr Genet 2008;147B:1152–8.

128. Silverman JM, Buxbaum JD, Ramoz N, et al. Autism-related routines and rituals associated with a mitochondrial aspartate/glutamate carrier SLC25A12 polymor-phism. Am J Med Genet Part B, Neuropsychiatr Genet 2008;147:408–10.

129. Turunen JA, Rehnstrom K, Kilpinen H, et al. Mitochondrial aspartate/gluta-mate carrier SLC25A12 gene is associated with autism. Autism Res 2008;1:189–92.

130. Chien WH, Wu YY, Gau SS, et al. Association study of the SLC25A12 gene and autism in Han Chinese in Taiwan. Prog Neuro-Psychopharmacology Biol Psychi-atry 2010;34:189–92.

131. Maussion G, Carayol J, Lepagnol-Bestel AM, et al. Convergent evidence iden-tifying MAP/microtubule affinity-regulating kinase 1 (MARK1) as a susceptibility gene for autism. Hum Mol Genet 2008;17:2541–51.

132. Fattal O, Link J, Quinn K, et al. Psychiatric comorbidity in 36 adults with mitochondrial cytopathies. CNS spectrums 2007;12:429–38.
133. Inczedy-Farkas G, Remenyi V, Gal A, et al. Psychiatric symptoms of patients with primary mitochondrial DNA disorders. Behav Brain functions 2012;8:9.
134. Anglin RE, Tarnopolsky MA, Mazurek MF, et al. The psychiatric presentation of mitochondrial disorders in adults. J Neuropsychiatry Clin Neurosci 2012;24:394–409.
135. Kessler RC, Chiu WT, Demler O, et al. Prevalence, severity, and comorbidity of 12-month DSM-IV disorders in the National Comorbidity Survey Replication. Arch Gen Psychiatry 2005;62:617–27.
136. Amore M, Tagariello P, Laterza C, et al. Subtypes of depression in dementia. Arch Gerontol Geriatr 2007;44(Suppl 1):23–33.
137. Davis JD, Tremont G. Neuropsychiatric aspects of hypothyroidism and treatment reversibility. Minerva Endocrinol 2007;32:49–65.
138. Rosenblatt A. Neuropsychiatry of Huntington's disease. Dialogues Clin Neurosci 2007;9:191–7.
139. Greden JF. The burden of disease for treatment-resistant depression. J Clin Psychiatry 2001;62(Suppl 16):26–31.
140. Miovic M, Block S. Psychiatric disorders in advanced cancer. Cancer 2007;110:1665–76.
141. Wallace DC. A new manifestation of Leber's disease and a new explanation for the agency responsible for its unusual pattern of inheritance. Brain 1970;93:121–32.
142. Stewart JB, Naylor GJ. Manic-depressive psychosis in a patient with mitochondrial myopathy - a case report. Med Sci Res 1990;18:265–6.
143. Ciafaloni E, Shanske S, Apostolski S, et al. Multiple deletions of mitochondrial DNA. Neurology 1991;41:207.
144. Suomalainen A, Majander A, Haltia M, et al. Multiple deletions of mitochondrial DNA in several tissues of a patient with severe retarded depression and familial progressive external ophthalmoplegia. J Clin Invest 1992;90:61–6.
145. Shanske AL, Shanske S, Silvestri G, et al. MELAS point mutation with unusual clinical presentation. Neuromuscul Disord 1993;3:191–3.
146. Sweeney MG, Bundey S, Brockington M, et al. Mitochondrial myopathy associated with sudden death in young adults and a novel mutation in the mitochondrial DNA leucine transfer RNA(UUR) gene. QJM 1993;86:709–13.
147. Kato T, Takahashi Y. Deletion of leukocyte mitochondrial DNA in bipolar disorder. J Affect Disord 1996;37:67–73.
148. Miyaoka H, Suzuki Y, Taniyama M, et al. Mental disorders in diabetic patients with mitochondrial transfer RNA(Leu) (UUR) mutation at position 3243. Biol Psychiatry 1997;42:524–6.
149. Onishi H, Kawanishi C, Iwasawa T, et al. Depressive disorder due to mitochondrial transfer RNALeu(UUR) mutation. Biol Psychiatry 1997;41:1137–9.
150. Gardner A, Johansson A, Wibom R, et al. Alterations of mitochondrial function and correlations with personality traits in selected major depressive disorder patients. J Affect Disord 2003;76:55–68.
151. Molnar MJ, Perenyi J, Siska E, et al. The typical MERRF (A8344G) mutation of the mitochondrial DNA associated with depressive mood disorders. J Neurol 2009;256:264–5.
152. Morava E, Gardeitchik T, Kozicz T, et al. Depressive behaviour in children diagnosed with a mitochondrial disorder. Mitochondrion 2010;10:528–33.

153. Koene S, Kozicz TL, Rodenburg RJ, et al. Major depression in adolescent children consecutively diagnosed with mitochondrial disorder. J Affect Disord 2009; 114:327–32.
154. Lertrit P, Noer AS, Byrne E, et al. Tissue segregation of a heteroplasmic mtDNA mutation in MERRF (myoclonic epilepsy with ragged red fibers) encephalomyopathy. Hum Genet 1992;90:251–4.
155. Anglin RE, Garside SL, Tarnopolsky MA, et al. The psychiatric manifestations of mitochondrial disorders: a case and review of the literature. J Clin Psychiatry 2012;73:506–12.
156. Goodnick PJ, Henry JH, Buki VM. Treatment of depression in patients with diabetes mellitus. J Clin Psychiatry 1995;56:128–36.
157. Wilkinson G, Borsey DQ, Leslie P, et al. Psychiatric disorder in patients with insulin-dependent diabetes mellitus attending a general hospital clinic: (i) two-stage screening and (ii) detection by physicians. Psychol Med 1987;17:515–7.
158. Barragan-Campos HM, Vallee JN, Lo D, et al. Brain magnetic resonance imaging findings in patients with mitochondrial cytopathies. Arch Neurol 2005;62: 737–42.
159. Suomalainen A, Majander A, Wallin M, et al. Autosomal dominant progressive external ophthalmoplegia with multiple deletions of mtDNA: clinical, biochemical, and molecular genetic features of the 10q-linked disease. Neurology 1997;48:1244–53.
160. Sabunciyan S, Kirches E, Krause G, et al. Quantification of total mitochondrial DNA and mitochondrial common deletion in the frontal cortex of patients with schizophrenia and bipolar disorder. J Neural Transm 2007;114:665–74.
161. Shao L, Martin MV, Watson SJ, et al. Mitochondrial involvement in psychiatric disorders. Ann N Y Acad Sci 2008;40:281–95.
162. Munakata K, Iwamoto K, Bundo M, et al. 3243A>G mutation and increased expression of LARS2 gene in the brains of patients with bipolar disorder and schizophrenia. Biol Psychiatry 2005;57:525–32.
163. Rollins B, Martin MV, Sequeira PA, et al. Mitochondrial variants in schizophrenia, bipolar disorder, and major depressive disorder. PloS One 2009;4:e4913.
164. Munakata K, Fujii K, Nanko S, et al. Sequence and functional analyses of mtDNA in a maternally inherited family with bipolar disorder and depression. Mutat Res 2007;617:119–24.
165. Kasahara T, Kubota M, Miyauchi T, et al. Mice with neuron-specific accumulation of mitochondrial DNA mutations show mood disorder-like phenotypes. Mol Psychiatry 2006;11:577–93, 523.
166. Hakonen AH, Heiskanen S, Juvonen V, et al. Mitochondrial DNA polymerase W748S mutation: a common cause of autosomal recessive ataxia with ancient European origin. Am J Hum Genet 2005;77:430–41.
167. Vawter MP, Tomita H, Meng F, et al. Mitochondrial-related gene expression changes are sensitive to agonal-pH state: implications for brain disorders. Mol Psychiatry 2006;11(615):663–79.
168. Whatley SA, Curti D, Marchbanks RM. Mitochondrial involvement in schizophrenia and other functional psychoses. Neurochem Res 1996;21:995–1004.
169. Altar CA, Jurata LW, Charles V, et al. Deficient hippocampal neuron expression of proteasome, ubiquitin, and mitochondrial genes in multiple schizophrenia cohorts. Biol Psychiatry 2005;58:85–96.
170. Karry R, Klein E, Ben Shachar D. Mitochondrial complex I subunits expression is altered in schizophrenia: a postmortem study. Biol Psychiatry 2004;55: 676–84.

171. Ben-Shachar D, Karry R. Neuroanatomical pattern of mitochondrial complex I pathology varies between schizophrenia, bipolar disorder and major depression. PloS One 2008;3:e3676.
172. Verhulst FC, van der Ende J, Ferdinand RF, et al. The prevalence of DSM-III-R diagnoses in a national sample of Dutch adolescents. Arch Gen Psychiatry 1997;54:329–36.
173. Burmeister M, McInnis MG, Zollner S. Psychiatric genetics: progress amid controversy. Nat Rev Genet 2008;9:527–40.
174. Goodwin FK, Jamison KR. Manic-depressive illness. New York: Oxford University Press; 1990.
175. Berrettini W. Genetic studies of bipolar disorders: new and recurrent findings. Mol Psychiatry 1996;1:172–3.
176. Uranova NA, Casanova MF, DeVaughn NM, et al. Ultrastructural alterations of synaptic contacts and astrocytes in postmortem caudate nucleus of schizophrenic patients. Schizophr Res 1996;22:81–3.
177. Uranova N, Orlovskaya D, Vikhreva O, et al. Electron microscopy of oligodendroglia in severe mental illness. Brain Res Bull 2001;55:597–610.
178. Cataldo AM, McPhie DL, Lange NT, et al. Abnormalities in mitochondrial structure in cells from patients with bipolar disorder. Am J Pathol 2010;177: 575–85.
179. Kato T, Takahashi S, Shioiri T, et al. Alterations in brain phosphorous metabolism in bipolar disorder detected by in vivo 31P and 7Li magnetic resonance spectroscopy. J Affect Disord 1993;27:53–9.
180. Kato T, Takahashi S, Shioiri T, et al. Reduction of brain phosphocreatine in bipolar II disorder detected by phosphorus-31 magnetic resonance spectroscopy. J Affect Disord 1994;31:125–33.
181. Frey BN, Stanley JA, Nery FG, et al. Abnormal cellular energy and phospholipid metabolism in the left dorsolateral prefrontal cortex of medication-free individuals with bipolar disorder: an in vivo 1H MRS study. Bipolar Disord 2007; 9(Suppl 1):119–27.
182. Dager SR, Friedman SD, Parow A, et al. Brain metabolic alterations in medication-free patients with bipolar disorder. Arch Gen Psychiatry 2004;61:450–8.
183. Brambilla P, Stanley JA, Nicoletti MA, et al. 1H magnetic resonance spectroscopy investigation of the dorsolateral prefrontal cortex in bipolar disorder patients. J Affect Disord 2005;86:61–7.
184. Anglin RE, Rosebush PI, Noseworthy MD, et al. Metabolite measurements in the caudate nucleus, anterior cingulate cortex and hippocampus among patients with mitochondrial disorders: a case-control study using proton magnetic resonance spectroscopy. CMAJ Open 2013;1:E48–55.
185. Floyd RA. Antioxidants, oxidative stress, and degenerative neurological disorders. Proc Soc Exp Biol Med Soc Exp Biol Med 1999;222:236–45.
186. Kuloglu M, Ustundag B, Atmaca M, et al. Lipid peroxidation and antioxidant enzyme levels in patients with schizophrenia and bipolar disorder. Cell Biochem Funct 2002;20:171–5.
187. Ranjekar PK, Hinge A, Hegde MV, et al. Decreased antioxidant enzymes and membrane essential polyunsaturated fatty acids in schizophrenic and bipolar mood disorder patients. Psychiatry Res 2003;121:109–22.
188. Ozcan ME, Gulec M, Ozerol E, et al. Antioxidant enzyme activities and oxidative stress in affective disorders. Int Clin Psychopharmacol 2004;19:89–95.
189. Andreazza AC, Frey BN, Erdtmann B, et al. DNA damage in bipolar disorder. Psychiatry Res 2007;153:27–32.

190. Wang JF, Shao L, Sun X, et al. Increased oxidative stress in the anterior cingulate cortex of subjects with bipolar disorder and schizophrenia. Bipolar Disord 2009;11:523–9.
191. Andreazza AC, Kauer-Sant'anna M, Frey BN, et al. Oxidative stress markers in bipolar disorder: a meta-analysis. J Affect Disord 2008;111:135–44.
192. Andreazza AC, Shao L, Wang JF, et al. Mitochondrial complex I activity and oxidative damage to mitochondrial proteins in the prefrontal cortex of patients with bipolar disorder. Arch Gen Psychiatry 2010;67:360–8.
193. Brown NC, Andreazza AC, Young LT. An updated meta-analysis of oxidative stress markers in bipolar disorder. Psychiatry Res 2014;218:61–8.
194. Steckert AV, Valvassori SS, Moretti M, et al. Role of oxidative stress in the pathophysiology of bipolar disorder. Neurochem Res 2010;35:1295–301.
195. Andreazza AC, Wang JF, Salmasi F, et al. Specific subcellular changes in oxidative stress in prefrontal cortex from patients with bipolar disorder. J Neurochem 2013;127:552–61.
196. Frey BN, Andreazza AC, Houenou J, et al. Biomarkers in bipolar disorder: a positional paper from the International Society for Bipolar Disorders Biomarkers Task Force. Aust N Z J Psychiatry 2013;47:321–32.
197. Kato T. Behavioral neurobiology of bipolar disorder and its treatment. In: Manji HK, Zarate CA, editors. Current topics in behavioral neurosciences. Heidelberg (Germany): Springer; 2011. p. 187–200.
198. Winokur G, Pitts FN Jr. Affective disorder: VI. A family history study of prevalences, sex differences and possible genetic factors. J Psychiatr Res 1965;3:113–23.
199. McMahon FJ, Stine OC, Meyers DA, et al. Patterns of maternal transmission in bipolar affective disorder. Am J Hum Genet 1995;56:1277–86.
200. Kato T, Winokur G, Coryell W, et al. Parent-of-origin effect in transmission of bipolar disorder. Am J Med Genet 1996;67:546–50.
201. Gershon ES, Badner JA, Detera-Wadleigh SD, et al. Maternal inheritance and chromosome 18 allele sharing in unilineal bipolar illness pedigrees. Am J Med Genet 1996;67:202–7.
202. Winokur G, Reich T. Two genetic factors in manic-depressive disease. Compr Psychiatry 1970;11:93–9.
203. Kato T, Kunugi H, Nanko S, et al. Association of bipolar disorder with the 5178 polymorphism in mitochondrial DNA. Am J Med Genet 2000;96:182–6.
204. Kato T, Kunugi H, Nanko S, et al. Mitochondrial DNA polymorphisms in bipolar disorder. J Affect Disord 2001;62:151–64.
205. Kazuno AA, Munakata K, Mori K, et al. Mitochondrial DNA haplogroup analysis in patients with bipolar disorder. Am J Med Genet Part B, Neuropsychiatr Genet 2009;150B:243–7.
206. Kirk R, Furlong RA, Amos W, et al. Mitochondrial genetic analyses suggest selection against maternal lineages in bipolar affective disorder. Am J Hum Genet 1999;65:508–18.
207. McMahon FJ, Chen YS, Patel S, et al. Mitochondrial DNA sequence diversity in bipolar affective disorder. Am J Psychiatry 2000;157:1058–64.
208. Munakata K, Tanaka M, Mori K, et al. Mitochondrial DNA 3644T–>C mutation associated with bipolar disorder. Genomics 2004;84:1041–50.
209. Marzuki S, Noer AS, Lertrit P, et al. Normal variants of human mitochondrial DNA and translation products: the building of a reference data base. Hum Genet 1991;88:139–45.
210. Tanaka M, Gong JS, Zhang J, et al. Mitochondrial genotype associated with longevity. Lancet 1998;351:185–6.

211. Mackey D, Howell N. A variant of Leber hereditary optic neuropathy character-ized by recovery of vision and by an unusual mitochondrial genetic etiology. Am J Hum Genet 1992;51:1218–28.

212. Kazuno AA, Munakata K, Nagai T, et al. Identification of mitochondrial DNA poly-morphisms that alter mitochondrial matrix pH and intracellular calcium dy-namics. PLoS Genet 2006;2:e128.

213. Li CT, Bai YM, Hsieh JC, et al. Peripheral and central glucose utilizations modu-lated by mitochondrial DNA 10398A in bipolar disorder. Psychoneuroendocri-nology 2015;55:72–80.

214. Washizuka S, Ikeda A, Kato N, et al. Possible relationship between mitochon-drial DNA polymorphisms and lithium response in bipolar disorder. Int J Neuro-psychopharmacol 2003;6:421–4.

215. Doyle GA, Dahl JP, Bloch PJ, et al. Association study of polymorphisms in the autosomal mitochondrial complex I subunit gene, NADH dehydrogenase (ubi-quinone) flavoprotein 2, and bipolar disorder. Psychiatr Genet 2011;21:51–2.

216. Washizuka S, Iwamoto K, Kazuno AA, et al. Association of mitochondrial com-plex I subunit gene NDUFV2 at 18p11 with bipolar disorder in Japanese and the National Institute of Mental Health pedigrees. Biol Psychiatry 2004;56:483–9.

217. Xu C, Li PP, Kennedy JL, et al. Further support for association of the mitochon-drial complex I subunit gene NDUFV2 with bipolar disorder. Bipolar Disord 2008;10:105–10.

218. Berrettini WH, Ferraro TN, Goldin LR, et al. Chromosome 18 DNA markers and manic-depressive illness: evidence for a susceptibility gene. Proc Natl Acad Sci U S A 1994;91:5918–21.

219. Berrettini W. Linkage of bipolar disorder to chromosome 18 DNA markers. Mol Psychiatry 1997;2:391–2.

220. Berrettini WH, Ferraro TN, Goldin LR, et al. A linkage study of bipolar illness. Arch Gen Psychiatry 1997;54:27–35.

221. Stine OC, Xu J, Koskela R, et al. Evidence for linkage of bipolar disorder to chro-mosome 18 with a parent-of-origin effect. Am J Hum Genet 1995;57:1384–94.

222. Segurado R, Detera-Wadleigh SD, Levinson DF, et al. Genome scan meta-analysis of schizophrenia and bipolar disorder, part III: bipolar disorder. Am J Hum Genet 2003;73:49–62.

223. Turecki G, Grof P, Cavazzoni P, et al. Lithium responsive bipolar disorder, unili-neality, and chromosome 18: a linkage study. Am J Med Genet 1999;88:411–5.

224. Lewis CM, Levinson DF, Wise LH, et al. Genome scan meta-analysis of schizo-phrenia and bipolar disorder, part II: Schizophrenia. Am J Hum Genet 2003;73:34–48.

225. Forabosco P, Ng MY, Bouzigon E, et al. Data acquisition for meta-analysis of genome-wide linkage studies using the genome search meta-analysis method. Hum Hered 2007;64:74–81.

226. de Coo R, Buddiger P, Smeets H, et al. Molecular cloning and characterization of the active human mitochondrial NADH: ubiquinone oxidoreductase 24-kDa gene (NDUFV2) and its pseudogene. Genomics 1995;26:461–6.

227. Hattori N, Suzuki H, Wang Y, et al. Structural organization and chromosomal localization of the human nuclear gene (NDUFV2) for the 24-kDa iron-sulfur sub-unit of complex I in mitochondrial respiratory chain. Biochem Biophys Res Com-mun 1995;216:771–7.

228. Washizuka S, Kametani M, Sasaki T, et al. Association of mitochondrial complex I subunit gene NDUFV2 at 18p11 with schizophrenia in the Japanese popula-tion. Am J Med Genet Part B, Neuropsychiatr Genet 2006;141B:301–4.

229. Iwamoto K, Bundo M, Kato T. Altered expression of mitochondria-related genes in postmortem brains of patients with bipolar disorder or schizophrenia, as revealed by large-scale DNA microarray analysis. Hum Mol Genet 2005;14: 241–53.

230. Kato T. The role of mitochondrial dysfunction in bipolar disorder. Drug News Perspect 2006;19:597–602.

231. Kato T. Role of mitochondrial DNA in calcium signaling abnormality in bipolar disorder. Cell Calcium 2008;44:92–102.

232. Washizuka S, Kakiuchi C, Mori K, et al. Expression of mitochondria-related genes in lymphoblastoid cells from patients with bipolar disorder. Bipolar Disord 2005;7:146–52.

233. Kakiuchi C, Ishiwata M, Kametani M, et al. Quantitative analysis of mitochondrial DNA deletions in the brains of patients with bipolar disorder and schizophrenia. Int J Neuropsychopharmacol 2005;8:515–22.

234. Kato T, Stine OC, McMahon FJ, et al. Increased levels of a mitochondrial DNA deletion in the brain of patients with bipolar disorder. Biol Psychiatry 1997;42:871–5.

235. Fuke S, Kametani M, Kato T. Quantitative analysis of the 4977-bp common deletion of mitochondrial DNA in postmortem frontal cortex from patients with bipolar disorder and schizophrenia. Neurosci Lett 2008;439:173–7.

236. Clay Montier LL, Deng JJ, Bai Y. Number matters: control of mammalian mitochondrial DNA copy number. J Genet Genomics 2009;36:125–31.

237. Iwamoto K, Kakiuchi C, Bundo M, et al. Molecular characterization of bipolar disorder by comparing gene expression profiles of postmortem brains of major mental disorders. Mol Psychiatry 2004;9:406–16.

238. Park H, Davidson E, King MP. The pathogenic A3243G mutation in human mitochondrial tRNALeu(UUR) decreases the efficiency of aminoacylation. Biochemistry 2003;42:958–64.

239. Rossmanith W, Karwan RM. Impairment of tRNA processing by point mutations in mitochondrial tRNA(Leu)(UUR) associated with mitochondrial diseases. FEBS Lett 1998;433:269–74.

240. Yasukawa T, Suzuki T, Ueda T, et al. Modification defect at anticodon wobble nucleotide of mitochondrial tRNAs(Leu)(UUR) with pathogenic mutations of mitochondrial myopathy, encephalopathy, lactic acidosis, and stroke-like episodes. J Biol Chem 2000;275:4251–7.

241. Siciliano G, Tessa A, Petrini S, et al. Autosomal dominant external ophthalmoplegia and bipolar affective disorder associated with a mutation in the ANT1 gene. Neuromuscul Disord 2003;13:162–5.

242. Spelbrink JN, Li FY, Tiranti V, et al. Human mitochondrial DNA deletions associated with mutations in the gene encoding Twinkle, a phage T7 gene 4-like protein localized in mitochondria. Nat Genet 2001;28:223–31.

243. Van Goethem G, Dermaut B, Lofgren A, et al. Mutation of POLG is associated with progressive external ophthalmoplegia characterized by mtDNA deletions. Nat Genet 2001;28:211–2.

244. Sun X, Wang JF, Tseng M, et al. Downregulation in components of the mitochondrial electron transport chain in the postmortem frontal cortex of subjects with bipolar disorder. J Psychiatry Neurosci 2006;31:189–96.

245. Konradi C, Eaton M, MacDonald ML, et al. Molecular evidence for mitochondrial dysfunction in bipolar disorder. Arch Gen Psychiatry 2004;61:300–8.

246. Kubota M, Kasahara T, Iwamoto K, et al. Therapeutic implications of downregulation of cyclophilin D in bipolar disorder. Int J Neuropsychopharmacol 2010;13:1355–68.

247. Karlsgodt KH, Sun D, Jimenez AM, et al. Developmental disruptions in neural connectivity in the pathophysiology of schizophrenia. Dev Psychopathol 2008; 20:1297–327.
248. Lewis DA, Levitt P. Schizophrenia as a disorder of neurodevelopment. Annu Rev Neurosci 2002;25:409–32.
249. Sullivan PF. The genetics of schizophrenia. PLoS Med 2005;2:e212.
250. Lyons MJ, Huppert J, Toomey R, et al. Lifetime prevalence of mood and anxiety disorders in twin pairs discordant for schizophrenia. Twin Res 2000;3: 28–32.
251. Lyons MJ, Bar JL, Kremen WS, et al. Nicotine and familial vulnerability to schizophrenia: a discordant twin study. J Abnorm Psychol 2002;111:687–93.
252. Tsuang MT, Stone WS, Faraone SV. Genes, environment and schizophrenia. Br J Psychiatry Suppl 2001;40:s18–24.
253. Kremen WS, Lyons MJ, Boake C, et al. A discordant twin study of premorbid cognitive ability in schizophrenia. J Clin Exp Neuropsychol 2006;28: 208–24.
254. Owen MJ, Craddock N, O'Donovan MC. Suggestion of roles for both common and rare risk variants in genome-wide studies of schizophrenia. Arch Gen Psychiatry 2010;67:667–73.
255. Mowry BJ, Gratten J. The emerging spectrum of allelic variation in schizophrenia: current evidence and strategies for the identification and functional characterization of common and rare variants. Mol Psychiatry 2013;18: 38–52.
256. Verge B, Alonso Y, Valero J, et al. (mtDNA) and schizophrenia. Eur Psychiatry 2011;26:45–56.
257. Verge B, Alonso Y, Miralles C, et al. New evidence for the involvement of mitochondrial inheritance in schizophrenia: results from a cross-sectional study evaluating the risk of illness in relatives of schizophrenia patients. J Clin Psychiatry 2012;73:684–90.
258. Ben-Shachar D. Mitochondrial dysfunction in schizophrenia: a possible linkage to dopamine. J Neurochem 2002;83:1241–51.
259. Clay HB, Sillivan S, Konradi C. Mitochondrial dysfunction and pathology in bipolar disorder and schizophrenia. Int J Dev Neurosci 2011;29:311–24.
260. Shimizu A, Kurachi M, Yamaguchi N, et al. Morbidity risk of schizophrenia to parents and siblings of schizophrenic patients. Jpn J Psychiatry Neurol 1987;41: 65–70.
261. Goldstein JM, Faraone SV, Chen WJ, et al. Sex differences in the familial transmission of schizophrenia. Br J Psychiatry 1990;156:819–26.
262. Goldstein JM, Faraone SV, Chen WJ, et al. Genetic heterogeneity may in part explain sex differences in the familial risk for schizophrenia. Biol Psychiatry 1995;38:808–13.
263. Goldstein JM, Cherkerzian S, Tsuang MT, et al. Sex differences in the genetic risk for schizophrenia: history of the evidence for sex-specific and sex-dependent effects. Am J Med Genet Part B, Neuropsychiatr Genet 2013; 162B:698–710.
264. Wolyniec PS, Pulver AE, McGrath JA, et al. Schizophrenia: gender and familial risk. J Psychiatr Res 1992;26:17–27.
265. Reed SC, Urbaitis JC, National Institute of Mental Health (U.S.). The psychoses: family studies [by] Sheldon C. Reed [et al.] with the collaboration of John C. Urbaitis, Robert H. Israel [and] Anna Wendt Finlayson. Philadelphia: Saunders; 1973.

266. Bellodi L, Bussoleni C, Scorza-Smeraldi R, et al. Family study of schizophrenia: exploratory analysis for relevant factors. Schizophr Bull 1986;12:120–8.
267. Nimgaonkar VL, Wessely S, Murray RM. Prevalence of familiality, obstetric complications, and structural brain damage in schizophrenic patients. Br J Psychiatry 1988;153:191–7.
268. Nasrallah HA, Wilcox JA. Gender differences in the etiology and symptoms of schizophrenia genetic versus brain injury factors. Ann Clin Psychiatry 1989;1:51–3.
269. Pulver AE, Brown CH, Wolyniec P, et al. Schizophrenia: age at onset, gender and familial risk. Acta Psychiatr Scand 1990;82:344–51.
270. Pulver AE, Liang KY. Estimating effects of proband characteristics on familial risk: II. The association between age at onset and familial risk in the Maryland schizophrenia sample. Genet Epidemiol 1991;8:339–50.
271. Kendler KS, McGuire M, Gruenberg AM, et al. The Roscommon Family Study. I. Methods, diagnosis of probands, and risk of schizophrenia in relatives. Arch Gen Psychiatry 1993;50:527–40.
272. Nanko S, Moridaira J. Reproductive rates in schizophrenic outpatients. Acta Psychiatr Scand 1993;87:400–4.
273. Fananas L, Bertranpetit J. Reproductive rates in families of schizophrenic patients in a case-control study. Acta Psychiatr Scand 1995;91:202–4.
274. Nimgaonkar VL, Ward SE, Agarde H, et al. Fertility in schizophrenia: results from a contemporary US cohort. Acta Psychiatr Scand 1997;95:364–9.
275. Srinivasan TN, Padmavati R. Fertility and schizophrenia: evidence for increased fertility in the relatives of schizophrenic patients. Acta Psychiatr Scand 1997;96: 260–4.
276. McGrath JJ, Hearle J, Jenner L, et al. The fertility and fecundity of patients with psychoses. Acta Psychiatr Scand 1999;99:441–6.
277. Haukka J, Suvisaari J, Lonnqvist J. Fertility of patients with schizophrenia, their siblings, and the general population: a cohort study from 1950 to 1959 in Finland. Am J Psychiatry 2003;160:460–3.
278. Svensson AC, Lichtenstein P, Sandin S, et al. Fertility of first-degree relatives of patients with schizophrenia: a three generation perspective. Schizophr Res 2007;91:238–45.
279. Doi N, Hoshi Y. Persistence problem in schizophrenia and mitochondrial DNA. Am J Med Genet Part B, Neuropsychiatr Genet 2007;144B:1–4.
280. Doi N, Hoshi Y, Itokawa M, et al. Persistence criteria for susceptibility genes for schizophrenia: a discussion from an evolutionary viewpoint. PloS One 2009;4: e7799.
281. Inagaki T, Ishino H, Seno H, et al. Psychiatric symptoms in a patient with diabetes mellitus associated with point mutation in mitochondrial DNA. Biol Psychiatry 1997;42:1067–9.
282. Fattal O, Budur K, Vaughan AJ, et al. Review of the literature on major mental disorders in adult patients with mitochondrial diseases. Psychosomatics 2006; 47:1–7.
283. Bamne MN, Talkowski ME, Moraes CT, et al. Systematic association studies of mitochondrial DNA variations in schizophrenia: focus on the ND5 gene. Schizophr Bull 2008;34:458–65.
284. Martorell L, Segues T, Folch G, et al. New variants in the mitochondrial genomes of schizophrenic patients. Eur J Hum Genet 2006;14:520–8.
285. Marchbanks RM, Ryan M, Day IN, et al. A mitochondrial DNA sequence variant associated with schizophrenia and oxidative stress. Schizophr Res 2003;65: 33–8.

286. Naneishvili BR, Zurabashvili ZA. The ultrastructure of formed white blood elements (neutrophils) in schizophrenia. Folia haematologica 1976;103: 160–5.

287. Inuwa IM, Peet M, Williams MA. QSAR modeling and transmission electron microscopy stereology of altered mitochondrial ultrastructure of white blood cells in patients diagnosed as schizophrenic and treated with antipsychotic drugs. Biotech Histochem 2005;80:133–7.

288. Kung L, Roberts RC. Mitochondrial pathology in human schizophrenic striatum: a postmortem ultrastructural study. Synapse 1999;31:67–75.

289. Kolomeets NS, Uranova NA. Synaptic contacts in schizophrenia: studies using immunocytochemical identification of dopaminergic neurons. Neurosci Behav Physiol 1999;29:217–21.

290. Somerville SM, Conley RR, Roberts RC. Striatal mitochondria in subjects with chronic undifferentiated vs. chronic paranoid schizophrenia. Synapse 2012; 66:29–41.

291. Somerville SM, Lahti AC, Conley RR, et al. Mitochondria in the striatum of subjects with schizophrenia: relationship to treatment response. Synapse 2011;65: 215–24.

292. Ben-Shachar D, Zuk R, Gazawi H, et al. Increased mitochondrial complex I activity in platelets of schizophrenic patients. Int J Neuropsychopharmacol 1999;2: 245–53.

293. Ben-Shachar D, Bonne O, Chisin R, et al. Cerebral glucose utilization and platelet mitochondrial complex I activity in schizophrenia: a FDG-PET study. Prog neuro-psychopharmacology Biol Psychiatry 2007;31:807–13.

294. Dror N, Klein E, Karry R, et al. State-dependent alterations in mitochondrial complex I activity in platelets: a potential peripheral marker for schizophrenia. Mol Psychiatry 2002;7:995–1001.

295. Prince JA, Blennow K, Gottfries CG, et al. Mitochondrial function is differentially altered in the basal ganglia of chronic schizophrenics. Neuropsychopharmacology 1999;21:372–9.

296. Maurer I, Zierz S, Moller H. Evidence for a mitochondrial oxidative phosphorylation defect in brains from patients with schizophrenia. Schizophr Res 2001;48: 125–36.

297. Cavelier L, Jazin EE, Eriksson I, et al. Decreased cytochrome-c oxidase activity and lack of age-related accumulation of mitochondrial DNA deletions in the brains of schizophrenics. Genomics 1995;29:217–24.

298. Bubber P, Tang J, Haroutunian V, et al. Mitochondrial enzymes in schizophrenia. J Mol Neurosci 2004;24:315–21.

299. Anglin RE, Rosebush PI, Mazurek MF. Treating psychiatric illness in patients with mitochondrial disorders. Psychosomatics 2010;51:179 [author reply: 179–80].

300. Anglin R, Rosebush P, Mazurek M. Psychotropic medications and mitochondrial toxicity. Nat Rev Neurosci 2012;13:650.

301. Goldstein JM, Faraone SV, Chen WJ, et al. Gender and the familial risk for schizophrenia. Disentangling confounding factors. Schizophr Res 1992;7:135–40.

302. Lindholm E, Cavelier L, Howell WM, et al. Mitochondrial sequence variants in patients with schizophrenia. Eur J Hum Genet 1997;5:406–12.

303. Ueno H, Nishigaki Y, Kong QP, et al. Analysis of mitochondrial DNA variants in Japanese patients with schizophrenia. Mitochondrion 2009;9:385–93.

304. Kazuno AA, Munakata K, Mori K, et al. Mitochondrial DNA sequence analysis of patients with 'atypical psychosis'. Psychiatry Clin Neurosci 2005;59: 497–503.

305. Levinger L, Morl M, Florentz C. Mitochondrial tRNA 3' end metabolism and human disease. Nucleic Acids Res 2004;32:5430–41.
306. Gentry KM, Nimgaonkar VL. Mitochondrial DNA variants in schizophrenia: association studies. Psychiatr Genet 2000;10:27–31.
307. Mulcrone J, Whatley SA, Ferrier IN, et al. A study of altered gene expression in frontal cortex from schizophrenic patients using differential screening. Schizophr Res 1995;14:203–13.
308. Middleton FA, Mirnics K, Pierri JN, et al. Gene expression profiling reveals alterations of specific metabolic pathways in schizophrenia. J Neurosci 2002;22:2718–29.
309. Prabakaran S, Swatton JE, Ryan MM, et al. Mitochondrial dysfunction in schizophrenia: evidence for compromised brain metabolism and oxidative stress. Mol Psychiatry 2004;9:684–97, 643.
310. Amar S, Shamir A, Ovadia O, et al. Mitochondrial DNA HV lineage increases the susceptibility to schizophrenia among Israeli Arabs. Schizophr Res 2007;94:354–8.
311. Magri C, Gardella R, Barlati SD, et al. Mitochondrial DNA haplogroups and age at onset of schizophrenia. Am J Med Genet Part B, Neuropsychiatr Genet 2007;144B:496–501.
312. Suzuki T, Koizumi J, Shiraishi H, et al. Mitochondrial encephalomyopathy (MELAS) with mental disorder. CT, MRI and SPECT findings. Neuroradiology 1990;32:74–6.
313. Odawara M, Arinami T, Tachi Y, et al. Absence of association between a mitochondrial DNA mutation at nucleotide position 3243 and schizophrenia in Japanese. Hum Genet 1998;102:708–9.
314. Lacey CJ, Salzberg MR. Obsessive-compulsive disorder with mitochondrial disease. Psychosomatics 2008;49:540–2.
315. Grados MA. Obsessive-compulsive disorder after traumatic brain injury. Int Rev Psychiatry 2003;15:350–8.
316. Gromb S, Lasseuguette K, Olivera A. Obsessive compulsive disorder secondary to head injury. J Clin Forensic Med 2002;9:89–91.
317. Thobois S, Jouanneau E, Bouvard M, et al. Obsessive-compulsive disorder after unilateral caudate nucleus bleeding. Acta Neurochir 2004;146:1027–31 [discussion: 1031].
318. Irle E, Exner C, Thielen K, et al. Obsessive-compulsive disorder and ventromedial frontal lesions: clinical and neuropsychological findings. Am J Psychiatry 1998;155:255–63.
319. Berthier ML, Kulisevsky J, Gironell A, et al. Obsessive-compulsive disorder associated with brain lesions: clinical phenomenology, cognitive function, and anatomic correlates. Neurology 1996;47:353–61.
320. Swoboda KJ, Jenike MA. Frontal abnormalities in a patient with obsessive-compulsive disorder: the role of structural lesions in obsessive-compulsive behavior. Neurology 1995;45:2130–4.
321. Chinnery P, Majamaa K, Turnbull D, et al. Treatment for mitochondrial disorders. Cochrane Database Syst Rev 2006;(1):CD004426.
322. Pfeffer G, Majamaa K, Turnbull DM, et al. Treatment for mitochondrial disorders. Cochrane Database Syst Rev 2012;(4):CD004426.
323. Kerr DS. Treatment of mitochondrial electron transport chain disorders: a review of clinical trials over the past decade. Mol Genet Metab 2010;99:246–55.
324. Chen RS, Huang CC, Chu NS. Coenzyme Q10 treatment in mitochondrial encephalomyopathies. Short-term double-blind, crossover study. Eur Neurol 1997;37:212–8.

325. Glover EI, Martin J, Maher A, et al. A randomized trial of coenzyme Q10 in mitochondrial disorders. Muscle Nerve 2010;42:739–48.

326. Rodriguez MC, MacDonald JR, Mahoney DJ, et al. Beneficial effects of creatine, CoQ10, and lipoic acid in mitochondrial disorders. Muscle Nerve 2007;35: 235–42.

327. Tarnopolsky MA, Roy BD, MacDonald JR. A randomized, controlled trial of creatine monohydrate in patients with mitochondrial cytopathies. Muscle Nerve 1997;20:1502–9.

328. Klopstock T, Querner V, Schmidt F, et al. A placebo-controlled crossover trial of creatine in mitochondrial diseases. Neurology 2000;55:1748–51.

329. De Stefano N, Matthews PM, Ford B, et al. Short-term dichloroacetate treatment improves indices of cerebral metabolism in patients with mitochondrial disorders. Neurology 1995;45:1193–8.

330. Duncan GE, Perkins LA, Theriaque DW, et al. Dichloroacetate therapy attenuates the blood lactate response to submaximal exercise in patients with defects in mitochondrial energy metabolism. J Clin Endocrinol Metab 2004;89: 1733–8.

331. Stacpoole PW, Kerr DS, Barnes C, et al. Controlled clinical trial of dichloroacetate for treatment of congenital lactic acidosis in children. Pediatrics 2006;117:1519–31.

332. Liet JM, Pelletier V, Robinson BH, et al. The effect of short-term dimethylglycine treatment on oxygen consumption in cytochrome oxidase deficiency: a double-blind randomized crossover clinical trial. J Pediatr 2003;142:62–6.

333. Enns GM, Kinsman SL, Perlman SL, et al. Initial experience in the treatment of inherited mitochondrial disease with EPI-743. Mol Genet Metab 2012;105:91–102.

334. Martinelli D, Catteruccia M, Piemonte F, et al. EPI-743 reverses the progression of the pediatric mitochondrial disease–genetically defined Leigh Syndrome. Mol Genet Metab 2012;107:383–8.

335. Sadun AA, Chicani CF, Ross-Cisneros FN, et al. Effect of EPI-743 on the clinical course of the mitochondrial disease Leber hereditary optic neuropathy. Arch Neurol 2012;69:331–8.

336. Chicani CF, Chu ER, Miller G, et al. Comparing EPI-743 treatment in siblings with Leber's hereditary optic neuropathy mt14484 mutation. Can J Ophthalmol 2013; 48:e130–133.

337. Neustadt J, Pieczenik SR. Medication-induced mitochondrial damage and disease. Mol Nutr Food Res 2008;52:780–8.

338. Cordero MD, Moreno-Fernandez AM, Gomez-Skarmeta JL, et al. Coenzyme Q10 and alpha-tocopherol protect against amitriptyline toxicity. Toxicol Appl Pharmacol 2009;235:329–37.

339. Moreno-Fernandez AM, Cordero MD, Garrido-Maraver J, et al. Oral treatment with amitriptyline induces coenzyme Q deficiency and oxidative stress in psychiatric patients. J Psychiatr Res 2012;46:341–5.

340. Souza ME, Polizello AC, Uyemura SA, et al. Effect of fluoxetine on rat liver mitochondria. Biochem Pharmacol 1994;48:535–41.

341. Curti C, Mingatto FE, Polizello AC, et al. Fluoxetine interacts with the lipid bilayer of the inner membrane in isolated rat brain mitochondria, inhibiting electron transport and F1F0-ATPase activity. Mol Cell Biochem 1999;199:103–9.

342. Kato T, Inubushi T, Kato N. Prediction of lithium response by 31P-MRS in bipolar disorder. Int J Neuropsychopharmacol 2000;3:83–5.

343. Hongpaisan J, Winters CA, Andrews SB. Calcium-dependent mitochondrial superoxide modulates nuclear CREB phosphorylation in hippocampal neurons. Mol Cell Neurosci 2003;24:1103–15.

344. Nair A, Vaidya VA. Cyclic AMP response element binding protein and brain-derived neurotrophic factor: molecules that modulate our mood? J Biosci 2006;31:423–34.

345. Cipriani A, Reid K, Young AH, et al. Valproic acid, valproate and divalproex in the maintenance treatment of bipolar disorder. Cochrane Database Syst Rev 2013;(10):CD003196.

346. Mancuso M, Orsucci D, Filosto M, et al. Drugs and mitochondrial diseases: 40 queries and answers. Expert Opin Pharmacother 2012;13:527–43.

347. Finsterer J, Segall L. Drugs interfering with mitochondrial disorders. Drug Chem Toxicol 2010;33:138–51.

348. Ponchaut S, Veitch K. Valproate and mitochondria. Biochem Pharmacol 1993; 46:199–204.

349. Haas R, Stumpf DA, Parks JK, et al. Inhibitory effects of sodium valproate on oxidative phosphorylation. Neurology 1981;31:1473–6.

350. Lin CM, Thajeb P. Valproic acid aggravates epilepsy due to MELAS in a patient with an A3243G mutation of mitochondrial DNA. Metab Brain Dis 2007;22: 105–9.

351. Balijepalli S, Boyd MR, Ravindranath V. Inhibition of mitochondrial complex I by haloperidol: the role of thiol oxidation. Neuropharmacology 1999;38:567–77.

352. Whatley SA, Curti D, Das Gupta F, et al. Superoxide, neuroleptics and the ubiquinone and cytochrome b5 reductases in brain and lymphocytes from normals and schizophrenic patients. Mol Psychiatry 1998;3:227–37.

353. Burkhardt C, Kelly JP, Lim YH, et al. Neuroleptic medications inhibit complex I of the electron transport chain. Ann Neurol 1993;33:512–7.

Index

Note: Page numbers of article titles are in **boldface** type.

Neurol Clin 34 (2016) 295–311
http://dx.doi.org/10.1016/S0733-8619(15)00111-5
0733-8619/15/$ – see front matter © 2016 Elsevier Inc. All rights reserved.

neurologic.theclinics.com

Moving?

Make sure your subscription moves with you!

To notify us of your new address, find your **Clinics Account Number** (located on your mailing label above your name), and contact customer service at:

Email: journalscustomerservice-usa@elsevier.com

800-654-2452 (subscribers in the U.S. & Canada)
314-447-8871 (subscribers outside of the U.S. & Canada)

Fax number: 314-447-8029

Elsevier Health Sciences Division
Subscription Customer Service
3251 Riverport Lane
Maryland Heights, MO 63043

*To ensure uninterrupted delivery of your subscription, please notify us at least 4 weeks in advance of move.

Printed and bound by CPI Group (UK) Ltd, Croydon, CR0 4YY

03/10/2024

01040491-0011